Moreton Morrell Site

£12.99

611.

KT-568-900

Essential Histology

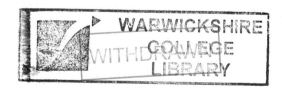

Essential Histology

Second Edition

David H. Cormack, PhD

Professor
Division of Anatomy
Department of Surgery
Faculty of Medicine
University of Toronto
Toronto, Canada

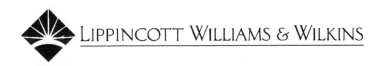
LIPPINCOTT WILLIAMS & WILKINS

Editor: Robert Anthony
Managing Editor: Eric Branger
Marketing Manager: Aimee Sirmon
Project Editor: Jennifer Pirozzoli
Indexer: David H. Cormack
Cover Illustration: Terry Watkinson
Compositor: Maryland Composition
Printer: Courier

530 Walnut Street
Philadelphia, Pennsylvania 19106

351 West Camden Street
Baltimore, Maryland 21201-2436 USA

The publisher is not responsible (as a matter of product liability, negligence or otherwise) for any injury resulting from any material contained herein. This publication contains information relating to general principles of medical care which should not be construed as specific instructions for individual patients. Manufacturers' product information and package inserts should be reviewed for current information, including contraindications, dosages and precautions.

Printed in the United States of America

Library of Congress Cataloging-in-Publication Data

Cormack, David H.
    Essential histology / David H. Cormack.—2nd ed.
      p. ; cm.
    Includes bibliographical references and index.
    ISBN 0-7817-1668-3
     1. Histology. I. Title.
    [DNLM: 1. Histology. QS 504 C811e 2001]
    QM551 .C638 2001
    611'.018—dc21

                2001029215

The publishers have made every effort to trace the copyright holders for borrowed material. If they have inadvertently overlooked any, they will be pleased to make the necessary arrangements at the first opportunity.

To purchase additional copies of this book, call our customer service department at **(800) 638-3030** or fax orders to **(301) 824-7390**. For other book services, including chapter reprints and large quantity sales, ask for the Special Sales department.

For all other calls originating outside of the United States, please call **(301)714-2324**.

Visit Lippincott Williams & Wilkins on the Internet: http://www.lww.com. Lippincott Williams & Wilkins customer service representatives are available from 8:30 am to 6:00 pm, EST, Monday through Friday, for telephone access.

00 01 02 03 04
1 2 3 4 5 6 7 8 9 10

Preface to the Second Edition

Essential Histology is a core selection of histology relating microscopic and molecular details of tissues, cells, and key cellular products to medical cell biology. Its primary focus is tissue and organ function at the cellular level. Maintained from the first edition is the primary goal of presenting the essentials of histology concisely to medical students and others who are faced with the dual challenge of having a minimal background in medical cell biology and a restricted amount of time for study. Those who are entirely new to the subject will also find the logical progression from fundamentals to body systems adequately explained. The subject matter added to this edition remains appropriate for the time constraints experienced by most students who are studying histology.

The second edition of *Essential Histology* contains further molecular information to reflect its burgeoning importance. Keyed to the revised text are improved color plates for facilitating slide interpretation when supplementary atlases are not available. In relating histology further to medical disorders, I have endeavoured to keep this edition fully congruent and synergistic with my other text, *Clinically Integrated Histology* (Lippincott-Raven, 1998).

DAVID H. CORMACK

Acknowledgments

The invaluable assistance of B. H. Smith in providing the color photomicrographs for this book is duly acknowledged. I thank D. Irwin and T. Watkinson for their artwork, generous contributors of other illustrations, and the Lippincott, Williams & Wilkins Company for expert guidance and assistance. Certain illustrations appeared previously in Ham's Histology, 9th edition, by D.H. Cormack (Philadelphia, J.B. Lippincott, 1987) and Introduction to Histology, by D.H. Cormack (Philadelphia, J.B. Lippincott, 1984). Valuable contributions from the following sources are gratefully acknowledged.

Figure 1-14: Courtesy of P.J. Lea and M.J. Hollenberg
Figure 2-2: Miyai K, Steiner JW. Exp Mol Pathol 4:525, 1965
Figure 2-2, *inset*: Courtesy of V.I. Kalnins
Figure 2-7A: Courtesy of D. Osmond and S. Miller
Figure 2-7B: Stanners CP, Till JE. Biochim Biophys Acta 37:406, 1960
Figure 2-12, *left*: Miller OL, Beatty BR. Science 164:955, 1969
Figure 2-13: Courtesy of L. Chouinard
Figure 2-15, *left*: Courtesy of V.I. Kalnins and M. Wassman
Figure 2-17: Courtesy of V.I. Kalnins
Figure 2-18A: Courtesy of L. Arsenault
Figure 2-18B: Courtesy of S. Marie
Figure 2-19: DuPraw EJ. DNA and Chromosomes. New York, Holt, Rinehart & Winston, 1970
Figure 2-22: Courtesy of I. Teshima
Figure 2-23: Moore KL, Barr ML. Lancet 2:57, 1955
Plate 2-2: Courtesy of I. Teshima
Figure 3-1: Courtesy of M. Weinstock
Figure 3-2: Courtesy of S. Ito
Figure 3-4A: Cormack DH, Ambrose EJ. J Royal Microscop Soc 81:11, 1962
Figure 3-4B: Courtesy of L. Arsenault
Figure 3-5A and C: Courtesy of P.J. Lea and M.J. Hollenberg
Figure 3-5B and D: Courtesy of K. Visser
Figure 3-6: Courtesy of A. Jézéquel
Figure 3-6, *upper inset*: Courtesy of E. Yamada
Figure 3-7, *top*: Cardell R. Anat Rec 180:309, 1974
Figure 3-9A: Courtesy of A.R. Hand
Figure 3-11: Courtesy of C. Nopajaroonsri and G. Simon
Figure 3-13A: Perry MM, Gilbert AB. J Cell Sci 39:257, 1979
Figure 3-14. Hirokawa N, Heuser J. Cell 30:395, 1982
Figure 3-15: Courtesy of M.J. Phillips
Figure 3-16: Cardell R. Int Rev Cytol 48:221, 1977
Figure 3-17: Courtesy of J.A. Connolly
Figure 3-18A: Courtesy of M. Sandig
Figure 3-18B: Courtesy of V.I. Kalnins
Figure 3-19: Dirksen ER. In Hafez ESE, ed. Scanning Electron Microscopic Atlas of Mammalian Reproduction. Tokyo, Igaku Shoin, 1975
Figure 3-21: Sturgess J. Morphological characteristics of the bronchial mucosa in cystic fibrosis. In Quinton P, Martinez R, eds. Fluid and Electrolyte Transport in Exocrine Glands in Cystic Fibrosis. San Francisco, San Franciso Press, 1982
Figure 3-22A: Courtesy of J. Sturgess

Figure 12-4*B*: Courtesy of A. Chalvardjian
Figure 12-8: Courtesy of C. P. Leblond
Figures 13-2, *bottom*, and 13-3*B*: Courtesy of C.P. Leblond
Figure 13-5: Courtesy of E. Freeman
Figure 13-6: Weinstock M, Leblond CP. J Cell Biol 60:92, 1974
Figure 13-7: Courtesy of H. Warshawsky
Figure 13-10: Modified from Anderson JE: Grant's Atlas of Anatomy, ed 7. Baltimore, Williams & Wilkins, 1978, with permission
Figure 13-12: Courtesy of S. Ito, R. Winchester, and D.W. Fawcett
Figure 13-15*C*: Courtesy of H. Cheng, J. Merzel, and C.P. Leblond
Figure 13-16: Bjerknes M, Cheng H. Anat Rec 199:565, 1981
Figure 13-17*A*: Courtesy of Y. Clermont
Figure 13-21*A*: Courtesy of M. Phillips and J.W. Steiner
Figure 13-23: Courtesy of A. Blouin
Figure 13-24: Jones AL, Schmucker DL. Gastroenterology 73:833, 1977
Figure 14-5*A*: Courtesy of J. Sturgess
Figure 14-5*B*: Sturgess JM. Am Rev Respir Dis 115:819, 1977
Figures 14-11 and 14-12: Courtesy of E.R. Weibel
Figure 15-6*A*: Tisher CC. Anatomy of the kidney. In: Brenner BM, Rector FC, eds. The Kidney, vol 1. Philadelphia, WB Saunders, 1976
Figure 15-8: Courtesy of E. Rau
Figure 15-10*B*: After D.M. Morison
Figure 16-4: Courtesy of K. Kovacs and E. Horvath
Figure 16-9: Courtesy of S. Carmichael
Figure 16-10: Courtesy of W. Wilson
Figure 16-11: Courtesy of K. Kovacs and E. Horvath
Figure 17-2: Patten BM. Foundations of Embryology. New York, McGraw-Hill, 1958, with permission
Figures 17-4 and 17-5: Modified from Moore KL. The Developing Human: Clinically Oriented Embryology, ed 2. Philadelphia, WB Saunders, 1977, with permission
Figure 18-3: Clermont Y. Am J Anat 112:35, 1963
Figure 18-5: Courtesy of J. Sturgess
Figure 18-7: Courtesy of K. Kovacs, E. Horvath, and D. McComb
Figure 19-7: Noback CR, Demarest RJ. The Human Nervous System: Basic Principles of Neurobiology, ed 2. New York, McGraw-Hill, 1975, with permission
Figure 19-10: After J.C.B. Grant
Figure 19-11: Courtesy of K. Money and J. Laufer
Figure 19-12: Courtesy of C.P. Leblond and Y. Clermont
Plate 19-1*A* and *B*: Courtesy of C. Park
Plate 19-1*C*: Courtesy of J. Holash and P.A. Stewart

Contents

Essential Histology

Second Edition

CHAPTER 1

Introduction to Histology

OBJECTIVES

The information in this chapter should enable you to do the following:

- Define histology
- Explain the term **basic tissue**
- Recognize which components in a histologic section represent cells, extracellular matrix, or body fluids
- Draw a cross section of a cell and show which parts of it can be seen in histologic sections
- Use a microscope properly and study sections effectively
- Distinguish between basophilic and acidophilic staining and cite examples of each
- Interpret in three dimensions what you observe in sections
- Summarize the main similarities and differences between a light microscope and an electron microscope

Histology means the **science of the tissues** (Gk. *histos*, web or tissue; *logia*, branch of learning). By establishing the significance of distinctive microscopic features of cells and tissues, histologic studies elucidate the relationships between microscopic structure and function.

BASIC TISSUES

The word **tissue** (L. *texere*, to weave) was first used in an anatomical context by Bichat, a French surgeon who was impressed by the different textures found in the body parts he dissected. As a result, he described the body as being made up of a variety of different **tissues**. Instead of the many distinct tissues that Bichat originally proposed, only four basic tissues are currently recognized, each with variants. All body parts are made up of basic tissues and their variants in distinctive combinations. The first part of this book introduces the cell and the four basic tissues, i.e., epithelial tissue, connective tissue, nervous tissue, and muscle. The remainder describes the body's various organ systems, constructed of basic tissues, which perform essential functions for the body as a whole.

1

NONCELLULAR CONSTITUENTS OF TISSUES

Cells are essentially soft and gelatinous. If the body were composed entirely of cells, it would be too weak to support its weight. However, cells of connective tissue produce **intercellular (extracellular) matrix** constituents (L. *inter*, between; L. *extra*, outside of), some of which are remarkably strong. Bone tissue, for example, produces a hard extracellular matrix that is reinforced internally in the same way as concrete. Hence, in some respects, the body resembles a building made of extracellular matrix that is inhabited by various kinds of cells. These cells must also be supplied with nutrients and oxygen, and adequate arrangements are required for disposal of toxic byproducts. For these purposes, the body depends on yet another component, its **body fluids**. These include blood plasma, which is a complex fluid that circulates within the confines of the blood vascular system, and a few other extracellular fluids that will be considered in due course. The three primary components that make up the body tissues are 1) cells, 2) extracellular matrix, and 3) body fluids. The first step in recognizing various tissues is to appreciate the microscopic appearance of their individual cells and to learn how to identify the various extracellular matrix constituents. In addition, it is helpful to learn how to recognize the sites where body fluids were present during life. But before we consider the microscopic appearance of these primary tissue components, we should outline how tissues are prepared for routine light microscopy.

PREPARATION OF HISTOLOGIC SECTIONS

Much of our detailed knowledge of body structure comes from a study of small representative samples cut into very thin slices termed tissue **sections**. Light microscopic sections need to be thin enough to transmit plenty of light, which comes from underneath and must pass through the specimen, the objective lens, and then the eyepiece lens, before reaching the eye. In general, the thinner the section, the less is the likelihood that its components will appear superimposed. The optimal thickness of light microscopic sections (5 to 8 μm) is less than the diameter of a typical cell. Histologic sections are routinely prepared by the **paraffin technique.** Alternate procedures for preparing tissues are also described.

Paraffin Sections

The standard paraffin technique consists of the following stages.

Tissue Sampling

Tissue blocks (tissue samples cut <1 cm in each dimension) may be obtained through biopsy (diagnostic sampling), surgical excision, or postmortem dissection. To avoid misleading structural deterioration, postmortem samples should be taken as soon as possible, and to minimize tissue distortion, dissection instruments should be kept extremely sharp. Tissue blocks must be immersed in fixative immediately after removal.

Fixing

Chemical fixation, required to avoid unnecessary distortion, crosslinks certain proteins and denatures others through dehydration. The resulting coagulation of tissue proteins has a hardening effect on soft tissues. Fixation needs to be rapid enough to curtail release from dead cells of enzymes capable of digesting tissue constituents. If degradation by such enzymes is allowed to continue, it ruins microscopic detail, causing **postmortem degeneration.** Fixatives also lock into position a number of carbohydrate- and fat-containing macromolecules that otherwise would be lost during tissue processing. Moreover, fixation kills bacteria and other disease-causing agents, and its antiseptic action decreases risk of contamination when infected tissues are handled. Fixation can also enhance tissue staining. Special fixatives are used for some tissue components, but a 4% aqueous solution of formaldehyde, buffered to neutral pH, is suitable for routine work.

Dehydrating

Paraffin embedding replaces tissue water with paraffin wax, enabling the block to be cut readily. Because paraffin is not water soluble, water is removed from the fixed tissue by passing it through successively stronger solutions of ethyl alcohol, allowing enough time for thorough reagent penetration at each stage. Because paraffin is insoluble in alcohol, the next stage, clearing, involves replacing alcohol with a paraffin solvent that is miscible with alcohol.

Clearing

Xylene is routinely used for clearing tissues. The alcohol-permeated block is passed through several changes of this solvent to replace alcohol with xylene.

Embedding

The xylene-permeated block is passed through several changes of warm paraffin wax, which is soluble in xylene. Once the tissues become completely saturated, melted wax occupies spaces formerly occupied by water. On cooling, the wax hardens. Thin shavings can then be cut off the embedded tissues.

Sectioning

Surplus wax is trimmed away and the block is mounted on a cutting device called a **microtome**. The edges of the thin shavings (**sections**) coming off the microtome knife adhere to one another, producing a long ribbon from which single sections may readily be detached (Fig. 1-1).

Staining and Mounting

Aqueous solutions are usually used in staining. Prior to this, the wax must be dissolved and replaced with water. For this, the slide with the attached section is passed first through xylene to remove paraffin, then through

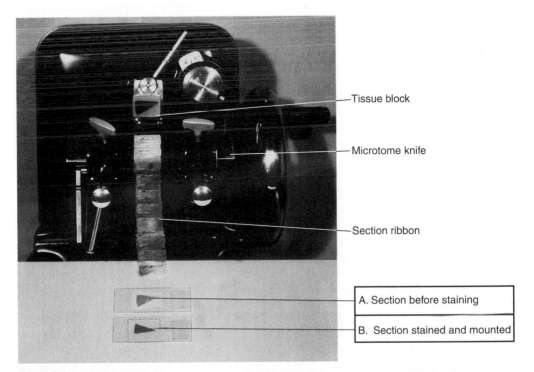

Figure 1-1
Paraffin sections are cut on a microtome for light microscopy.

absolute alcohol to remove xylene, followed by alcohols of decreasing strength and eventually, water. When prepared for staining, the section appears as in Figure 1-1, label *A*. After staining, the section is passed through alcohol solutions of increasing strength, absolute alcohol, and xylene. It is then covered with mounting medium dissolved in xylene. This medium minimizes refraction of the light passing through the section. Once a protective coverslip has been added and xylene has evaporated around its edges, dried mounting medium bonds the coverslip firmly to the slide (see Fig. 1-1, label *B*).

Frozen Sections

If sections need to be examined without delay, **tissue freezing** becomes a preferable means of preparation. Frozen sections are particularly appropriate 1) if the course of a surgical procedure depends on rapid histologic assessment of the nature or spread of a diseased tissue, or 2) if a study of undenatured proteins or lipids in tissues requires avoidance of extraction or harsh fixation. Virtually everything present in living tissues remains represented in frozen sections, but these sections require prompt observation because their constituents are not preserved (subsequent fixation, though sometimes used, compromises certain advantages of the method). Moreover, frozen sections need to be cut slightly thicker (5 to 10 μm) than paraffin sections, and they are laborious to prepare in large batches.

The first step in preparing frozen sections is to freeze the block of fresh tissue as rapidly as possible, using liquid nitrogen. Sections are cut inside a refrigerated cabinet called a **cryostat**, which maintains the microtome knife at a subzero temperature. They are then suitably stained for tissue diagnosis or further microscopic observation.

Semithin Sections

Greater resolution is obtainable if light microscopic sections (**semithin sections**) are cut at 0.5 to 2 μm. This requires the use of an epoxy or acrylic resin as the embedding medium. Toluidine blue is usually used to stain these sections.

LIGHT MICROSCOPY

Microscopes 1) produce enlarged images of small objects and 2) reveal details. Whereas enlarging an optical image is called **magnification**, disclosing its fine details is called **resolution**.

The simplified light path in a monocular microscope is shown in Figure 1-2. Unlike the coarse and fine focusing knobs of older microscopes, which raise or lower the microscope tube and its 10× (magnification) **eyepiece (ocular)**, focusing adjustments on modern, binocular microscopes move the stage instead. The microscope stage is a flat plate with a central opening for the condenser that collects light from the lamp filament. At each magnification, the aperture of the iris diaphragm that regulates the diameter of the light beam entering the condenser should be restricted to two-thirds open. To obtain optimal illumination of the slide clipped to the stage, condenser height should also be adjusted. Temporary withdrawal of the top lens of the condenser from the optical path may be necessary when scanning power is used. Interchangeable **objectives** on a revolving disk at the lower end of the microscope tube provide magnifications of 10×, 40×, and 100×, respectively. The 10× objective, known as the **low-power objective**, provides tenfold magnification. Because the eyepiece enlarges the resulting image by a further factor of 10, total magnification with the low-power objective is ×100. Likewise, the 40× objective, called the **high-power objective**, together with the 10× eyepiece, gives a total magnification of ×400. The 100× objective, which is called the **oil-immersion objective**, used in combination with the 10× eyepiece, gives a total magnification of ×1000. When the oil-immersion objective is being used, however, it is necessary to replace the air

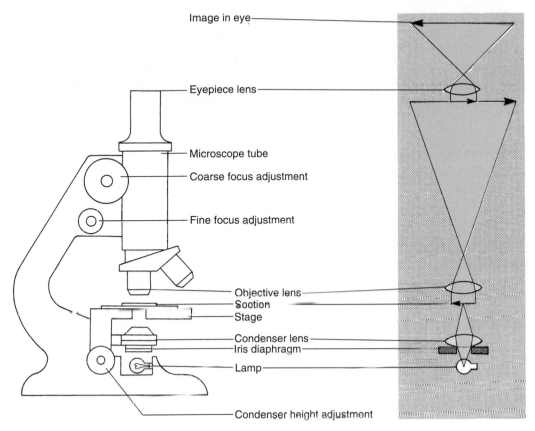

Figure 1-2
Optical components and imaging path of a light microscope (simplified).

between the objective lens and the coverslip with immersion oil of appropriate refractive index. Focus is unobtainable with this objective if the requirement for oil is overlooked. The need for extreme caution when using the oil-immersion objective is noted below.

Modern microscopes have an additional objective that is known as the **scanning lens** because of its low magnification. Such a very low power objective ensures that a relatively large area of the slide comes into view. The *extent* (i.e., diameter) of a given field of view *decreases* in direct proportion to the magnification used. The amount of *detail* that is obtained, however, *increases* with effective magnification up to a maximum of about ×1400.

STUDYING HISTOLOGIC SECTIONS

Before each slide is positioned on the microscope stage, it should be held up to the light and inspected directly, without magnification. Rapid confirmation of the surface of the slide bearing the section serves as a precaution against getting the slide upside down (labels are sometimes inadvertently mounted on the wrong side) and may reveal dirt or oil on the coverslip. Preliminary direct observation often helps in recognition of tissues by those experienced in interpreting histologic sections.

Low-Power Magnification

Most beginners enthusiastically grasp an opportunity to examine tissues under the highest possible magnification. The main advantage of starting at scanning or low-power magnification is that relatively large areas can be seen each time. Also, the slide may be surveyed thoroughly by racking it back and forth in a systematic manner. Meaningful details confined to certain areas may be found only in low-power searches of entire sections. Initial surveys under low power also pinpoint areas for observation under higher magnification.

High-Power Magnification

Swinging the high-power objective into position to examine areas selected under low power should not be a problem. However, if adequate focus cannot be obtained, the slide may be upside down and the section lies too far away to be brought into focus.

Oil-Immersion Magnification

To obtain focus at this magnification, the objective must be brought uncomfortably close to the coverslip over the section. Most oil-immersion objectives are therefore spring-loaded in design. Nevertheless, to avoid damaging the objective or breaking the coverslip, focusing should be done in a cautious manner. Before the oil-immersion objective is swung into place to observe an area preselected under high power, a small drop of immersion oil is placed on the coverslip. Unless it is known that the microscope is parfocal, the free end of the oil-immersion objective, viewed *from one side of the microscope*, is then brought into contact with the oil through use of the coarse focus adjustment. Once contact is established, as indicated by a brief flash of light, focusing is completed through use of the fine focus adjustment. However, if focusing requires a number of turns, make sure that part of the section is aligned with the tiny objective aperture, in which case some color should be visible. Considerable caution is necessary until some experience has been gained.

Cleaning Lenses

If the field of view appears irregularly clouded, distorted, or covered with specks, 1) the coverslip may be dirty, 2) the objective lens may be smeared with immersion oil (this is fairly common in the case of the 40× objective), 3) an eyepiece lens may be dirty, or 4) the top lens of the condenser may be dirty. If the distortion or specks turn when an eyepiece is rotated, the problem is a dirty eyepiece lens. An effective way to clean this lens is to breathe on it lightly and polish it *very gently* with lens paper. Oil on a coverslip or objective may be removed with lens paper (moistened, if required, with a drop of xylene).

HISTOLOGIC STAINS

Tissue components are difficult to distinguish with an ordinary light microscope because their optical densities are so similar. However, many of them can be rendered visible through the selective absorption of dyes. **Histologic stains** reveal tissue components either by coloring them selectively or by increasing their optical densities to different extents. **Electron microscopic stains** increase the electron density of particular tissue components without imparting any colors.

Sections are commonly stained with 1) a dye that imparts a bright color to certain components and 2) a counterstain that imparts a contrasting color to the remainder. **H&E-stained sections** are stained with hematoxylin and eosin. **Hematoxylin** is a dye called **hematein** (obtained from the logwood tree) used in combination with Al^{3+} ions. **Eosin** imparts a pink to red color to most components not stained a bluish purple by hematoxylin. However, many factors influence H&E staining, and the colors obtained depend on staining expertise and the stain batches used.

Basophilic and Acidophilic Staining

Basophilic components take up **basic stains**, whereas **acidophilic** components take up **acid stains.**

Both kinds of stains represent neutral salts. The **acid radical** of a salt is capable of combining with hydrogen to form an *acid*, whereas its **basic radical** is capable of combining with a hydroxyl group to form a *base*. If the color-imparting part of a dye molecule resides in its acid radical, the dye is an **acid stain**; if it lies in the basic radical, the dye is a **basic stain.** Hematoxylin is a basic stain because its color-imparting constituent (hematein + Al^{3+} ions) is its basic radical. Components stained by hematoxylin are therefore described as **basophilic.** Because eosin is an acid stain, components stained by eosin are correspondingly described as **acidophilic** or **eosinophilic.**

Another basis for stain classification is whether the color-imparting constituent is 1) the positively charged cation or 2) the negatively charged anion of the salt. If the color is imparted by the acid radical, which in ionic form bears a negative charge, the stain is an **anionic stain.** Conversely, if the color is imparted by the positively charged (cationic) basic radical, the stain is a **cationic stain.** Thus, acid stains such as eosin are anionic stains, and basic stains such as hematoxylin are cationic stains.

Stains can provide two different colors if their anion imparts one color to acidophilic components and their cation imparts another color to basophilic components. Such **neutral stains** are used primarily to stain blood cells. Alternative staining methods have been devised for tissue components that have weak affinity for ordinary stains. These special methods will be described in the context of the tissues for which they are used.

Interpreting the Colors Seen in Histologic Sections

The composition of tissue components is, of course, more relevant than their colors when stained. However, in a few instances these colors do indicate chemical composition. In **histochemical staining,** established color reactions are used to detect specific chemical groups in tissue components. An example (the PAS reaction) is given later in this chapter. However, histochemical staining is a special case; ordinary stains such as hematoxylin and eosin yield only nonspecific information about the chemical composition of components that they color, as we shall now explain.

Tissue components stain with a basic stain such as hematoxylin, or with an acid stain such as eosin, only if they carry a sufficient number of charged sites to enable them to bind colored dye radicals bearing the opposite charge. Basophilic components possess anionic (negative) sites, and bind the colored cations of hematoxylin (hematein complexed with Al^{3+} ions), whereas acidophilic components possess cationic (positive) sites, and bind the colored anions of eosin. However, the anion- or cation-binding sites are usually present on more than one sort of molecule, and their relative numbers vary according to fixation and staining conditions, so the resulting colors are seldom consistent. Basic and acid stains therefore provide a general indication of chemical composition, but this is not very specific.

Students should guard against becoming over-dependent on colors for routine tissue identification because these can vary. Furthermore, the importance of colors in this connection is often exaggerated. Color-blind students can become proficient at recognizing stained tissues, and stained sections may be usefully compared with black and white photomicrographs. Indeed, such comparisons are helpful preparation for the study of electron micrographs, which are always taken in black and white because an electron beam possesses no color spectrum. In tissue recognition, ample use should always be made of any additional confirming evidence such as size, location, shape, number, and association with other components.

In black and white photomicrographs, blue to purple staining appears as black tones whereas pink to red staining appears as shades of gray. Hence, darker tones indicate hematoxylin staining and lighter tones indicate eosin staining. Contrast between comparable depths of blue and red may be enhanced optically through the use of suitable color filters.

Unstained tissue components are hard to distinguish with an ordinary light microscope because they have comparable optical densities, i.e., they obstruct light to a similar extent. The degree to which they change the *phase* of light, however, varies. By disclosing phase differences as optical density differences, the **phase contrast microscope** reveals various components as gradations of black and white even without fixation or staining, allowing tissues to be observed in the living state.

Our next consideration is interpretation of what is seen in H&E-stained sections.

RECOGNIZING CELLS IN SECTIONS

A cell that has been sectioned through its middle typically appears as a more or less round structure (Fig. 1-3). Even before ways were devised to produce stained sections, it was known from microscopic studies that animal cells were rounded, jelly-like components, each with a central part differing in refractive index from the part surrounding it. The central part was called the cell **nucleus** (L. *nux,* nut) because it resembled a nut in its shell, and terms that related to the nucleus were given the prefix *karyo* (Gk. *karyon,* nut), an example being **karyolysis**, which is one of the nuclear changes associated with cell death.

The outer part of the cell is termed *cytoplasm* (see Fig. 1-3), a word derived from the Greek *kytos,* which means something that is hollow or covers, and *plasma*, which means something that is molded. Thus the cytoplasm is essentially molded around the nucleus. At the outer boundary of the cytoplasm lies the **cell membrane,** known also as the **plasmalemma**, a membrane so thin that cross sections of it may be observed only with the electron microscope. An impression of the approximate position of the cell membrane is nevertheless gained where the membrane takes an oblique course through a histologic section and thus appears as a slanting expanse.

Each of the 200 or so distinct cell types in the body has its characteristic distribution, size, shape, and special functions. Tissue sections with cells of uniform appearance are appropriate for observing individual cells. The example we will be using is the *hepatocyte* (Gk. *hepar*, liver), the chief cell type in the liver. The first thing to consider is how hepatocytes appear at different magnifications.

Magnification and Section Thickness Determine Microscopic Detail

Histologic sections have to be scanned in their entirety to overcome the inherent limitation that only restricted areas are observable at each moment. The field of view obtained with the low-power objective, for example, is approximately 1.5 mm in diameter, which is roughly the area enclosed by a letter *o* as printed on this page. The unit of length used in light microscopy is the micrometer (μm), 1 μm being equal to 0.001 mm, so the area seen under low power has a diameter of 1500 μm. When higher-powered objectives are used, the field of view is reduced in direct proportion to the magnification used, as summarized in Table 1-1. Another pertinent consideration is the relation between section thickness and cell diameter. An easily remembered approximation is that the thickness of a typical paraffin section (5 to 8 μm) is roughly the diameter of a red blood cell (7 μm). Hence, two or three serial sections (meaning consecutive sections) need to be observed to see every part of a hepatocyte roughly 20 μm in diameter. With these matters in mind, we shall now consider what can be seen in H&E-stained liver sections at different magnifications.

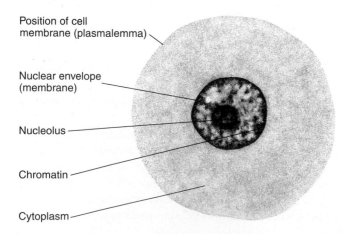

Position of cell
membrane (plasmalemma)

Nuclear envelope
(membrane)

Nucleolus

Chromatin

Cytoplasm

Figure 1-3
Parts of a cell as seen with a light
microscope.

TABLE 1-1.

FIELDS OF VIEW OBTAINED AT DIFFERENT MAGNIFICATIONS			
	Low Power	High Power	Oil Immersion
Eyepiece	× 10	× 10	× 10
Objective	× 10	× 40	× 100
Magnification	× 100	× 400	× 1000
Diameter of field of view	1500 μm	375 μm	150 μm

First, apart from a few large holes (each representing the lumen of a large blood vessel), a liver section held up to the light appears more or less evenly pink. The low-power objective nevertheless discloses that what seems a uniformly pink substance is not really solid at all. Instead, it contains radiating rows of cells, and these rows anastomose and are separated by long narrow spaces. At this magnification, the pink-staining rows appear to contain tiny purple dots (Plate 1-1A). The purple structures are the nuclei of hepatocytes, and the pink-staining substance of the rows is their cytoplasm. The lighter slit-like spaces between the rows are blood passageways.

Next, a rapid examination under high power will confirm the above-mentioned points, and the oil-immersion objective may be used to observe the finest details (Plate 1-1B). In the **nuclei** of these cells, the components, illustrated in Figure 1-3, can be seen. These are 1) the **nuclear envelope** or **membrane**, 2) the **nucleolus**, 3) **chromatin granules** (Gk. *chroma*, color), and 4) the unstained component in which the chromatin and nucleolus appear suspended. The blue to purple staining of the nuclei (see Plate 1-1) and the basophilia of the cytoplasm (which, as will be explained, is an active site of protein synthesis) are both due to an abundance of **nucleic acids**. The nucleic acids are important negatively charged macromolecules whose name reflects the fact that they were initially isolated from nuclei. Their strong affinity for hematoxylin reflects their high density of PO_4^{3-} groups. In general, however, the **cytoplasm** stains pink because cytoplasmic proteins are mostly acidophilic. Their acidophilia is enhanced by eosin staining at pH 5–6 since the number of positively ionized groups (e.g., NH_3^+) on fixed protein molecules is increased at acid pH. Because the cell membrane is too thin to be visible with a light microscope, *cell boundaries* are often hard to recognize, but some are discernible as indistinct pink lines demarcating the borders between contiguous cells. Such borders, the positions of which are indicated by arrows in Plate 1-1B, indicate the dimensions of individual hepatocytes. Finally, a note of caution—nuclear membranes are fairly conspicuous in H&E-stained sections, and because most nucleoli appear as isolated bodies inside these nuclei, beginners sometimes make the mistake of thinking that nuclei are entire cells and that nucleoli are their nuclei.

Composite Drawings Usually Represent Summaries of Histologic Information

Certain important features or parts of cells or tissues may be inadequately represented in single sections, or components of interest may not stain optimally with the stains that are used. Composite drawings that effectively combine information gathered from the use of various histologic techniques and direct observation of living cells and tissues are usually used to supplement photomicrographs. Students should not expect their sections to disclose all the features depicted in such detailed drawings. Artwork also has the potential to depict histologic structure in three dimensions. It is sometimes difficult to appreciate three-dimensional internal organization from a single microscopic section of a body part, especially if its organization is complex or the plane of section is not known. Single sections may be insufficient or even misleading for understanding the organization of the

structures from which they were obtained. Visualizing body parts in three dimensions (i.e., not restricting structural perception to a single plane) is important enough to warrant further discussion.

INTERPRETING HISTOLOGIC SECTIONS IN THREE DIMENSIONS

The inherent difficulties of understanding three-dimensional organization from random single sections become apparent if we use thin slices of hard-boiled egg as an analogy. On seeing only the slice
labeled *A* in Figure 1-4, anyone unaware of the organization of an egg might think it spherical without perceiving that it possesses a yolk. The slice labeled *B* would disclose a yolk, but would suggest
that an egg was spherical. The third slice, *C*, would reveal the true shape of an egg but not the presence of a yolk. Slice *D* is the only one with sufficient information for correct conceptualization of
the structure of an egg. The corresponding section of a cell would similarly fully disclose its internal organization.

In contrast, the liver has a more or less uniform internal organization. A liver section cut in any
plane is accordingly fairly representative of the organ as a whole. However, such uniformity of structure is more often the exception than the rule. Elucidation of the complicated internal organization
of certain organs and structures of the body requires the preparation of consecutive (**serial**) sections.

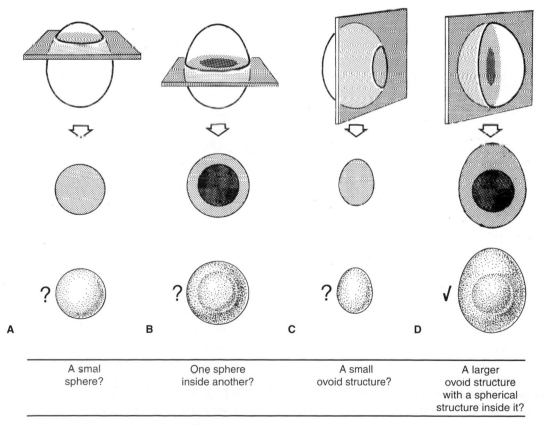

A	B	C	D
A smal sphere?	One sphere inside another?	A small ovoid structure?	A larger ovoid structure with a spherical structure inside it?

Figure 1-4
Three-dimensional visualization of a structure depends on the plane of section.

Photographic enlargements of such sections may be mounted on a backing of appropriate thickness and assembled as large-scale models called **reconstructions**. These models may then be dismantled in a manner that reveals their detailed internal structure.

If our interpretation of the internal organization of the liver were restricted to two dimensions, it might be concluded from the section seen in Plate 1-1 that most hepatocytes would be arranged in single rows. Yet hepatocytes could not carry out many of their functions unless they were more than one cell deep, and a comparison between Plate 1-1 and Figure 1-5 shows that a single-row appearance may in fact be derived from arrangements that are several cells deep.

Three-dimensional visualization is particularly important when matching the shapes seen in sections with corresponding shapes in anatomical parts. Before discussing this further, we need to consider the variety of planes in which histologic sections may be cut.

Histologic Sections: Planes of Section

A tissue sample or anatomic structure of greater length than width may be cut in any one of three planes (Fig. 1-6). Thus, a cut that is parallel to the longest dimension produces a **longitudinal section**, and a cut that is perpendicular to this plane produces a **transverse (cross) section**. Any cut made at an angle between these two planes results in an **oblique section**. However, some body parts and most cells are round in shape. A spherical structure cut through its middle produces a transverse section, but if only its surface is grazed, a **grazing section** is obtained instead. Such a shaving from a rounded surface just touches and incorporates a tiny area of the surface, so it is alternatively known as a **tangential section** (L. *tangere*, to touch).

Next, we shall consider how some representative body parts usually appear in sections, depending on the plane of section.

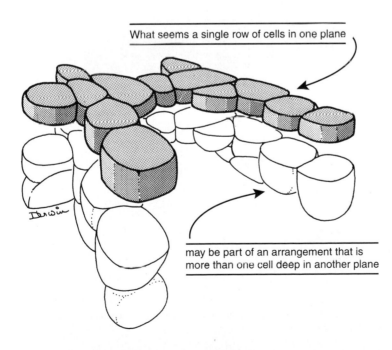

What seems a single row of cells in one plane

may be part of an arrangement that is more than one cell deep in another plane

Figure 1-5
Three-dimensional interpretation of a section requires consideration of what lay above and below the plane of section.

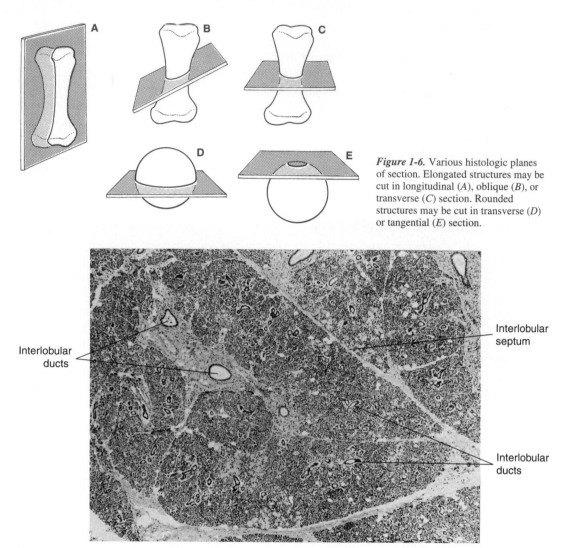

Figure 1-6. Various histologic planes of section. Elongated structures may be cut in longitudinal (*A*), oblique (*B*), or transverse (*C*) section. Rounded structures may be cut in transverse (*D*) or tangential (*E*) section.

Figure 1-7
Low-power photomicrograph of a salivary gland (the submandibular) showing a lobule surrounded by fibrous septa, with tubular ducts cut mostly in transverse or oblique section.

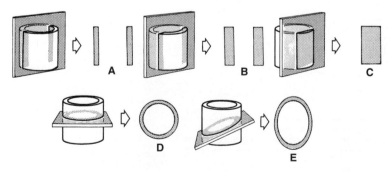

Figure 1-8
Planes of section of straight tubes. (*A–C*) Longitudinal sections, cut at various levels relative to the lumen. *C* does not include the lumen. (*D*) Transverse section. (*E*) Oblique section.

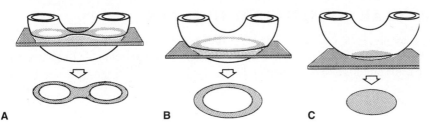

Figure 1-9
Planes of section of curved tubes. *A* and *B* include the lumen; *C* does not.

Microscopic Appearance of Tubes

Dissections indicate that the body abounds with tubes of various diameters. Many of the tubes observed in histologic sections are blood vessels or their accompanying lymphatics (the tubes that carry lymph). Furthermore, exocrine glands have ducts, i.e., conducting tubules for their secretions. Ducts are prominent in the gland illustrated in Figure 1-7. Tubes are seldom difficult to recognize if cut in transverse section, as in Figure 1-8D. But, if they are cut longitudinally (Fig. 1-8 *A-C*), obliquely (Fig. 1-8*E*), or at a site where they curve (Fig. 1-9), the observer needs to think in three dimensions for their recognition as tubes.

Microscopic Appearance of Partitions

Most glands and glandular organs are supported by internal fibrous partitions made primarily of intercellular fibers (see Fig. 1-7); such partitions are known as **septa** (L. *saeptum*, wall). Even if the individual compartments of a subdivided gland have similar dimensions, some may appear larger or smaller than others, depending on the plane of section. This effect is demonstrated by cutting oranges in different planes and observing the cut surface of their segments (Fig. 1-10).

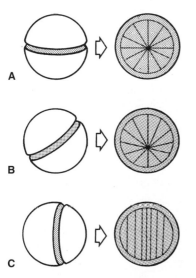

Figure 1-10
An orange sectioned in different planes, showing its partitions. (*A*) Transverse section. (*B*) Oblique section. (*C*) Longitudinal section (off-center). In *B* and *C*, segments appear unequal in size.

MACROMOLECULAR CONSTITUENTS OF CELLS

Besides containing water and ions, cells are made up of four major classes of organic constituents: 1) proteins, 2) carbohydrates, 3) fats (lipids), and 4) nucleic acids. Constituents (1) to (3) are considered here; nucleic acids are discussed in Chapter 2.

Proteins

Protein molecules are made up of one or more chains of amino acids, each amino acid having an amino ($-NH_2$) and a carboxyl ($-COOH$) group. Plants synthesize their amino acids and proteins from nitrogen, carbon dioxide, and water, but animals are unable to do this and depend on dietary proteins obtained either from plants or from animals directly or indirectly sustained by plants. Digestion degrades proteins to their constituent amino acids. These are absorbed into the blood and carried to body parts where cells incorporate them into their own proteins.

Proteins are doubly essential for cells. First, metabolic reactions (biochemical reactions that maintain cell viability) are regulated by catalytic proteins known as **enzymes**. Second, an essential constituent of every part of the cell is **structural protein.** For example, cytoplasmic microtubules and filaments are assembled from structural protein subunits, and distinctive membrane proteins are closely associated with phospholipid bilayers in the various membranes of the cell. Subdivision of the cell interior by intracellular membranes makes metabolic reactions more efficient by segregating the enzymes, along with their substrates, in separate subcompartments.

Stored Carbohydrates

Hepatocytes convert excess blood glucose into **glycogen**. Because intracellular stores of this polysaccharide remain unstained by eosin or hematoxylin, H&E-stained cells containing intracellular deposits of glycogen are characterized by empty-looking cytoplasmic spaces with ragged edges (see Plate 1-1*B*). The presence of glycogen in cells may be confirmed by the periodic acid-Schiff staining reaction.

The **periodic acid-Schiff (PAS) reaction** is a two-staged histochemical procedure. First, the 1,2-glycol groups present in polysaccharide chains are oxidized by periodic acid, yielding aldehyde groups. Then Schiff reagent, which is decolorized basic fuchsin, is used to reveal the aldehyde groups, with which it forms a bright magenta (purple) complex. Glycogen-storing hepatocytes stain positively with the PAS procedure.

Glycogen is not the only tissue macromolecule bearing polysaccharide chains. To confirm that a PAS-positive constituent represents glycogen, an additional step is required. Because glycogen is susceptible to digestion by salivary diastase, a control section is incubated with saliva before PAS staining to establish whether this treatment extracted the reactive constituent from the section. Instead of indicating glycogen, PAS staining unimpaired by previous diastase digestion indicates polysaccharide chains of **glycoproteins** or **proteoglycans** (and, to some extent, glycolipids). Thus, thyroglobulin (the macromolecular hormone precursor synthesized and stored in the thyroid gland) is PAS positive (**Plate 1-2**) yet unextractable with diastase because it is a glycoprotein. Plate 1-2 compares the colors typically obtained with H&E and PAS staining.

Stored Fat (Lipid)

In H&E-stained sections, the cytoplasm of hepatocytes may also exhibit empty spaces of a different kind. Unlike the ragged-edged, irregular spaces that characterize glycogen, such spaces are rounded with smooth edges (Plate 1-3). They remain when droplets of **fat**, the other main storage product in cells, become extracted during the dehydrating and clearing stages of the paraffin technique. An excessive content of fat droplets in hepatocytes, or a single large fat droplet, as in Plate 1-3, indicates a **fatty liver**, a change usually brought on by heavy alcohol consumption.

Fat extraction renders paraffin sections unsuitable for showing stored lipids. However, these lipids are retained if frozen sections are prepared instead. Stored lipids may be demonstrated readily in thawed frozen sections by using a fat-soluble stain, e.g., a Sudan dye (see Plate 1-3*B*).

LOCALIZATION OF SPECIFIC TISSUE CONSTITUENTS

Individual molecular constituents of tissues may be specifically localized by fluorescence or confocal microscopy or through in situ hybridization.

Fluorescence Microscope

This microscope is equipped with an illumination source that emits some ultraviolet light. Appropriate optical filters screen out all wavelengths that are unnecessary to elicit fluorescence in the preparation. The retina is shielded from damaging ultraviolet light by a protective optical filter positioned below the eyepiece. This filter transmits visible light but blocks ultraviolet light.

Immunofluorescent Staining

Fluorescent dyes (e.g., fluorescein with green fluorescence or lissamine rhodamine with red fluorescence) can be used to label and trace specific antibodies. Because a labeled antibody interacts specifically with its corresponding antigenic protein, a specific **fluorescent-labeled antibody** may be used to localize a given protein. In **direct** immunofluorescent staining, a labeled antibody is itself used to localize the target protein. In **indirect** immunofluorescent staining, fluorescent-labeled **anti-immunoglobulin,** directed against the unlabeled primary antibody and produced in another species, is used instead. This indirect method is more sensitive because of the total amount of antibody bound in the two stages of staining.

Confocal Microscope

The three-dimensional distribution of a specific constituent of a living tissue is more accurately established by searching through a number of **optical sections** (*optical planes* analogous to *CT scans* of the tissue) with a microscope capable of precise depth discrimination. The confocal microscope scans the tissue with a narrow laser beam that is precisely focused to the appropriate depth. Whereas structural details that lie in the plane of the scan are disclosed, details that do not lie within the thin focal plane of the scanning beam are not represented in the image. The computer component of the confocal microscope can display compilations of serial optical section images three-dimensionally, and fluorescence images recording the distribution of fluorescent markers may be compared directly with the corresponding optical images.

Blotting Techniques and In Situ Hybridization

The specifications for the unique molecular structures of proteins typically pass from genomic DNA → specific messenger RNAs (**mRNA**) → specific proteins (see Chapter 2). Availability of radioactive or fluorescent-labeled DNA fragments, oligonucleotides (synthetic probes), and specific antibodies enables the detection of specific DNA sequences, expressed genes, or specific proteins in individual cells. Techniques widely used for identifying cells that produce particular proteins include the following:

Northern Blots

Gene expression involves production of specific mRNAs. Under certain conditions, a single-stranded mRNA molecule recognizes its complementary DNA sequence and selectively hybridizes with it. Single-stranded segments of labeled DNA accordingly are employed as **DNA probes** to detect the presence of **complementary mRNA** strands, either in blots (**Northern blots,** Fig. 1-11) or in situ. Radioautographic detection of radioactivity is described in Chapter 2. The specific DNA probe may be a DNA fragment prepared from the isolated gene, or it may be synthesized in vitro from a gene-specific mRNA template, using reverse transcriptase which produces single-stranded **cDNA** (the *c* denotes *complementary* or *copy*) representing genomic DNA minus its introns. DNA:mRNA hybridization makes it possible to quantitate specific mRNA transcripts in cells, and thereby to establish which genomic DNA sequences are being transcribed. It detects specific gene expression in given cell types.

fin Sections. Unless cells are fixed immediately, oxygen deprivation liberates destructive enzymes that, during life, are segregated from the remainder of the cell in membranous vesicles called **lysosomes**. The released enzymes digest cells from within (**postmortem degeneration**).

Shrinkage Artifact

Many of the reagents used for preparing paraffin sections cause marked tissue shrinkage. Uneven shrinkage causes contiguous components to separate and creates the illusion that they are separated by empty spaces (Fig. 1-12A). Empty-looking spaces are always suspect because they may not have existed during life.

Precipitate

Any particles in sections should also be viewed with suspicion. For example, precipitates may form in tissues fixed with formalin (i.e., formaldehyde solution) that is acidic because of insufficient buffering (Fig. 1-12B). Also, once exposed to acidic formalin, hemoglobin (the chief protein in red blood cells) may precipitate as an artificial granular brown pigment (**formalin pigment**). Blood stains show a strong tendency to precipitate if drying occurs during staining.

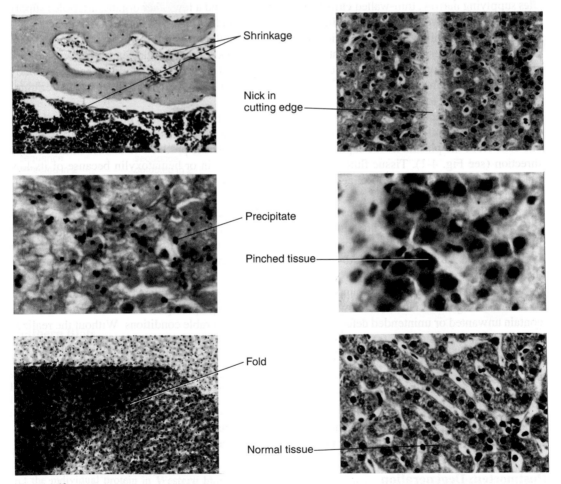

Figure 1-12
Artifacts frequently encountered in histological sections.

Wrinkles or Folds

Sections can buckle or fold when they are being attached to slides (Fig. 1-12*C*).

Microtome Knife Nicks

In the cutting of embedded tissues, accidental nicks in the cutting edge can produce straight lines across the sections. The lines represent imperfections along which the structural detail is distorted (Fig. 1-12*D*).

Rough Handling

Inadvertent rough handling greatly distorts the microscopic appearance of tissues. Sites where the tissues were pinched by forceps or crushed by dull scissors are shown in Figure 1-12*E*, which may be compared with undistorted tissue in Figure 1-12*F*.

ELECTRON MICROSCOPY

An electron microscope is necessary for the observation of tiny structural details in cells and tissues for the following reason. The amount of requisite separation between two adjacent details in the specimen to allow these to be distinguished as separate features is known as **resolution**. The smaller the distance between the tiniest discernible features in a light microscope (LM), the more detailed is its image. However, details that are less than 0.2 μm apart cannot be distinguished as separate entities, even with a well-equipped LM. The critical distance of 0.2 μm represents the **limit of resolution** of the LM, the maximal resolving power of which is restricted by the wavelength of light (the source of illumination). Because of this absolute limitation, magnifications exceeding $\times$1,400 are unobtainable with the LM.

The **electron microscope** (EM) uses an electron beam instead of light rays, and electromagnetic coils instead of glass lenses. Generated electrons are first accelerated and then focused by the electromagnetic fields of these coils. The **electron beam** produced is of shorter wavelength than a light beam, so it can achieve greater magnification and resolution. Modern EMs provide magnifications of up to $\times$50,000 or so, and this makes it possible to resolve biological details only 1 nm apart.

Transmission Electron Microscope

The type of EM used in most routine work is in some ways comparable to an LM. Its electron beam is transmitted through the section, so it is called a **transmission electron microscope** (TEM). The electron path is compared with the simplified light path of an LM in Figure 1-13 . Electrons emitted by the **cathode** (generally a heated tungsten filament) are accelerated toward the **anode** by a large voltage difference. The stream of electrons passing through a central aperture in the anode becomes shaped into an electron beam by an electromagnetic **condenser lens** corresponding to that of an LM. However, electrons cannot travel far unless they are in a high vacuum, and this limitation, along with the fact that accelerated electrons are highly damaging, precludes use of the EM for studying living cells. The electrons that remain unscattered by electron-blocking (**electron-dense**) regions of the EM section reach the **objective lens.** The enlarged image that this lens produces is further magnified by a **projection lens** corresponding to an LM eyepiece. The final image is projected onto a fluorescent viewing screen or the film for a **transmission electron micrograph.**

Preparation of TEM Sections

Tissue blocks are generally fixed in glutaraldehyde and postfixed in osmic acid. Following dehydration in alcohol, they are transferred to propylene oxide, which is miscible with the resinous embedding medium. Because accelerated electrons do not penetrate deeply into tissues, TEM sections are extremely thin (60-80 nm).

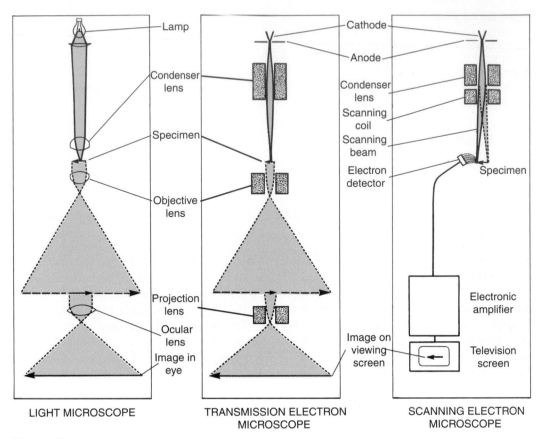

LIGHT MICROSCOPE   TRANSMISSION ELECTRON   SCANNING ELECTRON
                       MICROSCOPE   MICROSCOPE

Figure 1-13
Imaging paths of the transmission and scanning electron microscopes and light microscope. Optical path of the light microscope is inverted and simplified to facilitate comparison.

A hard embedding medium (e.g., an epoxy resin) is therefore necessary. The tissue block is infiltrated with the unpolymerized resin and gentle heat is applied to harden the resin. Sections are cut on a plate glass edge or diamond knife, mounted on a device called an **ultramicrotome**. Salts of metals with high atomic numbers (heavy metals) are suitable EM stains because such metals scatter electrons and therefore appear electron-dense. Components of cells and tissues have varying affinities for heavy metals, and this selective uptake increases contrast in the image. The metals commonly used are osmium (as osmic acid, which acts as a stain as well as a fixative), uranium (as uranyl acetate), and lead (as lead hydroxide).

Transmission Electron Micrographs

The energy of the accelerated electrons reaching the fluorescent screen of a TEM is converted into visible light. A more permanent record is obtained when this energy acts on a photographic emulsion to produce silver grains. Printing of such EM negatives as enlarged **electron micrographs** not only discloses fine details in the image but also leads to the reversal of black and white. Parts of an EM section that scatter electrons appear white in EM negatives because insufficient electrons remain in these areas for grain formation in the emulsion. The same areas are reversed to black when the negatives are printed. Hence, the *black* regions in printed electron micrographs represent the *electron-dense* regions in EM sections.

Whereas focusing up and down helps to show whether a given component of an LM section lies in a different plane from another, everything in an EM section lies in a single plane of focus, a limitation that should always be taken into account in interpreting transmission electron micrographs. Furthermore, in contrast to the complete disclosure of entire cells by two or three LM sections, approximately 400 EM sections are required to achieve this end.

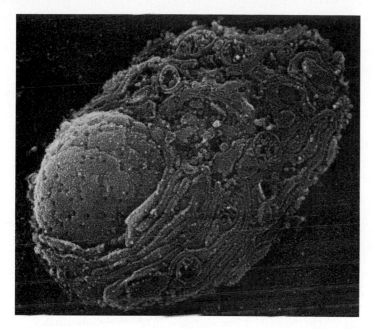

Figure 1-14
Scanning electron microscopes can reveal nuclear and cytoplasmic membranes of cells in three dimensions (chondrocyte, ×12,000).

Scanning Electron Microscope

Knowledge of the fine structure (**ultrastructure**) of cells and tissues largely depends on availability of the relevant transmission electron micrographs. However, in cases where surface features are more relevant than internal structure, a **scanning electron microscope** (SEM) may be used (see Fig. 1-13). It is not necessary for the electron beam of the SEM to pass through the specimen. Instead, it scans the surface. Reflected electrons and secondary electrons emitted from the thin heavy metal coating applied to the specimen's surface are converted into electrical signals that provide a televised image of the scanned surface. Photographic prints of these images (**scanning electron micrographs**) show surface projections and recesses much as they would be seen in three dimensions (Fig. 1-14).

Electron Microscopic Measurements

Electron microscopic measurements are metric. One *micrometer* (μm) represents 0.001 millimeter, and 1 *nanometer* (nm) (Gk. *nanos,* dwarf) represents 0.001 μm (i.e., one millionth of a millimeter). The *Angström unit* (Å), formerly used, represents 0.1 nm; hence 1 nm = 10 Å. EM sections, which are much thinner (60 to 80 nm) than LM sections (5 to 8 μm), are sometimes referred to as **thin sections.**

Summary

Histology relates the microscopic structure of cells and tissues to tissue functions. The four basic tissues are epithelial, connective, nervous, and muscle tissue. The body is made up of cells, extracellular matrix, and body fluids.

The basic parts of the cell are the cytoplasm, which surrounds the nucleus and is bounded by the cell membrane, and the nucleus, which contains chromatin and a nucleolus and is bounded by the nuclear envelope. Cells contain structural and enzymatic proteins, generally with some stored carbohydrate (PAS-positive glycogen) or stored lipid (which becomes extracted from paraffin sections but is retained in frozen sections).

Some constituents of the extracellular matrix form fibers, providing strength and elasticity; the others are amorphous and hold tissue fluid. The chief body fluids are 1) blood, which consists of plasma and cells and circulates in vessels; 2) tissue (interstitial) fluid, which occupies intercellular spaces and permits nutrients, gases, and metabolites to exchange between the blood and tissue cells; and 3) lymph, which is excess protein-containing tissue fluid collected by lymphatics.

Hematoxylin, a blue basic stain, is positively charged (cationic), whereas eosin, a red acid stain, is negatively charged (anionic). However, the colors that these two stains impart are essentially nonspecific indicators of chemical composition. Basic (positive) stains bind to multiple PO_4^{3-} groups on nucleic acids, and, to a lesser extent, multiple SO_3^- groups on certain interstitial matrix macromolecules. Acid (negative) stains bind to positive sites (e.g., NH_3^+) on fixed proteins.

The histologic planes of section are longitudinal, transverse, oblique, and grazing (tangential). Distinguishable arrangements in sections include tubules, partitions, and rows of cells, but their recognition may require thinking in three dimensions.

Increasing magnification diminishes the field of view. The amount of detail seen increases with LM magnifications up to $\times 1,400$ or so. LM sections are 5 to 8 μm thick (1 μm = 0.001 mm). Maximal resolution of the LM is 0.2 μm; for greater resolution an EM is required.

The transmission EM, with magnifications up to $\times 50,000$, is capable of resolving details 1 nm apart (1 nm = 0.001 μm). EM sections, 60 to 80 nm thick, are stained with heavy metals, which scatter electrons. Black areas in electron micrographs are electron-dense, and everything in an EM section focuses in a single plane.

Bibliography

Light Microscopy

Barer R. Lecture Notes on the Use of the Microscope. Oxford, Blackwell, 1968.

Dixon K. Principles of some tinctorial and cytochemical methods. In Champion RH, Gilman T, Rook AJ, Sims RT, eds. An Introduction to the Biology of the Skin. Oxford, Blackwell, 1970.

Gaunt PN, Gaunt WA. Three-Dimensional Reconstruction in Biology. Baltimore, University Park Press, 1978.

James J. Light Microscopic Techniques in Biology and Medicine. The Hague, Martinus Nijhoff, 1976.

Krstí RV. Illustrated Encyclopedia of Human Histology. Berlin, Springer-Verlag, 1984.

Pawley JB, ed. Handbook of Biological Confocal Microscopy. New York, Plenum, 1990.

Pearse AGE. Histochemistry: Theoretical and Applied, ed 3, vols 1 and 2. Boston, Little, Brown & Co, 1968.

Shuman H, Murray JM, DiLullo C. Confocal microscopy: An overview. BioTechniques 7:154, 1989.

Skawamura A, Jr, ed. Fluorescent Antibody Techniques and Their Application, ed 2. Baltimore, University Park Press, 1977.

Taylor D, Nederlof M, Lanni F, Waggoner A. The new vision of light microscopy. Am Sci 80:322, 1992.

Wilson T, ed. Confocal Microscopy. London, Academic Press, 1990.

Electron Microscopy

Agar AW, Alderson RH, Chescoe D. Principles and practice of electron microscope operations. In: Glauert AM, ed. Practical Methods in Electron Microscopy, vol 2. Amsterdam, North Holland, 1974.

Bullock GR. The current status of fixation for electron microscopy: a review. J Microsc 133:1, 1984.

Everhart TE, Hayes TL. The scanning electron microscope. Sci Am 226(1):54, 1972.

Frank J. Three-dimensional imaging techniques in electron microscopy. BioTechniques 7:164, 1989.

Glauert AM. Fixation, dehydration and embedding of biological specimens. In: Glauert AM, ed. Practical Methods in Electron Microscopy, vol 3, pt 1. Amsterdam, North Holland, 1975.

Hayat MA. Basic Electron Microscopy Technics. New York, Van Nostrand Reinhold, 1972.

Hayat MA. Introduction to Biological Scanning Electron Microscopy. Baltimore, University Park Press, 1978.

Hayat MA. Correlative Microscopy in Biology: Instrumentation and Methods. Orlando, Academic Press, 1987.

Lewis PR, Knight DP. Staining methods for sectioned material. In: Glauert AM, ed. Practical Methods in Electron Microscopy, vol 5. Amsterdam, North Holland, 1977.

Maunsbach AB, Afzelius BA. Biomedical Electron Microscopy: Illustrated Methods and Interpretations. San Diego, Academic Press, 1999.

Reid N. Ultramicrotomy. In: Glauert AM, ed. Practical Methods in Electron Microscopy, vol 3, pt 2. Amsterdam, North Holland, 1975.

Severs NJ. Freeze-fracture cytochemistry: review of methods. J Electron Microsc Tech 13:175, 1989.

Van Aelst AC, Wilms HJ. A scanning electron microscopic method for intracellular and extracellular structure. Stain Technol 63:327, 1988.

Wischnitzer S. Introduction to Electron Microscopy, ed 2. New York, Pergamon Press, 1970.

CHAPTER 2

Cell Nucleus

OBJECTIVES

The contents of this chapter should enable you to do the following:

* Describe a cell nucleus and nucleolus and state their functions
* Discuss the composition and functional properties of two different forms of chromatin
* Explain what is meant by a cell cycle
* Outline the body's various arrangements for cell renewal
* Describe four stages of mitosis
* Define diploid, haploid, polyploid, and aneuploid
* Differentiate between mitotic cells and any dead cells also present in a section

Within each typical body cell is a distinct compartment called the **cell nucleus**, the contents of which are segregated from the cytoplasm by a double-limiting membrane known as the **nuclear envelope** or **nuclear membrane**. Serving as a master control center, the nucleus contains almost all the cell's deoxyribonucleic acid (DNA); however, a small proportion of DNA in slightly different form is also present in the mitochondria. The DNA stored within the nucleus is essential to the cell because its genes encode the amino acid sequences of the various proteins that the cell must produce to stay alive. Furthermore, the nucleus is the part of the cell where the process of decoding these genetic instructions begins.

Each newly formed cell requires an entire set of genes. Before dividing, the mother cell therefore has to replicate all the DNA molecules present in its nucleus. Both of the progeny cells from the usual kind of division (**mitosis**) receive the same full complement of DNA that in the previous division was passed on to their mother cell. But in **meiosis**, which is the special division process that produces germ cells for reproduction, only half the usual amount of DNA enters each germ cell, and the full complement of DNA necessary for the next generation is attained upon fertilization. Mitosis, which is relatively uncomplicated, is described in this chapter. Because meiosis is more complex, it is appropriately described in the context of female reproduction (see Chapter 17).

Mitosis represents only a short proportion of a cell's total lifespan. Over the remainder, typical cells carry out useful functions for the body as a whole. We shall first consider nuclear appearance when such activities are in progress.

NUCLEAR ORGANIZATION

Figure 2-1 illustrates the nucleus of hepatocytes in H&E-stained sections, observed under oil immersion. At the nuclear boundary, a bluish-purple line indicates the position of the **nuclear envelope** or **nuclear membrane**. The one or more large, deeply stained masses within the nucleus are **nucleoli**, and the many small, dark-staining granules are **chromatin**. Dark bluish-purple staining of these components indicates an abundance of nucleic acids.

The **nucleolus** has a conspicuous appearance in large nuclei that have well-dispersed chromatin. A few such nuclei may exhibit two or more nucleoli (see Fig. 2-1, cell at right), whereas other nuclei appear to lack nucleoli because these are not represented in the plane of section. In most cases, however, the nucleolus appears as a single rounded and darkly stained mass. Its deep basophilic staining is chiefly due to nucleolus-associated chromatin (see Fig. 2-2). Small nuclei usually contain so much condensed chromatin that it obscures the nucleolus in LM sections (see Fig. 2-1, lining cell of sinusoid).

The above features are common to most nuclei. However, shapes, sizes, and numbers of nuclei are not identical in all cell types, and this variability is sometimes useful for cell identification. Most cells possess a rounded, loosely packed nucleus resembling that of a hepatocyte, but some have a relatively small nucleus with tightly packed contents, as for example in the cells lining the blood spaces (sinusoids) of the liver. A few kinds of cells possess a nucleus of distinctive shape, e.g., neutrophils, which are white blood cells with a deeply indented (**segmented**) nucleus (see Fig. 6-5). Occasionally, certain cells that ordinarily possess a single nucleus acquire a second one, thereby becoming **binucleated** (e.g., a minority of hepatocytes and muscle cells in the heart). Certain other cell types always have several nuclei (i.e., more than two) and so are described as **multinucleated**, e.g., osteoclasts (cells that erode bone) and skeletal muscle cells. A few cell types have a single nucleus that is exceptionally large because it contains multiple amounts of DNA, e.g., megakaryocytes (the cells that produce blood platelets) and a small proportion of hepatocytes (see Fig. 2-20*B*). Finally, two cellular elements of blood possess no nucleus at all—red blood cells (erythrocytes) and blood platelets (the cytoplasmic fragments of megakaryocytes) persist for some time without a nucleus, but lack the nuclear DNA necessary for continuing protein synthesis and do not divide.

Genetic Sequences

Precise specifications exist for synthesizing proteins. With the exception of a few mitochondrial proteins, their molecular structure is specified by nuclear DNA sequences called **genes**. An example of a gene would be a series of DNA base sequences that collectively specify the amino acid sequence

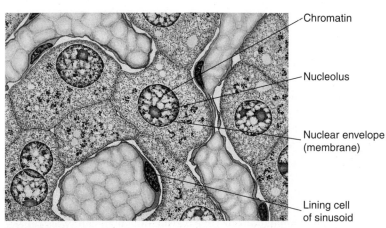

Chromatin

Nucleolus

Nuclear envelope (membrane)

Lining cell of sinusoid

Figure 2-1
Light microscopic appearance of interphase nuclei, showing their chromatin granules and abundant extended chromatin (hepatocytes, H&E). Hepatic sinusoid-lining cells have nuclei that are packed with condensed chromatin.

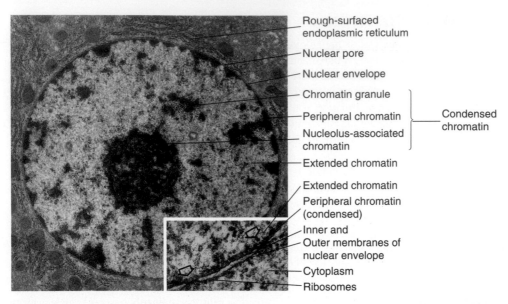

Rough-surfaced
endoplasmic reticulum

Nuclear pore

Nuclear envelope

Chromatin granule

Peripheral chromatin

Nucleolus-associated
chromatin

Condensed
chromatin

Extended chromatin

Extended chromatin

Peripheral chromatin
(condensed)

Inner and
Outer membranes of
nuclear envelope

Cytoplasm

Ribosomes

Figure 2-2
Electron micrograph of an interphase nucleus (hepatocyte, ×14,000). (*Inset*) Nuclear envelope seen under higher magnification. *Arrows* indicate nuclear pores.

of a constituent polypeptide of a protein. A more comprehensive definition of a gene is a series of nucleotide base sequences arranged along the same nucleic acid molecule (DNA in every case except retroviruses) that collectively encode a functional RNA molecule. Although each DNA molecule contains a great deal of genetic information, it does not consist entirely of genes. Stretches of genetically meaningless DNA can lie between one gene and the next, and in many cases irrelevant nucleotide sequences are interposed within the gene sequence itself. The amino acid-specifying segments of such a "discontinuous" gene are termed **exons** because they are **expressed** by the cell. The extraneous interrupting sequences are termed **introns** because they are physically **included** among the gene sequence, even though they are not expressed. Within the nucleus, each DNA molecule is coiled, supercoiled, and looped in an elaborate manner so as to constitute a thread-shaped structure called a **chromosome**. During mitosis (Gk., thread-like condition), each chromosome becomes microscopically visible as an individual thread that stains intensely with hematoxylin (Gk. *chroma*, color; *soma*, body). During the greater part of the cell's lifespan, however, chromosomes are typically indistinguishable as separate entities because they exist in a partly condensed and partly extended state that gives them the collective appearance of **chromatin granules** instead of individual threads. Moreover, most extended regions of chromosomes represent sites where genetic instructions are being used for protein synthesis, as we shall now describe.

Protein synthesis occurs in two stages. First, the information content of a gene is **transcribed** (copied) from DNA. This process, which occurs within the nucleus, produces a coded intermediate message, composed of the bases that make up RNA. The coded RNA message then reaches the cytoplasm, where its instructions are **translated** (decoded), directly specifying the amino acid sequence of the polypeptide being synthesized. The two stages of protein synthesis are discussed in more detail later in this chapter.

Different cell types express different combinations of genes, even though all cell types (in any given species) possess the same genetic information encoded in their DNA. In other words, the same gene complement becomes expressed in a variety of ways. Furthermore, acquisition of new structural or functional characteristics by a cell commonly reflects change in regulation of gene expression. Genetically regulated acquisition of specialized structural or functional attributes is termed **cell differentiation**. Successful manipulation of differentiation depends on an understanding of how sequential gene activation leads to differentiation.

Nuclear Envelope

The nuclear envelope is the limiting structure that compartmentalizes the contents of the nucleus, segregating them from the cytoplasm. Readers who are not familiar with the fine details of nuclear structure should compare Figure 2-2 with Figure 2-1, which shows the appearance of comparable nuclei at the LM level. Intense basophilia of the nuclear periphery is due to adherent chromatin, which is known as **peripheral chromatin** because of its peripheral position (Figs. 2-2 and 2-3). The nuclear envelope is too thin to be resolved with the LM. The EM shows that it is a double structure composed of two membranes (hence the name *envelope*) with a narrow intermembranous space (see Figs. 2-2, *inset*, and 2-3). The nuclear envelope is also provided with unique bidirectional access sites called **nuclear pores**, and its inner membrane is reinforced by a thin, finely fibrillar **nuclear lamina**. This membrane-supporting layer is made up of three polypeptides, called **lamins**, that are arranged as a meshwork of fine filaments (**intermediate filaments**, see Chapter 3). Peripheral chromatin adheres to the inner aspect of the nuclear lamina. The outer membrane of the nuclear envelope is studded with electron-dense particles called **ribosomes**; it is continuous with a cytoplasmic membranous system termed the **rough-surfaced endoplasmic reticulum**, described in Chapter 3. More information on the electron microscopic appearance and structure of membranes in general may be found in Chapter 3, under the heading Cell Membrane.

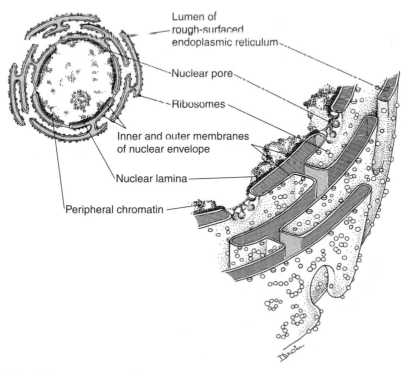

Lumen of
rough-surfaced
endoplasmic reticulum

Nuclear pore

Ribosomes

Inner and outer membranes
of nuclear envelope

Nuclear lamina

Peripheral chromatin

Figure 2-3
Interconnections between nuclear envelope and rough-surfaced endoplasmic reticulum. Inner and outer membranes of the nuclear envelope are continuous with each other around perimeters of nuclear pores.

Nuclear Pores

Certain macromolecules pass between the nucleus and cytoplasm by way of **nuclear pores**, which are gated transport sites on the nuclear surface (indicated by arrows in Fig. 2-2, *inset*). As may be seen in Figure 2-3, inner and outer membranes of the nuclear envelope are continuous with each other at the circular periphery of a nuclear pore. Each nuclear pore is characterized by containing a **nuclear pore complex** with eightfold symmetry (Fig. 2-4). The nuclear pore complex is believed to be made up of anchored coaxial rings with a medial spoke assembly that supports a central regulated aqueous pore or transporter that is ATP-dependent. The nuclear pore complex regulates access of large macromolecules to the nuclear compartment and also macromolecular exit from it. However, proteins (and other molecules) with a molecular weight <50,000 can diffuse across the nuclear pore complex in either direction. Nucleoproteins accumulate in the nucleus because they possess **nuclear localization signals** that bring about their active transport into the nucleus.

Chromatin and Nuclear Matrix

When a cell is not dividing, some of the chromatin domains are in an extended condition whereas others are highly condensed. The condensed regions collectively constitute **condensed chromatin (heterochromatin)**, which is intensely basophilic and electron-dense. Aggregates of such condensed regions are visible as **chromatin granules** associated with the nuclear envelope (**peripheral chromatin**, see Figs. 2-2 and 2-3) and nucleolus (**nucleolus-associated chromatin**, see Fig. 2-2). Other aggregates of condensed chromatin lie dispersed throughout the nucleus. Gene transcription is suppressed in condensed chromatin. Transcriptionally active DNA is present only in **extended chromatin (euchromatin)**, a much less electron-dense form of chromatin (see Fig. 2-2) that cannot be resolved in the LM. Representing extended chromatin domains of chromosomes, it occupies the

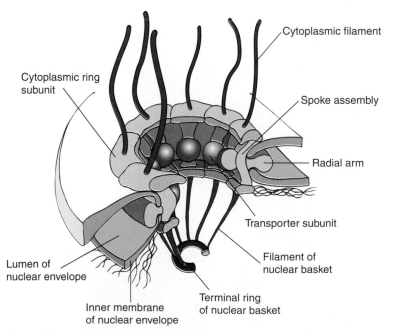

Figure 2-4
Detailed model of the nuclear pore complex. The attached cytoplasmic filaments and nuclear basket appear to be anchoring devices. The nuclear basket is firmly anchored to the nuclear matrix.

unstained regions of the nucleus. Hence, the unstained background represents the site where DNA is being transcribed; it contains extended chromatin, nucleoproteins, and the three forms of RNA (which are described later in this chapter). When a cell is not dividing, some of the nucleoproteins serve as attachment sites for DNA, and others are associated with enzymes that participate in DNA transcription and replication. Such proteins and the nuclear lamina to which they are attached therefore have skeletal, transcriptional, and/or replicative roles and are recognized as functionally important components of the supporting framework of the nucleus, which is known as the **nuclear matrix** or **nucleoskeleton**.

Further cell differentiation and hormonal induction of gene expression involve a changing of position of chromosomal gene-bearing domains within the nucleus. This repositioning brings the chromosomal domains with genes that are to be transcribed into close apposition with nuclear pores and the nuclear lamina.

DNA Codons

The two long polynucleotide chains of each DNA molecule are intertwined, forming a double helix (Fig. 2-5). The backbone of each chain is made up of alternating phosphate and deoxyribose sugar groups; a nitrogenous base extends as a side chain from each sugar group toward the interior of the double helix. The four bases of DNA are represented in Figure 2-5 as **A** for **adenine, T** for **thymine, C** for **cytosine**, and **G** for **guanine**. A salient feature shown in this diagram is specific obligatory pairing of bases in one chain with complementary bases in the other: adenine (A) always pairs with thymine (T), and cytosine (C) always pairs with guanine (G). As we shall see, precise matching of these complementary base pairs, known as **complementary base pairing**, enables an exact replica of each DNA molecule to be synthesized when DNA replicates.

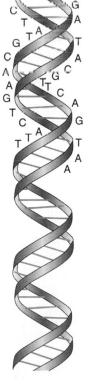

Figure 2-5
Two polynucleotide chains constitute the double helix of the DNA molecule. Obligatory base pairing occurs between A (adenine) and T (thymine), and also between G (guanine) and C (cytosine).

Nuclear DNA has genetic instructions for maintaining the cell's various vital functions. Genetic information is essentially a compilation of short code words that lie discontinuously encrypted in an immensely long, jumbled string of words. The interrupted, linear gene sequences in DNA are made up of triplet **codons** (code words) each *composed of three bases*. In most cases, gene sequences specify amino acids and their order of incorporation into polypeptides. At least one codon exists for each amino acid.

Interphase DNA Organization

Although chromosomes are condensed and recognizable at mitosis, without special methods they are unrecognizable as separate entities during interphase. This is because in interphase they exist in a partly extended and partly condensed state that results in the overall appearance of **chromatin granules. Chromatin** is a macromolecular complex, composed mostly of **DNA** together with **histones**, gene-regulatory **proteins**, and a small, variable proportion of **RNA**. Granules of **condensed chromatin** (see Fig. 2-2) are electron-dense aggregates of the chromosome regions that are not being transcribed. **Extended chromatin**, which is less electron-dense, is characterized by narrow chromatin fibers with a diameter indicative of several orders of DNA coiling. The organization of these fibers is conceptualized as the DNA double helix (2 nm wide) wound over a series of tiny spool-like structures called **nucleosomes.** The string of nucleosomes is coiled into a superhelix (30-nm wide) with the EM appearance of a chromatin fiber.

The currently accepted way in which the DNA is arranged in a **chromatin fiber** is shown in Figure 2-6. During mitosis, DNA is maximally compacted by tight looping and winding of the chromatin fiber, with the result that the long DNA molecule becomes accommodated by a relatively short, rod-like structure, the **mitotic chromosome** (Fig. 2-6, *top*).

Helical winding of the DNA molecule for two turns around the spool-like cores of nucleosomes achieves the first order of compaction. The core of each nucleosome is an octamer of four different histones; the fifth histone sequentially interconnects each adjacent nucleosome, stabilizing the distinctive linear array. These levels of organization characterize condensed and extended interphase chromatin, including chromatin that is transcriptionally active. The second order of compaction of interphase DNA is due to supercoiling of the chromatin fiber. In this configuration, called a **solenoid**, approximately six nucleosomes constitute each helical turn. In addition, **looped domains** of chromatin fiber with the supercoiled (solenoidal) configuration are present in both interphase chromatin and mitotic chromosomes. During DNA synthesis, these loops replicate as discrete entities when reeled through replication complexes bound to the nuclear matrix. Their average length and numbers indicate that most of them are sites of more than one gene. Such loops are observable in suitably prepared mitotic chromosomes (see Fig. 2-19). Their proximal ends are anchored in the supporting framework (chromosomal scaffold) by DNA topoisomerase II, one of the enzymes involved in chromatin compaction.

In any given cell type, certain genes are not expressed. All the cell's genes nevertheless have to be copied when the nuclear DNA replicates in preparation for cell division.

DNA Replication

When DNA replicates, DNA topoisomerase I produces a temporary nick in a DNA strand. This enables a short length of the double helix to unwind at a time. Each unwound portion of polynucleotide chain then acts as a template for DNA polymerase-mediated polymerization of a complementary new strand alongside it. The base sequence of the newly formed strand is complementary to that of the template strand. In each double-stranded DNA molecule produced, one strand is obtained directly from the original molecule and the complementary strand is synthesized anew.

Sequential **mismatch proofreading mechanisms** enable cells to detect most DNA replication errors (i.e., DNA base-pairing mistakes) and then rectify them. Also, **base excision-repair** and **nucleotide excision-repair** mechanisms are able to excise and replace DNA segments that are defective (e.g., DNA segments damaged by ultraviolet light, ionizing radiation, reactive metabolites, or other mutagenic agents). In some species, DNA polymerase itself possesses intrinsic proofreading capabilities. DNA base-pairing errors that are left unrectified are known as **mutations.**

Nuclear DNA replicates several hours before mitosis so each thread-like mitotic chromosome contains *two* complete DNA molecules. DNA synthesis is discussed further under Cell Cycle.

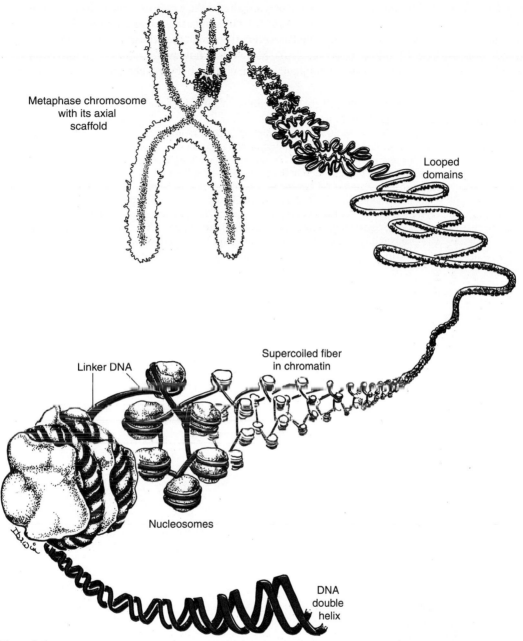

Figure 2-6
The several orders of DNA coiling and compaction in interphase chromatin and mitotic chromosomes.

Radioautographic Detection of DNA Replication

One strand of each replicating DNA molecule is synthesized anew from deoxyribonucleoside triphosphates. Cells that incorporate such DNA precursors are therefore undergoing DNA synthesis. If one of the DNA precursors is radioactively labeled, cells that are undergoing DNA synthesis may be specifically identified through use of an applied histological technique called **radioautography**. The deoxyribonucleoside **thymidine** is the precursor used because it becomes incorporated solely into DNA. **Tritiated thymidine** (thymidine labeled with tritium, a radioisotope of hydrogen) is used almost universally for radioautographic detection of DNA synthesis. Silver grains are found over the chromosomes of cells that have incorporated this precursor, as labeled **thymine**, into their new DNA strands and then entered mitosis (see Fig. 2-7*B*). More often, however, grains are found over nuclei of cells that have incorporated labeled thymine into their DNA but have not yet entered mitosis (see Fig. 2-7*A*).

Radioautography has been helpful for establishing cell lineages and has facilitated our detailed understanding of certain cell functions.

In general, cells handle low concentrations of radioisotopes (or radioisotope-labeled precursors) in similar ways to the unlabeled molecules. Sites of incorporation of radioactivity into tissues are established with either the LM or the EM (depending on the resolution required) by applying a coating of photographic emulsion because ionizing radiation affects the emulsion in the same manner as light.

The coated preparations are stored for several weeks in the dark to permit ionizing radiation to act on silver bromide crystals in the emulsion. Following the usual course of photographic developing and fixing, radiation-affected crystals appear in the LM as characteristic black dots (**grains**) that lie above sites from which radiation emanated (Fig. 2-7). Such preparations are called **radioautographs** (Gk. *radio,* ray-like; *autos,* self; *graphō,* to write). The grains indicate sites of incorporation of the radioisotope (Fig. 2-7, *top*).

The next section outlines the roles of DNA and RNA in protein synthesis.

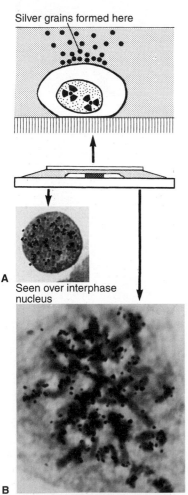

A Seen over interphase nucleus

Figure 2-7
Tritiated thymidine incorporation in S phase (nuclear DNA replication) is readily detectable by radioautography.

B Seen over mitotic chromosomes

TRANSCRIPTION AND TRANSLATION

RNA molecules resemble DNA molecules, except that 1) the sugar groups of RNAs are D-ribose, not 2-deoxy-D-ribose as in DNA, and 2) the base uracil of RNA replaces the base thymine of DNA. Furthermore, RNA exists in three distinct forms known as **messenger RNA, ribosomal RNA,** and **transfer RNA,** all with essential roles in protein synthesis.

Complementary base pairing during DNA replication ensures that a T is incorporated wherever an A is present in the template strand. Likewise, a G is added wherever there is a C, an A wherever there is a T, and a C wherever there is a G. Complementary base pairing occurs also in DNA **transcription** (information copying from DNA to RNA). DNA needs to be in its extended (euchromatin) configuration to be transcribed. Moreover, the information for any given gene is confined to a single strand of the DNA double helix (Fig. 2-8); the apposed strand conveys only complementary

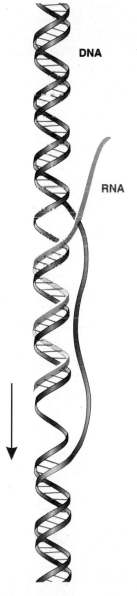

DNA

RNA

Figure 2-8
One polynucleotide chain in the DNA double helix acts as the template during its transcription into RNA.

information. A key difference between DNA replication and gene transcription is that during complementary base pairing, *RNA incorporates the base uracil* (U) in place of thymine (T). The base composition of RNA is therefore C, G, A and U, and where A is present in transcribable DNA, U becomes incorporated into the transcript (Fig. 2-9).

Messenger RNA

The amino acid sequence of each constituent polypeptide of a protein is specified by a series of three-nucleotide codons that lie along the length of a DNA strand. In some cases, the codon series is interrupted, i.e., discontinuous. To convey specifications from the nucleus to the cytoplasm, which is where protein molecules are synthesized, the information encoded in DNA is copied (**transcribed**) into a form of RNA called **messenger RNA** (mRNA). The other forms of RNA collaborate in polypeptide synthesis according to the specifications transcribed into mRNA.

Messenger RNA Processing

Some genetic sequences are interrupted by several irrelevant series of base sequences. The scattered intervening nongenetic groups of nucleotide sequences are known as **introns**. The newly transcribed RNA molecules, which are termed **precursor RNA molecules** or **primary RNA transcripts**, may therefore contain extraneous and gene-encoded sequences (Fig. 2-10). The intron-encoded extraneous segments are excised. The remaining segments (**exons**) are then spliced together to form a con-

DNA   **RNA**

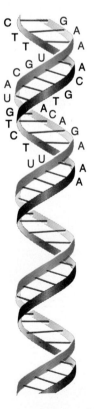

Figure 2-9
When one polynucleotide chain in the DNA double helix becomes transcribed into RNA, uracil (U) becomes incorporated into the polymerizing RNA molecule at sites where adenine (A) lies along the DNA template.

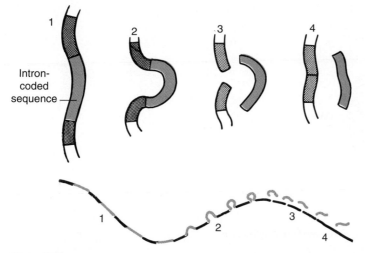

Figure 2-10

In mRNA processing, intron-coded sequences are excised from the primary mRNA transcripts. (*1*) An intron-coded sequence interrupts the genetically encoded sequence. (*2*) Discontinuous parts of the genetically encoded sequence become closely approximated through lateral looping of the intron-coded sequence. (*3*) The intron-coded sequence is excised. (*4*) Discontinuous parts of the genetically encoded sequence become spliced together, producing the mature mRNA molecule.

tinuous linear series, producing a mature mRNA molecule. This **RNA processing** occurs inside the nucleus prior to translation.

From the nuclear compartment of the cell, mRNA molecules pass to the cytoplasm, where their genetic information is decoded. The polypeptides they specify are assembled on **ribosomes**, which are nonmembranous cytoplasmic organelles consisting largely of **ribosomal RNA**.

Ribosomal RNA

A **ribosome** is a cytoplasmic electron-dense particle made up of a large subunit and a small subunit, each composed of ribosomal RNA (rRNA) complexed with protein as ribonucleoprotein. The rRNA is transcribed (in precursor form) from genes found only in the nucleolus. Its base composition is not variable as in mRNA because its role in protein synthesis is not specific to any particular protein. Ribosomes provide the necessary sites for assembling amino acids into proteins according to the instructions on mRNA. For assembly to proceed, however, the third form of RNA, **transfer RNA**, is also necessary.

Transfer RNA

Each transfer RNA (tRNA) possesses 1) a recognition site for one of the 20 amino acids and 2) a codon that specifically recognizes the complementary codon in mRNA (Fig. 2-11). The unique molecular structure of tRNAs enables them to match the amino acids they transfer to the nucleotide sequence present in mRNA.

Polypeptide Assembly

The nucleotide sequence of mRNA is **translated** in the cytoplasm. Here, a small ribosomal subunit binds to the 5' end of the mRNA, then a large ribosomal subunit locks onto the small subunit. When the mRNA passes between the two subunits, much as thread passes through the eye of a needle, its

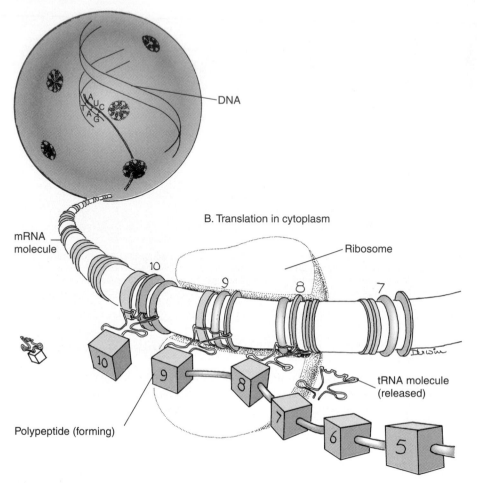

A. Transcription in nucleus

DNA

B. Translation in cytoplasm

mRNA
molecule

Ribosome

10

9   8   7

tRNA molecule
(released)

Polypeptide (forming)

Figure 2-11
Simplified schematic diagram of transcription (*A*) and translation (*B*). Amino acids assembling in the order transcribed
from a gene to mRNA are represented by blocks.

encoded information becomes translated. The leading (i.e., 5') end of the mRNA progressively
reaches other ribosomes so it is common to find a number of ribosomes spaced fairly regularly along
the molecule. Such an arrangement is termed a **polysome** (short form of **polyribosome**).

As a consequence of tRNA-mediated complementary base pairing, each ribosome assembles
amino acids in the order specified by the mRNA. A number of identical polypeptide chains can be
assembled concurrently, one by each ribosome through which the mRNA passes. As soon as the
amino acids become incorporated, their tRNAs are released and reused. Also, the same ribosomes
are used repeatedly in the synthesis of different proteins. Further details about protein synthesis may
be found in Chapter 3 in the sections on Ribosomes and Rough-Surfaced Endoplasmic Reticulum.

Hence, transcription occurs on extended chromatin in the nucleus, and translation takes place
on ribosomes in the cytoplasm.

Next, we consider where rRNA is formed and discuss how it becomes incorporated into ribosomes.

NUCLEOLUS

Ribosomal RNA is transcribed exclusively in **nucleoli**. Indeed, cells that are actively synthesizing proteins may often be recognized by the fact that their nucleoli appear large and prominent. Within each nucleolus, multiple copies of **nucleolar genes**, i.e., the genes that code for rRNA, lie on five different chromosomes in regions called **nucleolar organizers**. More than one nucleolus may therefore be present within the same nucleus. In most cases, however, only one or two large nucleoli are found in each cell. This is because the nucleolar organizer regions of the five chromosomes have a tendency to associate with one another, with the result that their gene product, rRNA, aggregates into one or two confluent masses.

Suitable special preparative techniques reveal nucleolar genes undergoing transcription. In Figure 2-12, numerous rRNA molecules (in precursor form) are being transcribed from nucleolar genes, which lie in a long, repetitive series along the DNA. As visualized by this technique, each transcriptionally active gene resembles a Christmas tree, the branches of which represent forming rRNA precursor. Short branches represent the precursor at an early stage of synthesis; longer ones are nearing completion. The rRNA precursor is processed into smaller molecules that become associated with protein and are incorporated into ribosomal subunits as ribonucleoprotein.

The appearance of the transcription product of nucleolar genes is helpful in interpreting the internal organization of the nucleolus.

Fine Structure of Nucleolus

In EM sections, the nucleolus typically appears as a moderately distinct, sponge-like network of electron-dense material (Fig. 2-13). It lies free in the interior of the nucleus, with no limiting membrane. Most of its electron-dense material has a granular appearance (see Fig. 2-13, *upper left*) and hence is termed the **pars granulosa.** This component represents an accumulation of rRNA-containing **ribonucleoprotein particles,** which subsequently leave the nucleus and become incorporated into ribosomes. The other main component of the nucleolus is a condensation of fine, tightly packed filaments collectively known as the **pars fibrosa.** This electron-dense component is newly transcribed rRNA still unassociated with protein. More difficult to discern in EM sections are slightly lighter-staining regions (labeled **nucleolar organizer** in Fig. 2-13) enclosed within the

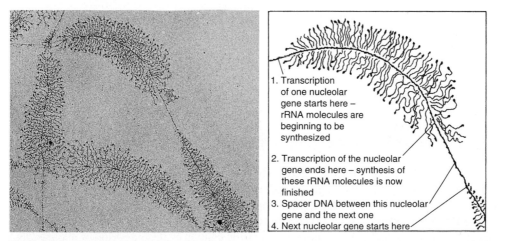

1. Transcription of one nucleolar gene starts here – rRNA molecules are beginning to be synthesized

2. Transcription of the nucleolar gene ends here – synthesis of these rRNA molecules is now finished
3. Spacer DNA between this nucleolar gene and the next one
4. Next nucleolar gene starts here

Figure 2-12
Electron micrograph of rRNA transcription from nucleolar genes and interpretive diagram (nucleolus isolated from a newt oocyte, ×25,000).

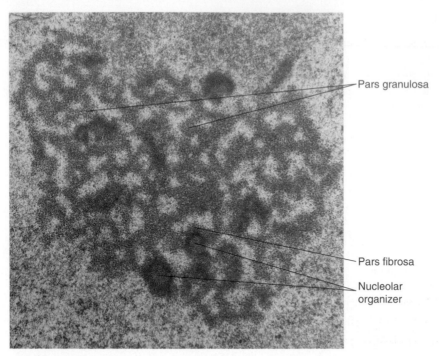

Figure 2-13
Electron micrograph of a nucleolus (mouse oocyte nucleus, ×26,000). Filamentous electron-dense material (the pars fibrosa) encloses the nucleolar organizer regions. The pars granulosa has a distinctive granular appearance.

electron-dense filamentous regions. These paler regions represent the nucleolar organizer regions of the chromosomes with nucleolar genes. Furthermore, each nucleolar gene (present as multiple copies in the extended chromatin in these regions) would correspond to a Christmas tree (see Fig. 2-12) with lateral branches (precursor rRNA molecules) that collectively constitute the pars fibrosa. When a cell undergoes mitosis (soon to be described), its nucleolus disappears in late prophase. Nucleoli reappear in the daughter cells by late telophase.

In the next part of the chapter, we consider dividing cells with their prerequisite period of DNA replication.

CELL CYCLE

A *cycle* is a sequence of events that occurs repeatedly. The concept that the life history of cells is essentially cyclical comes from studying cell types that divide repeatedly at regular intervals (*cycling cells*).

The life history of the cell, termed the **cell cycle,** is broadly divided into 1) **mitosis**, the stage of cell division, and 2) **interphase**, the stage between divisions (Fig. 2-14*A*). During one part of interphase, the cell replicates its nuclear DNA, producing a full gene complement for each of its daughter cells. The DNA replication period is determined radioautographically using tritiated thymidine. In mouse cells growing under in vitro conditions that keep them in cycle, the period of nuclear DNA synthesis, known as the **S phase** of the cell cycle (S for *synthesis*), begins about 8 hours after mito-

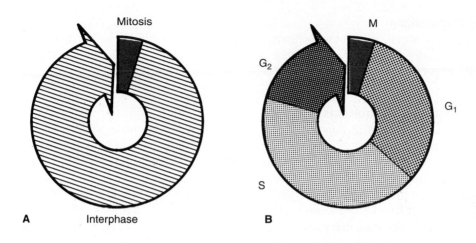

Figure 2-14
The cell cycle. (A) Mitosis and interphase. (B) Subdivisions of interphase.

sis and lasts 7 to 8 hours. The interval of 8 hours or so between mitosis and S is designated G_1 (G for *gap*), the first gap in the cell cycle. Another interval follows between the S phase and mitosis. This second gap, called G_2, lasts 4 hours or so in such cells. Hence, interphase consists of G_1, S, and G_2. An entire cell cycle is made up of the three stages of interphase plus **mitosis** (M), the shortest stage of the cycle, which takes 1–1.5 hour. Individual cell lines obtained from different species show considerable variation in duration of the cell cycle and length of its constituent stages, especially G_1, but cell cycle parameters remain fairly constant for any given cell line.

The situation is somewhat different in cells that carry out specialized functions for the body, because such cells generally are *not* in active cycle. *Specialized* functions are commonly performed by cells that are in an *extended G_1 phase*. The highest level of specialization, however, commonly requires that cells relinquish all capacity for further proliferation, so some highly differentiated cells have *left* the cell cycle and never return.

Not all the cells in a tissue specialize, however. Relatively undifferentiated cells may remain that are capable of dividing and producing specialized cells. Most of these unspecialized cells are not in active cycle. After leaving the cell cycle in G_1, they stay out of cycle until it becomes necessary for them to participate in producing specialized cells. This noncycling condition, which often lasts indefinitely but is not permanent, is termed the G_0 state (the *o* denotes that the cells are *out* of cycle). Since cells entering G_0 can be triggered back into cycle, they retain the potential for mitosis.

CELL RENEWAL

There is some truth in the generalization that in becoming highly specialized, cells may lose their capacity for proliferation. Unless replaced, however, specialized cells become depleted. In some instances, marked destruction or heavy losses stimulate the proliferation of less highly differentiated progenitors, which respond by going into cycle and generating the required numbers of specialized cells.

The body's various cell populations may be broadly classified according to their capacity for cell renewal, in the following manner.

Nonrenewing Populations

Some highly differentiated cells have entirely relinquished all capacity for mitosis, with serious consequences for those tissues that lack alternative ways of replacing their specialized cells. Adult cardiac muscle cells do not undergo renewal and therefore belong to this category.

Continuously Renewing Populations

Tissues that sustain major daily depletion of highly differentiated cells depend on continuous renewal to balance the deficit. Because of extreme specialization, however, these cells do not divide. Instead, less highly differentiated **progenitor cells**, produced in large numbers throughout life, generate the specialized cells that are needed.

Another class of cells present in this population category retains a comparatively undifferentiated state throughout adult life. These incompletely differentiated cells are mostly in the G_0 state. However, they can be triggered back into cycle at any time by cell depletion or heavy demands, and because they can give rise repeatedly to daughter cells whenever the need arises they are termed **stem cells**. Their daughter cells can either 1) *differentiate further* into progenitors of specialized cells or 2) *remain undifferentiated* as stem cells, maintaining the pool of stem cells through *self-renewal*. Under steady state conditions, mammalian stem cells undergo self-renewal divisions and differentiative divisions in roughly equal proportions. Most divisions (of either type) are symmetrical, i.e., one daughter cell is at the same stage of differentiation as the other. Some stem cells give rise to specialized cells of more than one type. Such stem cells are described as **pluripotential** or **multipotential** to indicate that several or many alternative differentiation pathways exist for their daughter cells. In contrast, **unipotential** stem cells are restricted to the production of a single specialized cell type. Continuously renewing populations derived from multipotential and pluripotential stem cells include the various types of blood cells and the gastrointestinal epithelium. In contrast, spermatozoa constitute a cell population that is continuously renewed from unipotential stem cells.

Potentially Renewable Populations

Although most types of cells that are highly differentiated do not divide, a few specialized cell types can go into cycle to compensate for severe depletion. Their potential for cell renewal is rarely evident until cell replacement becomes urgent, e.g., in hepatocytes, which go into cycle if parts of the liver are destroyed or removed. Once the original liver mass has been restored, the cycling hepatocytes become quiescent.

All these arrangements for somatic cell renewal depend on the process of mitosis, which will now be described.

MITOSIS

At the onset of mitosis, a typical human body cell (i.e., a **somatic cell**) contains 46 chromosomes. Because nuclear DNA replicates in the previous S phase, each mitotic chromosome contains two identical DNA molecules and hence is a *double* structure. As mitosis proceeds, these two molecules part company and one each enters each daughter cell. Initially, then, each mitotic chromosome is a double thread-like structure. Its two constituent threads are termed **chromatids** (Gk. *idio*, small or young), but essentially each chromatid is equivalent to a single (unreplicated) chromosome. Later in mitosis, these threads part company and are called **chromosomes**; the cell now contains 92 daughter chromosomes, each in the single configuration. Next, a set of daughter chromosomes migrates toward each pole, and when the cell splits into two, each progeny cell acquires the full complement of chromosomes.

The four stages of mitosis, lasting from 1 to 1–1.5 hours depending on the cell type, are **prophase, metaphase, anaphase,** and **telophase.** Before this process can begin it is necessary for the cell's paired centrioles to replicate.

Centriolar Replication

Between cell divisions, two tiny cytoplasmic organelles called **centrioles** lie near the middle of the cell (see Fig. 2-16A). Each centriole is a small cylindrical structure, with nine bundles of narrow tubular **microtubules** embedded in its walls (Fig. 2-15). Microtubules are hollow, polymerized assemblies of dimers of a protein called **tubulin** (see under Microtubules in Chapter 3), and in centrioles they are arranged in bundles of three (**triplets**) that are surrounded by fibrillar material.

During the course of the cell cycle, each of the centrioles replicates. Thus a cell in G_1 has a single pair of closely associated centrioles that lie perpendicular to each other (Fig. 2-16F). By G_2, each pre-existing centriole has a new centriole lying perpendicular to it, so the cell now possesses *two pairs* of centrioles (see Fig. 2-16A). When the cell enters mitosis, groups of microtubules grow from each centriole pair, forming a temporary structure called a **mitotic spindle.** The details are as follows.

Prophase

As the cell progresses into prophase, the two centriole pairs move toward opposite poles (ends) of the cell (Fig. 2-16B). This is because both arrays of **polar microtubules** that develop in association with the centriole pairs lengthen through polymerization at their distal, fast growing, **plus** end. Their continuing growth drives the centriole pairs farther apart, lengthening the mitotic spindle, until the end of anaphase.

Later in prophase, the nuclear envelope fragments and the nucleolus disappears (see Fig 2-16B). Chromosomes are first discernible as slender threads, then as darker-staining, wavy rods. They continue to shorten and thicken when the cell enters metaphase. This progressive change in mitotic chromosomes is described as chromatin **condensation.**

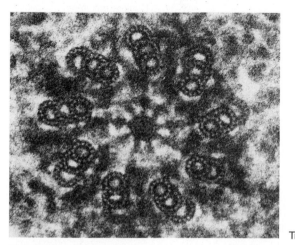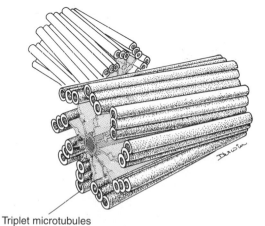

Triplet microtubules

Figure 2-15
Electron micrograph of a centriole in transverse section (chick tracheal epithelial cell, ×330,000) and interpretive diagram of a centriole pair. Nine triplet microtubules are arranged around an axial structure that resembles a cartwheel in this plane of section.

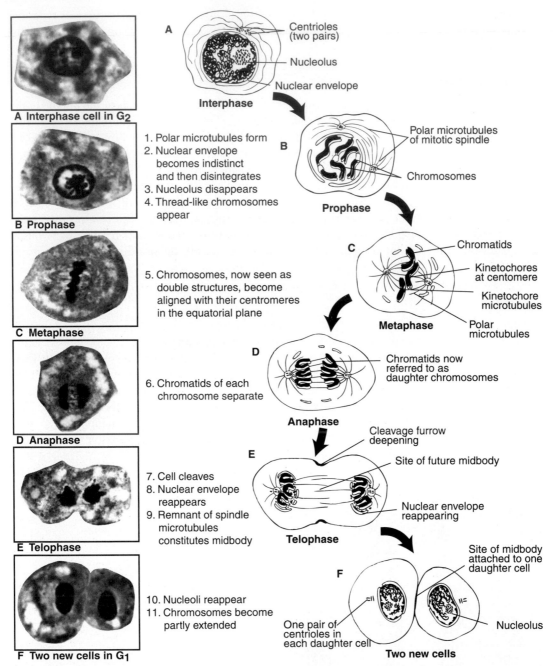

A Interphase cell in G₂

B Prophase

C Metaphase

D Anaphase

E Telophase

F Two new cells in G₁

A

Centrioles
(two pairs)

Nucleolus

Nuclear envelope

Interphase

1. Polar microtubules form
2. Nuclear envelope
   becomes indistinct
   and then disintegrates
3. Nucleolus disappears
4. Thread-like chromosomes
   appear

B

Polar microtubules
of mitotic spindle

Chromosomes

Prophase

5. Chromosomes, now seen as
   double structures, become
   aligned with their centromeres
   in the equatorial plane

C

Chromatids

Kinetochores
at centomere

Kinetochore
microtubules

Polar
microtubules

Metaphase

6. Chromatids of each
   chromosome separate

D

Chromatids now
referred to as
daughter chromosomes

Anaphase

7. Cell cleaves
8. Nuclear envelope
   reappears
9. Remnant of spindle
   microtubules
   constitutes midbody

E

Cleavage furrow
deepening

Site of future midbody

Nuclear envelope
reappearing

Telophase

10. Nucleoli reappear
11. Chromosomes become
    partly extended

F

Site of midbody
attached to one
daughter cell

Nucleolus

One pair of
centrioles in
each daughter cell

Two new cells

Figure 2-16
The interphase nucleus and the stages of mitosis as seen in hepatocytes (series at left).

Metaphase

The fact that mitotic chromosomes are essentially double structures is evident in metaphase, by which stage their two chromatids may be discerned in whole mounts (see Fig. 2-19 and **Plate 2-2**). The most striking feature of a metaphase cell, however, is the way all its chromosomes are arranged in a single transverse plane. This plane traverses the middle of the cell, perpendicular to the spindle axis. Equivalent in position to the world's equator, it is known as the **equatorial plane** (see Fig. 2-16C). By the time the chromosomes assume this particular arrangement, another group of microtubules is also involved. Until anaphase, the two chromatids of a mitotic chromosome remain joined at a region known as the **centromere** (Gk., central part) of the chromosome. Here, each chromatid has a microtubule attachment site called a **kinetochore** (Fig. 2-17). Kinetochores cannot be resolved with an LM, so the centromere region appears only as a constriction (see Fig. 2-21 and Plate 2-2).

In the latter part of prophase, groups of microtubules known as **kinetochore microtubules** become anchored laterally in the kinetochores (Fig. 2-17). The kinetochore region of each chromatid progressively captures the plus ends of kinetochore microtubules growing toward it from one pole of the spindle. Initially, the opposing forces moving sister chromatids to opposite poles balance each other because the two kinetochore complexes in each mitotic chromosome pull equally on antiparallel sets of kinetochore microtubules. As a result, the chromosomes assume a steady-state configuration, known as a **metaphase plate**, in which their centromeres lie equidistant from the poles, in the equatorial plane (see Fig. 2-16C and **Plate 2-1**).

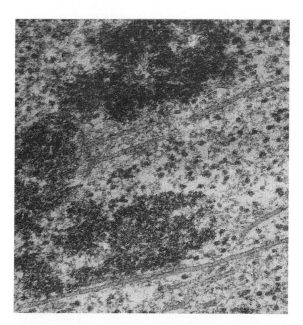

Figure 2-17
Electron micrograph showing the kinetochore region on a mitotic chromosome.

Anaphase

Early in the first part of anaphase (called **anaphase A**), mitotic chromosomes split at their centromeres. Their constituent chromatids, which from anaphase onward are referred to as *chromosomes*, separate and approach the two poles of the mitotic spindle (see Fig. 2-16D). Poleward movement involves both the activity of kinetochore regions and the presence of kinetochore microtubules, but the origins of the motive force that brings about chromosome movement are still unclear. Present evidence suggests that most of the poleward movement during anaphase is produced by the spindle microtubule-associated motor protein, **dynein** (considered further in Chap. 3 under Microtubules), which is closely associated with the kinetochore region. During the same stage (anaphase A), the kinetochore microtubules progressively disassemble at their kinetochore (plus) end without loss of kinetochore attachment. In **anaphase B**, the mitotic spindle attains its full length, presumably due to sliding of the two antiparallel sets of polar microtubules past each other in the region where they overlap in the mid-zone of the spindle. The cell then begins to constrict in its equatorial plane.

Telophase

In telophase, the developing constriction deepens into a **cleavage furrow** that pinches the cell into two (see Fig. 2-16E and F). The spindle microtubules that still interconnect the forming daughter cells constitute the **midbody** (Fig. 2-16E), a residual structure that may remain as a temporary appendage on a daughter cell after it has separated. Finally, the nuclear envelope and the nucleolus are both reconstituted in each daughter cell, and the daughter chromosomes acquire the partly extended condition that characterizes interphase (see Fig. 2-16F).

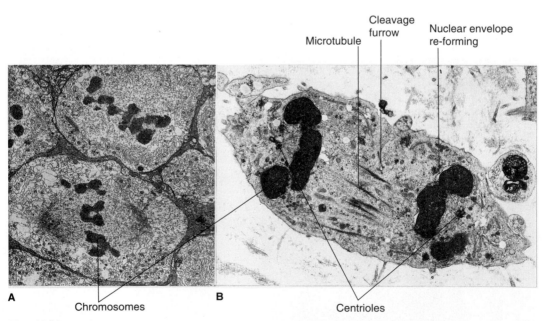

Figure 2-18
Electron micrographs of dividing cells at metaphase (*A*) and telophase (*B*). The spindle microtubules in *B* will remain as the midbody.

Recognizing Mitotic Cells

Mitotic cells may be recognized in sections by their distinctive chromosome arrangements. The general term for the various configurations that are seen is **mitotic figure.** Under low power, mitotic figures tend to stand out from the background as intensely stained, blue-to-purple blobs (Plate 2-1). However, they are not all equally easy to find. For example, a cell in prophase is hard to spot, whereas a metaphase plate is obvious if it is seen face on or from the side. The anaphase configuration is equally easy to find if the spindle was cut in longitudinal section. Beginners sometimes mistake a pair of adjacent interphase nuclei for a cell that is in late telophase. Unless two nuclei appear unusually close and seem to belong to relatively small (daughter) cells, they are unlikely to represent telophase.

Another potential source of confusion is that some mitotic figures may bear a superficial resemblance to nuclei of dead cells. Remember that during most of mitosis, the chromosomes are not confined within a nuclear envelope. So when trying to decide between a mitotic cell and a dead cell, bear in mind that a cluster of chromosomes generally has a spiky outline with protruding chromosomes (see Fig. 2-16C and E), whereas the nucleus of a dead cell is generally rounded or only slightly wrinkled.

In EM sections, mitotic chromosomes tend to be uneven in outline and appear as large fibrogranular masses (Fig. 2-18). This appearance is attributable to innumerable sections through the chromatin fiber that extend out as radial loops from the axis of each chromatid, a feature that is readily seen if a whole mitotic chromosome is viewed intact (Fig. 2-19).

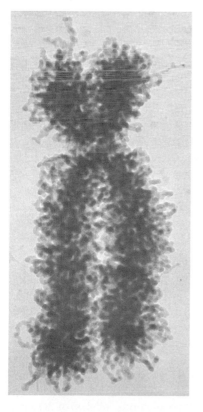

Figure 2-19
Electron micrograph of an intact metaphase chromosome 12 (isolated whole mount, ×60,400). The continuous chromatin fiber of each chromatid is seen extending laterally as multiple radial loops from the axial scaffold of the chromatid.

CLINICAL IMPLICATIONS

Interpreting Levels of Miotic Activity
The presence of mitotic figures in sections means that some cells were dividing when the tissue sample was obtained. Mitotic figures are not obvious in adult tissues unless cell renewal is continuous. However, an increased incidence of dividing cells is found 1) at sites where damaged tissues are undergoing repair or regeneration, and 2) at sites of mitogenic response to hormones and growth factors. A local abundance of dividing cells that does not appear to represent a normal response to some such stimulus may indicate an abnormal growth or tumor, and it potentially corroborates a diagnosis of cancer.

Some chemotherapeutic drugs and ionizing radiation interfere with mitosis by altering or damaging nuclear DNA, whereas certain other drugs interfere with the formation of a mitotic spindle. Thus the antimitotic actions of the vinca alkaloids, **vincristine** and **vinblastine**, are that they depolymerize microtubules and render the released tubulin subunits unavailable for spindle assembly by inducing them to form paracrystalline arrays. Antimitotic agents that are clinically valuable for inhibiting the proliferation of cancer cells also have adverse effects on the normal tissues that undergo continuous cell renewal.

Telomeres and Telomerase

When proliferating somatic cells have undergone a finite number of cell divisions (generally between 50 and 90), they enter a phase of proliferative senescence. Normal somatic cells accordingly have a limited and predetermined capacity for cell renewal. In contrast, cancer cells have the potential to proliferate indefinitely. A sustained capacity for cell division depends on the maintenance of a repetitive series of a distinctive DNA sequence at the free ends of chromosomes. The terminal regions of each chromosome that are made up of these tandomly repeated, species-specific short sequences (TTAGGG in humans) are known as **telomeres** (Gk. *telos*, end). Key features of telomeres include 1) irreparable breaks in each polynucleotide strand of the DNA double helix, and 2) looped-out configurations in some of their subterminal DNA sequences. Telomeres have the important role of stabilizing chromosome ends. Normal cells, however, lose telomeric sequences in each successive cell generation. Progressive loss of the terminal repetitive telomeric sequences is reversed only by **telomerase**, a ribonucleoprotein enzymatic complex with reverse transcriptase activity. This enzyme has the necessary intrinsic **complementary telomerase RNA template** for it to synthesize a single-stranded series of new telomeric repeats capable of maintaining stability of the chromosome ends. Telomerase levels, however, also tend to fall with successive divisions, a decline that leads to critical depletion of the terminal telomeric repeats. Since the DNA at the ends of chromosomes of cells with low levels of telomerase cannot replicate completely, aging normal cells eventually lose all ability to divide. In contrast, most cancer cells can produce enough telomerase to replace the lost telomeric repeats, ensuring ongoing proliferation. It has recently been found that raising the intracellular telomerase levels of normal human senescent somatic cells greatly prolongs their proliferative lifetime.

CHROMOSOME NUMBER AND IDENTIFICATION

Typical body cells (**somatic cells**) possess 46 chromosomes, but the **germ cells** that give rise to them have only 23. Of these 23 chromosomes, one determines the sex of the offspring and is called the **sex chromosome**, and the other 22 are known as **autosomes**. In female germ cells, which are called **ova**, the sex chromosome is invariably an X chromosome, whereas in male germ cells, termed **spermatozoa**, the sex chromosome can be either an X (the female sex chromosome) or a Y (the male sex chromosome). A male possesses 44 autosomes and the XY combination and is the result of fertilization by a spermatozoon that bears a Y chromosome, whereas a female has 44 autosomes and two X chromosomes and is the result of fertilization by a spermatozoon that bears an X chromosome.

In a somatic cell, each autosome derived from the mother is accompanied by a counterpart (**homologue**) from the father; the two chromosomes of the pair carry alternate forms (**alleles**) of the same

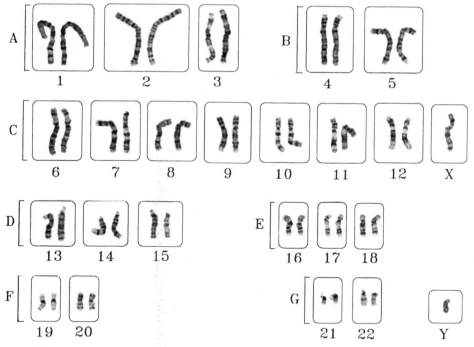

Figure 2-22
G-banded human karyotype (chromosomally normal male). Giemsa staining of the specially prepared chromosomes yields distinctive banded patterns for the chromosome pairs and sex chromosomes.

the 22 pairs of autosomes and the two sex chromosomes to be identified fairly unequivocally and hence facilitates the detection of chromosomal anomalies. A less laborious, recent innovation combines spectral imaging of chromosomes with computer-based recognition and distinctive color coding of the 22 chromosome pairs and sex chromosomes (**multicolor spectral karyotyping**). Following in situ hybridization with a variety of different fluorescent-labeled DNA probes specific for individual chromosomes, emission spectra indicative of the different chromosomal staining affinities are analyzed. Specifically identified chromosomes are then displayed with their computer-assigned colors. Automated karyotypic analyses based on specific recognition and color coding ("painting") of all chromosomes could greatly help detection of genetic defects and other cytogenetic abnormalities.

To complete our discussion of chromosomes, we shall consider an instance in which a chromosome stays fully condensed when the cell enters interphase. This exception to the general rule enables some useful information to be obtained about a person's chromosome constitution without the bother of preparing a karyotype.

Sex Chromatin

If the diploid cells of a person possess more than a single X chromosome, *all but one* of these X chromosomes remain *condensed* and hence virtually transcriptionally inactive throughout interphase. The most obvious example of this situation is a normal female with two X chromosomes, only one of which is expressed. However, there are also instances in which an *abnormal* complement of sex chromosomes accounts for there being more than one X chromosome. Such examples include the anomalous **XXX** constitution in females, and also the **XXY** constitution that occurs in the most com-

SEX CHROMATIN

Seen in female

XX

Figure 2-23
Sex chromatin in whole nuclei (cresyl-echt violet stained buccal epithelial cells from oral mucosa, oil immersion). Arrow indicates a mass of sex chromatin.

Not seen in male

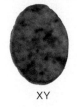

XY

mon form of **Klinefelter syndrome** in males. Representing the opposite extreme, females with **Turner syndrome** have the **XO** constitution (the *O* denoting the *absence* of a second sex chromosome); they therefore have no additional X chromosome to become condensed.

To investigate a person's X chromosome constitution, whole epithelial cells may be scraped from the inside of a cheek, and then suitably stained. Each extra X chromosome (one in a normal female and none in a normal male) appears under oil immersion as a separate, darkly stained mass adhering to the nuclear envelope (Fig. 2-23), indicated by arrow). Each tiny condensed chromosome is termed the **sex chromatin** or a **Barr body**. It stains more intensely and is somewhat larger and more smooth-edged than the usual kind of chromatin granule, yet it is a good deal smaller than the nucleolus. Even so, it may be recognized with certainty only if it lies at the periphery of the nucleus as in Figure 2-23. In many cells it is missed because of unfavorable orientation of the nucleus.

In any cell that contains two X chromosomes, it is a matter of chance whether the X chromosome that is condensed comes from the mother or from the father. The inactivation occurs early in embryonic life, however, and it is the same X chromosome that is perpetuated as the sex chromatin in all the cell's descendants. Accordingly, females are made up of two kinds of cells, with roughly half of these cells expressing their maternal X chromosome and the rest expressing their paternal X chromosome.

NUCLEAR APPEARANCES INDICATING CELL DEATH

A certain proportion of the cells encountered in a histologic section were degenerating or dead when the tissue was obtained. Because recognition of dying or dead cells is of substantial diagnostic value in histopathology, it is important to realize that the LM appearance of the nucleus is one of the most reliable indicators of whether cells were healthy when the tissue sample was taken. The three general nuclear signs of cell death are as follows.

Pyknosis

In most cell types, the nucleus of a dying cell shrivels into an intensely basophilic uniform mass, a change termed **pyknosis** (Gk., condensation). In situations in which it is difficult to distinguish between a pyknotic nucleus (Fig. 2-24*A*) and 1) a mitotic figure or 2) a nucleus tightly packed with condensed chromatin, it is helpful to examine the cytoplasm because the cytoplasm of a cell has died and may lack definition and have a "muddy" appearance.

Karyorrhexis

In a few cell types, the nucleus of a dying cell disintegrates into small, dark-staining fragments. This kind of degeneration is termed **karyorrhexis** (Gk. *rhexis*, breaking), and an example is shown in Figure 2-24*B*.

Karyolysis

A long-accepted third sign of cell death, known as **karyolysis** (Gk. *lysis*, dissolution), is gradual histological disappearance of the nucleus and its macromolecular contents, which literally fade

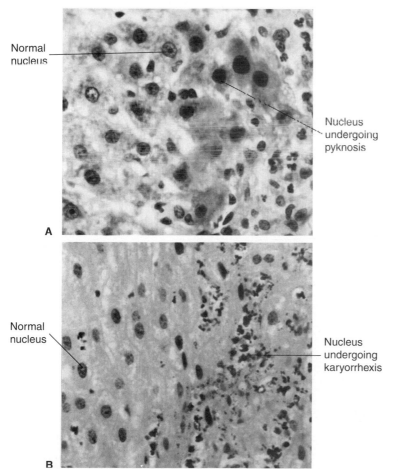

Figure 2-24
Nuclei of viable cells (shown at *upper left* in *A* and *B*), pyknotic nuclei (*A*), and karyorrhexic nuclei (*B*). Both panels show living and dead cancer cells.

away to nothing. This sign of cell death is seen in epidermal cells approaching the skin surface (Fig. 2-25).

Necrosis and Apoptosis

Pyknosis seen at sites where there is evidence of inflammation generally indicates accidental cell death caused by some extrinsic hazard. Such cell death is termed **necrosis** (Gk. *nekros*, dead). Cells can also perish under physiologically normal conditions, for example, when they become senescent. In such cases, cell death results from activation of an intrinsic program of self-destruction known as **apoptosis** (Gk. *apo*, away from, *ptōsis*, fall) or **programmed cell death**, i.e., abrupt pre-programmed termination of the cell's usual life span. Two key conditions that elicit the apoptotic response in normal cells are 1) substantial chromosomal damage and 2) dysregulation of the cell cycle. A significant difference found in cancer cells is that the apoptotic response is not an automatic consequence of equivalent levels of damage to the cell's nuclear DNA.

An early change considered to be indicative of apoptosis is loss of the asymmetric distribution of certain phospholipids in the cell membrane. The cell shrinks significantly when vital functions become compromised. Typically, the nucleus undergoes pyknosis and becomes darkly stained. The dying cell generally breaks into several pieces (**apoptotic bodies**) that are promptly phagocytosed. Because the constituent macromolecules are not widely disseminated, no evidence is seen of inflammatory reactions.

A critical stage of the apoptotic pathway is activation of a series of cytosolic cysteine proteases, structurally related to interleukin-1β-converting enzyme and known as **caspases**. The activated caspases catalyze a proteolytic cascade that not only severely damages cytoplasmic organelles but also activates endonucleases that go on to ravage the nuclear DNA, destructively fragmenting it into short stretches that are genetically meaningless (**DNA laddering**).

Unnecessary and potentially deleterious cells cleared from the body through activation of the apoptotic response include surplus or inappropriate neurons, self-reactive T cells, residual cytokine-producing T cells, and epithelial or endothelial cells that have lost their attachment.

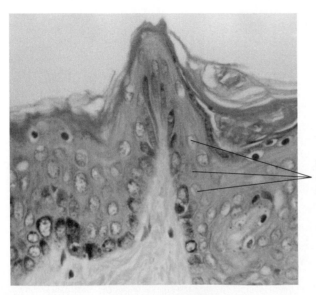

Nuclei undergoing karyolysis

Figure 2-25
Epidermal cell nuclei undergo karyolysis near the skin surface.

Summary

Each nuclear chromosome contains a DNA molecule that bears encoded genetic instructions. Nuclear DNA and its associated histones, RNA, and nucleoproteins constitute a macromolecular complex called chromatin. Condensed chromatin is intensely basophilic, electron-dense, and made up of chromosome regions that are transcriptionally inactive. Extended chromatin is comparatively diffuse, less electron-dense, and contains chromosome regions that are transcriptionally active. The cell replicates its nuclear DNA prior to cell division. This process can be detected by radioautography using tritiated thymidine, a radioactive precursor that becomes incorporated (as thymine) only into DNA.

The nuclear envelope is made up of two membranes. On the inner aspect of the inner membrane there is condensed chromatin, and on the outer aspect of the outer membrane there are ribosomes. Nuclear pores present in the nuclear envelope regulate the exchange of macromolecules between the nuclear and cytoplasmic compartments.

The nucleolus (there may be more than one per cell) is intensely basophilic because of associated chromatin, and it is large in cells that are actively synthesizing proteins. In EM sections, the nucleolus appears as a spongework of electron-dense ribonucleoprotein particles, with a poorly defined boundary. During mitosis, it is not seen. In interphase, it reappears in intimate association with the chromosomes that bear genes for rRNA. The nucleolus is the only site where rRNA is produced.

The genetic specifications for proteins are transcribed into mRNA in the nucleus and translated into polypeptides in the cytoplasm. Translation requires the participation of 1) ribosomes made of rRNA and protein and 2) tRNAs specific for individual amino acids. Ribosomes and tRNAs are both reutilized.

The cell cycle is made up of M (mitosis, typically 1 hour), G_1 (8 hours in mouse cells in vitro), S (DNA synthesis, 7 to 8 hours), and G_2 (4 hours in these cells). The duration of G_1 differs with cell type. In most specialized cells, G_1 is prolonged. Some cells leave the cell cycle in G_1 and enter G_0, then go back into cycle if the need arises. A few specialized cells (e.g., cardiac muscle and nerve cells) leave the cell cycle and do not divide again; such cell populations are devoid of mechanisms for cell renewal. Other cells, also too highly differentiated to divide, are continuously renewed from less highly differentiated progenitors arising from undifferentiated stem cells that persist throughout life. Stem cells may be multipotential (e.g., blood stem cells) or unipotential (e.g., spermatozoal stem cells). Their progeny can remain stem cells (self-renewal) or differentiate into progenitor cells. Only a few specialized cell types are able to proliferate when depleted.

During the S phase, chromosomes replicate and become double structures that contain two DNA molecules. By G_2, the centrioles also replicate, yielding two pairs. In mitotic prophase, a mitotic spindle forms between the centriole pairs, the nuclear envelope fragments, and the nucleolus disappears. At metaphase, the chromosomes condense and become aligned in the equatorial plane. At anaphase, their two chromatids separate. In telophase, the cell pinches into two and a nuclear envelope and nucleolus appear in each daughter cell. Sites showing an unexpectedly high incidence of mitotic figures may have clinical significance.

Mitotic chromosomes have an axial framework with radially extending chromatin loops. Interphase looped domains of chromatin are in a partly extended state; the intervening condensed domains amass and appear as chromatin granules. Karyotypes are made up of photographed mitotic chromosomes assembled in pairs according to their size, relative arm lengths, and banding patterns. Somatic cells of females possess 22 pairs of homologous autosomes with two X chromosomes. Males have the same autosomes with an XY combination. The total chromosome number, 46, is known as the diploid number. A few kinds of somatic cells, however, are polyploid, and germ cells are haploid. Some specific anomalies of chromosome number (particularly aneuploidy) are associated with clinical abnormalities. Finally, if there is more than one X chromosome per diploid cell (as in normal females), each extra X chromosome per diploid set remains condensed as sex chromatin (also known as a Barr body).

Necrotic or apoptotic cells can sometimes be recognized by the fact that their nucleus becomes solidly condensed and intensely basophilic (pyknosis). Other indications of cell death are nuclear fragmentation (karyorrhexis) or fading of the intact nucleus (karyolysis).

Bibliography

Interphase Nucleus

Akey CW. Interactions and structure of the nuclear pore complex revealed by cryo-electron microscopy. J Cell Biol 109:955, 1989.

Alberts B, Bray D, Lewis J et al. The cell nucleus. In: Molecular Biology of the Cell, ed 3, New York, Garland Publishing, 1994, p 336.

Burke B. The nuclear envelope and nuclear transport. Curr Opin Cell Biol 2:514, 1990.

Ciejek EM, Tsai M-J, O'Malley BW. Actively transcribed genes are associated with the nuclear matrix. Nature 306:607, 1984.

DeBoni U. The interphase nucleus as a dynamic structure. Int Rev Cytol 150:149, 1994.

Gerace L, Burke B. Functional organization of the nuclear envelope. Annu Rev Cell Biol 4:335, 1988.

Goessens G. Nucleolar structure. Int Rev Cytol 87:107, 1984.

Hancock R, Boulikas T. Functional organization in the nucleus. Int Rev Cytol 79:165, 1982.

Pardoll DM, Vogelstein B, Coffey DS. A fixed site of DNA replication in eukaryotic cells. Cell 19:527, 1980.

Chromosomes, Chromatin, and Protein Synthesis

Bavykin SG, Usachenko SI, Zalensky AO, Mirzabekov AD. Structure of nucleosomes and organization of internucleosomal DNA in chromatin. J Mol Biol 212:495, 1990.

Darnell JE. The processing of RNA. Sci Am 249(4):90, 1983.

Darnell JE. RNA. Sci Am 253(4):68, 1985.

De Boni U. Chromatin and nuclear envelope of freeze-fractured, neuronal interphase nuclei, resolved by scanning electron microscopy. Biol Cell 63:1, 1988.

Evan G. Regulation of gene expression. Br Med Bull 47:116, 1991.

Felsenfeld G. DNA. Sci Am 253(4):58, 1985.

Finch JT, Klug A. Solenoidal model for superstructure in chromatin. Proc Natl Acad Sci USA 73:1897, 1976.

Fisher PA. Chromosomes and chromatin structure: the extrachromosomal karyoskeleton. Curr Opin Cell Biol 1:447, 1989.

Hilliker AJ, Appels R. The arrangement of interphase chromosomes: structural and functional aspects. Exp Cell Res 185:297, 1989.

Kornberg RD, Klug A. The nucleosome. Sci Am 244(2):52, 1981.

Kornberg RD, Lorch Y. Chromatin structure and transcription. Annu Rev Cell Biol 8:563, 1992.

Marsden M, Laemmli UK. Metaphase chromosome structure: evidence for a radial loop model. Cell 17:849, 1979.

Miller OL. The nucleolus, chromosomes, and visualization of genetic activity. J Cell Biol 91:15S, 1981.

Moyzis R. The human telomere. Sci Am 265:48, 1991.

Paulson JR. Scaffold morphology in histone-depleted HeLa metaphase chromosomes. Chromosoma 97:289, 1989.

Rich A, Kim SH. The three-dimensional structure of transfer RNA. Sci Am 238(1):52, 1978.

Rogers AW. Techniques of Autoradiography, ed 3. Amsterdam, Elsevier, 1979.

Schultze B. Autoradiography at the Cellular Level. Physical Technics in Biological Research, vol 3B. New York, Academic Press, 1969.

Utsumi KR. A scanning electron microscopic study of chromosomes and nuclei. In: Scanning Electron Microscopy, vol 3. Chicago, SEM Inc, 1985, p 1121.

Williams MA. Autoradiography and immunocytochemistry. In Glauert AM, ed. Practical Methods in Electron Microscopy, vol 6, pt 1. Amsterdam, North Holland, 1978.

Cell Cycle, Apoptosis, and Mitosis

Barinaga M. Forging a path to cell death. Science 273:735, 1996.

Baserga R. The cell cycle. N Engl J Med 304:453, 1981.

Cross F, Roberts J, Weintraub H. Simple and complex cell cycles. Annu Rev Cell Biol 5:341, 1989.

Duke RC, Ojcius DM, Young JD. Cell suicide in health and disease. Sci Am 275(6):80, 1996.

Fulton C. Centrioles. In: Reinert J, Ursprung H, eds. Origin and Continuity of Cell Organelles, vol 2. New York, Springer-Verlag, 1971, p 170.

Gorbsky GJ, Sammack PJ, Borisy GG. Chromosomes move poleward in anaphase along stationary microtubules that coordinately disassemble from their kinetochore ends. J Cell Biol 104:9, 1988.

Hayden JH, Bowser SS, Rieder CL. Kinetochores capture astral microtubules during chromosome attachment to the mitotic spindle: Direct visualization in live newt lung cells. J Cell Biol 111:1039, 1990.

Jacobson MD, Weil M, Raff MC. Programmed cell death in animal development. Cell 88:347, 1997.

King KL, Cidlowski JA. Cell cycle and apoptosis: common pathways to life and death. J Cell Biochem 58:175, 1995.

Kroemer G, Petit P, Zamzami N, Vayssière JL, Mignotte B. The biochemistry of programmed cell death. FASEB J 9:1277, 1995.

McIntosh JR, McDonald KL. The mitotic spindle. Sci Am 261:48, 1989.

McIntosh JR, Hering GE. Spindle fiber action and chromosome movement. Annu Rev Cell Biol 7:403, 1991.

Mitchison TJ. Mitosis: basic concepts. Curr Opin Cell Biol 1:67, 1989.

Mitchison TJ. Mitosis: the kinetochore in captivity. Nature 348:14, 1990.

Murray AW, Kirschner MW. What controls the cell cycle. Sci Am 264:56, 1991.

Pfarr CM, Couc M, Grissom PM, Hays TS, Porter ME, McIntosh JR. Cytoplasmic dynein is localized to kinetochores during mitosis. Nature 345:263, 1990.

Rieder CL. Mitosis: towards a molecular understanding of chromosome behavior. Curr Opin Cell Biol 3:59, 1991.

Steuer ER, Wordeman L, Schroer TA, Sheetz MP. Localization of cytoplasmic dynein to mitotic spindles and kinetochores. Nature 345:266, 1990.

Vallee R. Mitosis: Dynein and the kinetochore. Nature 345:206, 1990.

Chromosome Identification, Polyploidy, and Sex Chromatin

Barr ML. The significance of the sex chromatin. Int Rev Cytol 19:35, 1966.

Brodsky WV, Uryvaeva JV. Cell polyploidy: its relation to tissue growth and function. Int Rev Cytol 50:275, 1977.

Comings DE. Mechanisms of chromosome banding and implications for chromosome structure. Annu Rev Genet 12:25, 1978.

Moore KL (ed). The Sex Chromatin. Philadelphia, WB Saunders, 1966. Schröck E, duManoir S, Veldman T, et al. Multicolor spectral karyotyping of human chromosomes. Science 273:494, 1996.

Sumner AT. The nature and mechanisms of chromosome banding. Cancer Genet Cytogenet 6:59, 1982.

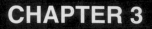

CHAPTER 3

Cell Cytoplasm

OBJECTIVES

After reading this chapter, you should be able to do the following:

- Summarize the structure of eight cytoplasmic organelles and relate it to their functions
- Draw a detailed diagram of the cell membrane and cell coat
- Recognize secretory cells in H&E-stained sections and electron micrographs
- Outline the steps involved in protein secretion
- Describe the different types of lysosomes and comment on their importance
- Summarize the similarities and differences between centrioles and cilia
- Name two energy-providing storage products and two pigments produced by cells

In contrast to the role of the nucleus, which is to store genetic instructions and direct and regulate what takes place in the cytoplasm, the role of the cytoplasm is to carry out the diverse processes that keep the cell alive and functioning on a daily basis. Besides executing a large number of metabolic reactions, the cytoplasm is the only part of the cell where proteins and other macromolecules are synthesized and the required energy for such activities is produced. This energy is derived chiefly through the oxidation from food-derived energy sources entering the cell by way of its limiting membrane, the cell membrane. Waste products pass in the opposite direction through the same membrane. The cell membrane is therefore the site of vital exchanges between the cell's interior and the immediate environment. Furthermore, it keeps the internal composition of the cell different from the external composition of the environment.

A number of **intracellular membranes** subdivide the cytoplasm into separate **compartments**. The content of each compartment can be different from that of other parts of the cell because it is segregated from them by a limiting membrane. This arrangement holds reactants and enzymes together in the same compartment, enabling them to interact effectively. The bounding membrane may even include requisite enzymes as an integral part of its structure. Furthermore, inappropriate reactions can be avoided by segregating the potential reactants, enzymes, and substrates, in different compartments.

FUNCTIONAL ROLE OF CYTOPLASM

Cells are characterized by having a number of functional properties that contrast them with inanimate objects. For example, they may react to certain organic and inorganic molecules and electrical signals, a property called **irritability**. Such stimuli may elicit transient changes in the ionic permeability of their cell membrane, changes that may spread over the entire cell surface as waves of excitation. The term used for the propagation of excitation is **conductivity**. If such stimuli induce shortening in some dimension, cells exhibit the property of **contractility**.

Cells absorb and utilize required nutrients and precursors for synthesizing their macromolecules and secretory products (**absorption** followed by **assimilation**). In addition, oxygen is necessary for the cell to produce energy through the oxidation of energy-rich substrates (**cell respiration**). Cell products with useful roles outside the cell are actively released to the exterior (**secretion**). Useless metabolic by-products are eliminated by diffusion across the cell membrane (**excretion**).

Finally, cells can increase their size by synthesizing an abundance of macromolecules (**growth**). Excessive, inefficient mass is typically avoided by division of the cell to form two daughter cells (**reproduction**), but the potential for cell division is lost in some cell types that attain a high degree of specialization.

INITIAL OVERVIEW OF CYTOPLASMIC CONSTITUENTS

Cells are able to carry out their diverse functional activities because the cytoplasm contains three different kinds of components. These are designated **cytoplasmic organelles, cytoplasmic inclusions, and the cytosol** or **cytoplasmic matrix.**

The distinctive design of the various cytoplasmic organelles enables them to carry out specific functions. Organelles with bounding membranes are classified as **membranous organelles**; the others are **nonmembranous organelles**. Listed in Table 3-1, their principal functions are as follows.

The cell membrane transports substances into and out of the cell, receives external signals, and discloses the cell's identity. Mitochondria are the chief source of energy expended in synthesizing macromolecules, transporting ions against diffusion gradients, cell movement and contraction, and other energy-consuming activities. The remainder of the membranous organelles play roles in the various stages of production and intracellular processing of proteins and lipids, including synthesis and release of those proteins, lipoproteins, and glycoproteins that are destined for secretion. Protein synthesis also involves ribosomes, which belong to the nonmembranous category of organelles.

The various other nonmembranous organelles, representing the cell's "bones" and "muscles", are collectively called the **cytoskeleton**. The main supporting elements in this group are thin rods called **microtubules** and a class of filaments known as **intermediate filaments**. The most obvious contractile elements are actin-containing **microfilaments**. Under appropriate conditions, these filaments interact with myosin, which is arranged as substantial **thick filaments** in muscle cells. Actin is involved in activities such as cell contraction, locomotion, and cytoplasmic constriction at the end of division.

Although the nonmembranous organelles do not have a membranous component, some of them are intimately *associated* with a membrane. Thus cilia and flagella are invested by extensions of the cell membrane, and certain filaments are attached to the cytoplasmic surface of the cell membrane without being considered a part of it.

Finally, microscopically visible intracellular accumulations of useful or superfluous materials are termed **cytoplasmic inclusions**. Examples of such inclusions are stored intracellular energy sources (e.g., polysaccharides and fats) and various pigments (see Table 3-1). Cytoplasmic inclusions are considered at the end of the chapter.

TABLE 3-1

COMPONENTS OF CYTOPLASM	
Cytosol (Cytoplasmic Matrix)	Filaments
Membranous Cytoplasmic Organelles	Microfilaments (= thin filaments)
Cell membrane or plasmalemma (with cell coat and microvilli)	Thick filaments
	Intermediate filaments
Mitochondria	*Cytoplasmic Inclusions*
Rough-surfaced endoplasmic reticulum	*Stored Foods*
Golgi apparatus	Glycogen
Secretory vesicles	Fat (lipid)
Lysosomes	*Exogenous Pigments*
Coated vesicles	Carotene
Endosomes	Carbon particles
Peroxisomes	*Endogenous Pigments*
Smooth-surfaced endoplasmic reticulum	Hemoglobin
Nonmembranous Cytoplasmic Organelles	Hemosiderin
Ribosomes	Bilirubin
Microtubules	Melanin
Microtubular assemblies	Lipofuscin (lipochrome pigment)
Centrioles	
Cilia	
Flagella	

CYTOSOL (CYTOPLASMIC MATRIX)

In between the organelles and inclusions lies the **cytosol** or **cytoplasmic matrix**. This cytoplasmic component contains many enzymes, other soluble proteins, ions, nutrients, and macromolecular precursors. Although the cytoplasmic matrix is often misrepresented as the unstructured, liquid part of the cytoplasm, it can assume a loosely organized gel structure and it contains a fragile supporting framework called a **microtrabecular lattice**. However, a high-voltage EM and special tissue culture preparations are required for the supporting framework to be seen. The microtrabecular lattice probably binds some soluble constituents of the matrix and holds the organelles in appropriate positions in the cytoplasm.

CELL MEMBRANE

Alternatively known as the **plasma membrane** or **plasmalemma**, the cell's limiting membrane (**cell membrane**) is 8 to 10 nm thick. At high magnifications, transverse sections of the cell membrane exhibit three fairly distinct layers: the extracellular and cytoplasmic borders, both of which are electron-dense, are separated by an electron-lucent layer of comparable thickness (Fig. 3-1). However, three layers are resolved only if high magnifications are used. This characteristic "railroad" pattern of staining is a reflection of the general molecular distribution in the cell membrane, details of which are given in the next section. A membrane that appears trilaminar at high magnification and as a single electron-dense line at lower magnifications is occasionally referred to as a **unit membrane**.

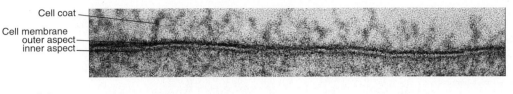

Figure 3-1
Electron micrograph of the cell membrane, showing the cell coat.

Intracellular membranes resemble the cell membrane in their cross-sectional appearance and underlying molecular organization. A distinctive feature of the cell membrane, however, is its morphologically indistinct, oligosaccharide-rich outer region, which is known as the **cell coat** or **glycocalyx** (see Figs. 3-1 and 3-2).

Molecular Distribution in Cell Membrane

Molecular organization of the cell membrane is essentially based on the presence of a **lipid bilayer** (Plate 3-1 and Fig. 3-3). This bimolecular layer contains **phospholipids**, together with some **glycolipids** and **cholesterol**. The presence of cholesterol stiffens the membrane. As indicated in Figure 3-3, the phospholipids and glycolipids are arranged with their uncharged region in the central core of the lipid bilayer, and their charged (polar) region adjacent to either the **cytoplasmic** (inner) surface or the **extracellular** (outer) surface of the membrane.

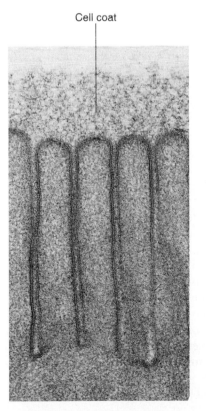

Figure 3-2
Electron micrograph of the cell membrane and cell coat on the luminal border of an absorptive epithelial cell (small intestine of cat, ×75,000). Parallel surface projections of the cell membrane below the cell coat are microvilli cut longitudinally.

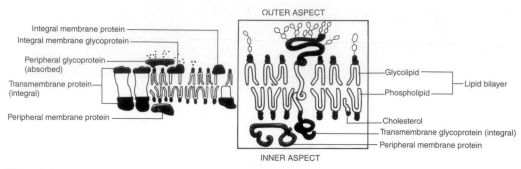

Figure 3-3
Molecular organization of the cell membrane. The central core of the membrane contains uncharged regions of its constituent lipid and protein molecules (indicated in *white*). Both membrane surfaces are characterized by the presence of charged regions on these molecules (indicated in *color*). The trilaminar appearance of the membrane in EM sections is widely attributed to the strong affinity between these charged groups and the heavy metals used as EM stains.

The other major macromolecular constituent of the cell membrane is its **proteins**. Two broad categories of membrane proteins, termed **integral** and **peripheral** membrane proteins, have characteristic distributions in the lipid bilayer (see Fig. 3-3 and Plate 3-1). **Integral membrane proteins** are characterized by having 1) **charged** regions that are located along the cytoplasmic or extracellular surfaces of the membrane and lie among the lipid polar groups; and 2) one or more **uncharged** regions (or covalently attached uncharged hydrocarbon chains) that in some cases traverse the lipid bilayer and in other cases anchor the protein in one of the two lipid layers. Such proteins are integral in the sense that disruptive chemical procedures are necessary to extract them from the membrane. They include **transmembrane proteins**, a term reserved for those proteins that span the lipid bilayer from one membranous surface to the other. In some transmembrane proteins, only a single uncharged region of the molecule traverses the bilayer. In multipass proteins, several uncharged regions traverse the bilayer. As a result, multipass proteins weave up and down a number of times through the bilayer in a pattern that has been likened to stitching. There are also integral membrane proteins that are anchored exclusively in the inner half or outer half of the bilayer. The other membrane proteins, known as **peripheral membrane proteins**, lack comparable uncharged regions or attached uncharged hydrocarbon chains and are not anchored in either layer of the lipid bilayer. Instead, they stay loosely associated with a membrane surface because weak electrostatic forces bind them to other membrane proteins. This peripheral association is reflected by the fact that neither solvents nor detergents are required to extract peripheral membrane proteins from the membrane. The weak forces that hold them in position are readily counteracted by altering the ionic strength or pH.

In the **fluid-mosaic membrane** model of Singer and Nicholson, the cell membrane proteins that are not restrained in any way are subject to lateral drift, much as icebergs drift freely in the sea. This mobility results from the fact that at body temperature, the lipid bilayer has fluid properties, although its viscosity increases with its cholesterol content. Certain integral membrane proteins, however, are anchored to an underlying stabilizing framework of structural proteins that lies in direct contact with the cytoplasmic surface of the cell membrane (see Plate 3-1). This **membrane cytoskeleton** is probably necessary for functional integrity of the cell membrane, because in the muscle cells of patients with muscular dystrophy (severe muscle degeneration), the protein **dystrophin**, a constituent of the stabilizing framework, is deficient. Dystrophin structurally resembles α-actinin and spectrin, two other membrane cytoskeletal proteins. It links the meshwork of microfilaments (i.e., actin filaments) present in the superficial zone of cytoplasm to a cell membrane glycoprotein complex that binds to extracellular laminin, which is an anchoring glycoprotein found in basement membranes.

The branched oligosaccharide chains that constitute external domains of cell membrane **glyco-proteins** and **glycolipids** coat the extracellular surface much as sugar coats a piece of candy. Here, oligosaccharide chains contribute to an indistinct layer termed the **cell coat** or **glycocalyx** (compare Fig. 3-1 with Plate 3-1). This peripheral layer of the membrane may be seen to advantage with the EM on the free surface of the epithelial lining of the small intestine (see Fig. 3-2). Tiny finger-like extensions (microvilli) present on this surface underlie a thick cell coat, certain glycoproteins of which function as digestive enzymes (see Chapter 13). In EM sections, the numerous oligosaccharide chains that constitute this layer appear as loosely tangled, fine filaments. In other cell types, however, the cell coat is typically a thin, fuzzy layer of low electron density (see Fig. 3-1). Its presence in EM sections is the only morphological evidence of asymmetrical molecular organization in the cell membrane.

Key Functional Roles of Cell Membrane

In interfacing cells with their immediate environment, the cell membrane performs a host of essential duties. Its molecular composition renders it essentially impermeable to large molecules that are not lipid soluble, but selectively permeable to many small molecules and ions. By preventing the loss of intracellular macromolecules and by excluding unwanted or potentially harmful substances from the cell, this membrane helps to maintain the cell's distinctive internal composition. It also supplies the cell with particular requirements and allows waste products to leave. Dissolved gases and other molecules with low molecular weight enter or leave the cell by passive diffusion across the cell membrane, but such movement occurs only toward sites of lower concentration. Ions can also move down concentration gradients through **gated channels**, which are selective ion channels that switch between open and closed configurations as required. In certain instances, however, molecules must be transported through the cell membrane against their diffusion gradients. For this purpose, **membrane transport proteins** in the cell membrane utilize energy derived from ATP (an energy-rich compound made by mitochondria) to move particular molecules in the necessary direction. A key cell membrane transport protein is **sodium—potassium ATPase**, which is an ion pump that withdraws sodium ions from the interior of the cell and concurrently brings in potassium ions from the surrounding tissue fluid. In addition to a full complement of ion channels and pumps, the cell membrane possesses **carrier proteins** that bring glucose and amino acids into the cell in the opposite direction to their concentration gradients. Furthermore, a special ingestion mechanism called **endocytosis** enables the cell to bring in macromolecules. Details of this process are given later in the chapter.

The cell membrane can also detect the presence of certain molecules in its immediate vicinity. Signaling integral transmembrane proteins termed **cell membrane receptors** specifically recognize a wide assortment of essential macromolecules and signal molecules that affect or regulate cell functions. Such molecules, called **ligands** because they bind selectively to receptors (L. *ligare*, to bind), include hormones, neurotransmitters, growth factors, and cell surface molecules of other cells. The cytoplasmic domain of some transmembrane receptors has regulated **protein-tyrosine kinase activity.** When such a receptor (often described as a **receptor PTK**) binds its signaling ligand (termed the **first messenger**), it phosphorylates tyrosyl residues in target proteins. In certain other cases, the receptor's regulated response to ligand binding involves interaction of its cytoplasmic domain with a **stimulatory G protein**, which leads to the production of a **second messenger, cyclic AMP.** The ligand-mediated action of another subset of G protein-linked receptors is to increase the concentration of free Ca^{2+} in the cytosol.

The distinctive sugar composition of the oligosaccharide chains in the cell coat is a key determinant in specific cell recognition and adhesion. Finally, the cell membrane of nerve and muscle cells is electrically excitable and able to carry out the specialized function of conduction.

MITOCHONDRIA

Many cell functions consume substantial quantities of energy. This energy is supplied in appropriate form by the cell's population of **mitochondria** (Gk. *mitos,* thread; *chondrion,* granule), so named because of their predominantly thread-like appearance in the LM (Fig. 3-4). These structures are up to several micrometers in length. Moreover, in living cells observed with a phase contrast microscope (a light microscope that converts otherwise invisible phase differences into visible amplitude differences), mitochondria often show signs of being translocated (e.g., slowly writhing about like

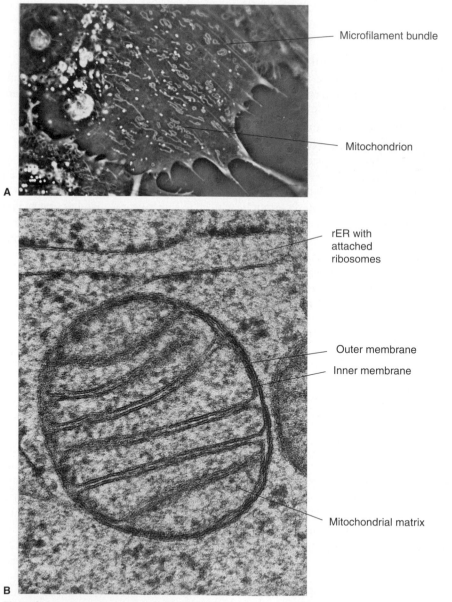

Figure 3-4
(*A*) Mitochondria (living cell under phase contrast, oil immersion). Microfilament bundles also are discernible.
(*B*) Transmission electron micrograph of a mitochondrion (hamster cell).

worms, as in Fig. 3-4*A*). At the EM level, an exclusive feature of the mitochondrion is that it is bounded by two unit membranes with an intervening **intermembranous space** (see Figs. 3-4 and 3-5). Whereas the **outer membrane** has a smooth outline, the **inner membrane** invaginates as a series of characteristic inward extensions called **cristae** (L. for crests) that permeate the interior of the organelle. The cristae are variable in number and generally are described as shelf-like with fenestrations. However, with improved methods of tissue preparation and the three-dimensional resolution now obtainable with the SEM, it is evident that many cell types, including some that were

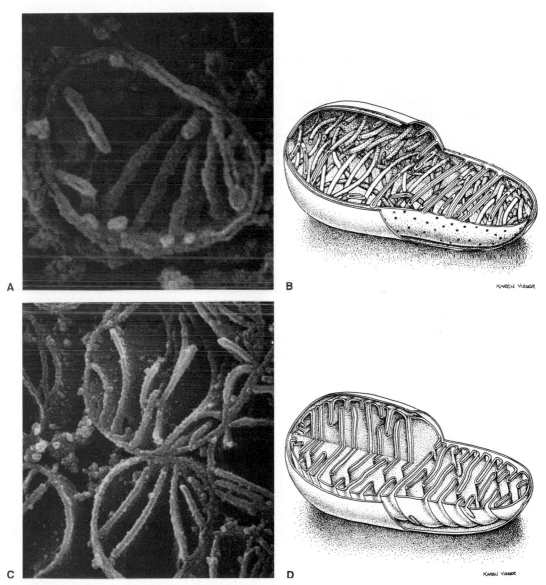

Figure 3-5
(*A*) High resolution scanning electron micrograph of a mitochondrion (rat hepatocyte, cytosol-extracted, ×60,000). (*B*) Interpretive drawing of the mitochondrion seen in *A*. Tubular cristae extend across a central cavity filled with mitochondrial matrix. (*C*) High resolution scanning electron micrograph of mitochondria (cell of brown fat, cytosol-extracted, ×36,000). (*D*) Interpretive drawing of a mitochondrion with shelf-like cristae. This interpretation is more consistent with micrograph (*C*) than with micrograph (*A*), yet both tissues were prepared identically.

thought to have shelf-like cristae, have mitochondrial cristae that are tubular (see Fig. 3-5A and B). Shelf-like cristae nevertheless exist in certain cell types, eg, adipocytes of brown fat. In EM sections, mitochondrial cristae can have an ambiguous appearance (see Fig. 3-4B), and this may have contributed to widespread acceptance that they are generally shelf-like, which now appears to be more the exception than the rule.

A slightly electron-dense material called the **mitochondrial matrix** fills the internal cavity of the mitochondrion (see Fig. 3-4B). This matrix contains DNA, RNA, ribosomes, and proteins, the significance of which is discussed later. In addition, it may contain a few electron-dense **matrix granules,** which consist mostly of calcium phosphate and are regarded as local accumulations of cations. Mitochondria are accordingly believed to play a role in keeping the cytosolic levels of calcium ions characteristically low.

The total numbers of mitochondria in cells reflect their overall energy requirements. Whereas metabolically inactive cells have relatively few mitochondria, active cells such as hepatocytes contain approximately 1000. Furthermore, in cells that expend a lot of energy, each mitochondrion contains more cristae. Mitochondria may be either evenly dispersed or concentrated at sites with high energy requirements. Mitochondria propagate, asynchronously and on an individual basis, by developing a cross partition and separating into two daughter mitochondria.

Mitochondria may represent present-day descendants of an aerobic bacterium-like organism that became incorporated into an incompletely evolved nucleated cell. The organism subsequently acquired the status of an essential organelle by adding valuable functions to those that had already evolved. Right from the start, mitochondria have been able to exist semi-autonomously because they possess their own DNA, RNA, and ribosomes. This intriguing hypothesis is corroborated by the findings that mitochondrial nucleic acids and ribosomes resemble their counterparts in bacteria and that mitochondrial DNA encodes a small number of mitochondrial proteins. The other mitochondrial proteins are encoded by the cell's nuclear DNA.

Mitochondrial Oxidative Phosphorylation Produces Adenosine Triphosphate

Mitochondria are uniquely equipped with the necessary enzymes for 1) obtaining energy from glucose, fatty acids, and amino acids, and 2) using this energy to synthesize the important energy-rich compound **adenosine triphosphate** (ATP) from its precursor, adenosine diphosphate (ADP). Mitochondria derive energy from these sources through oxidation, so the exclusive two-staged process by which they produce ATP is termed **oxidative phosphorylation.**

Hydrolytic degradation of ATP liberates essential energy for molecular transport across the cell membrane, macromolecular synthesis, muscular contraction, and other energy-consuming activities. The resulting ADP then undergoes re-phosphorylation to ATP. Mitochondria are the sites where most of this important energy currency is generated. Energy-providing substrates derived from digested food traverse both of the mitochondrial membranes and enter the matrix where enzymes responsible for their oxidation are situated. The released energy is immediately employed to phosphorylate ADP to ATP. The various enzymes that capture, pass on, and utilize energy released through oxidation constitute an integral part of the **inner membrane** and **cristae** of the organelle. Here they are arranged as integrated **functional complexes,** portions of which are discernible at the EM level, particularly when special EM preparative methods are used. Tiny knobs, known as **inner membrane spheres** or **elementary particles,** project inward into the mitochondrial matrix, supported on narrow stalks (see Fig. 3-5A and C). This unique arrangement of the membrane-bound enzymes ensures that the entire series of enzymatic reactions involved in oxidative phosphorylation proceeds efficiently and in the appropriate sequence. The ATP synthesized on these complexes passes out through both mitochondrial membranes to the cytosol and other organelles where it donates its store of energy.

RIBOSOMES

The cytoplasm contains a distinctive population of ribonucleoprotein particles known as ribosomes. Because ribosomes are 20 to 30 nm in diameter, they are not individually discernible with an LM, but in H&E-stained sections their relative abundance is to some extent revealed by cytoplasmic color. Thus, the cytoplasm of a cell that actively synthesizes proteins may appear blue to purple rather than pink. Termed **cytoplasmic basophilia,** the blue staining reflects the strong affinity between hematoxylin and the rRNA in ribosomes (see Chap. 1). In general, *diffuse* cytoplasmic basophilia indicates an abundance of free ribosomes, whereas *patchy* cytoplasmic basophilia indicates regions of closely packed rough-surfaced endoplasmic reticulum. However, such is not always the case because free ribosomes can be plentiful in the same regions as rough-surfaced endoplasmic reticulum, and some cells contain so much rough-surfaced endoplasmic reticulum that their cytoplasm is almost entirely basophilic.

Diffuse cytoplasmic basophilia reflecting an abundance of free ribosomes is noticeable in cells that proliferate and grow rapidly (e.g., cancer cells that are multiplying rampantly). Another example is the **basophilic erythroblast,** which actively synthesizes the globin component of hemoglobin. After staining with a blood stain, the cytoplasm of a basophilic erythroblast exhibits a diffuse bluish tinge (see Plate 7-1*B*), and the EM discloses that this staining is due to a high content of free ribosomes (Fig. 3-6).

The formation, subunit structure, and functional role of ribosomes are described in Chapter 2 under Nucleolus and Transcription and Translation. Besides existing as individual structures made up of a small and a large subunit, free ribosomes constitute strings called polysomes (polyribosomes). A **polysome** is a transitory structure in which a mRNA molecule is associated with a number of ribosomes. If the mRNA molecule is long, the polysome configuration is characteristically spiral (see Fig. 3-6, *inset*).

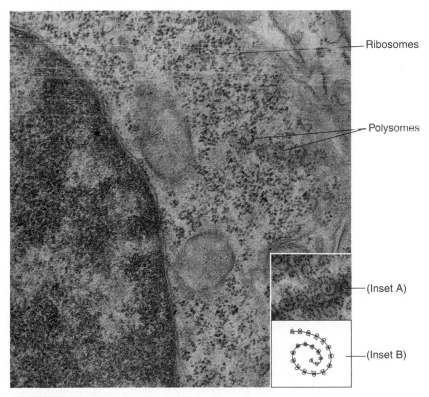

Ribosomes

Polysomes

(Inset A)

(Inset B)

Figure 3-6
Electron micrograph showing free ribosomes and polysomes (basophilic erythroblast, ×40,000). (*Insets*) A polysome is a linear series of ribosomes attached to an mRNA molecule.

As explained in Chapter 2 under Polypeptide Assembly, ribosomes represent the cell's exclusive site of amino acid incorporation into forming polypeptides. During passage of each mRNA between the ribosomal subunits, the amino acid specifications encoded in the mRNA nucleotide base sequence are translated. Each time the 5' leading end of the mRNA emerges, it engages further ribosomes that all begin assembling identical chains because they are translating the same encoded information. Because the length of the mRNA determines how many ribosomes attach, the number of ribosomes in the polysome gives some idea of the relative length of the polypeptide being assembled.

Each ribosomal subunit plays its respective role in the process, which typically occurs in less than 1 minute. First, the small subunit binds the necessary tRNA and latches onto the mRNA. The large subunit then attaches to the small subunit and implements peptide bonding, initiating the assembly process. When assembly is complete, the small and large subunits dissociate and then become individually available for further use. Hence ribosomes that are not actually in use exist largely as free subunits.

Cytosolic proteins, nucleoproteins, and certain mitochondrial proteins are synthesized by the ribosomes and polysomes that lie in the cytosol. In contrast, secretory, lysosomal, and integral membrane proteins are synthesized by membrane-bound ribosomes and polysomes that constitute an integral part of the rough-surfaced endoplasmic reticulum.

ROUGH-SURFACED ENDOPLASMIC RETICULUM

Sites of abundant rough-surfaced endoplasmic reticulum (rER) can appear as areas of local basophilia. This organelle is present in all cells, but is particularly prominent in protein-secreting cells, a classic example of which is the cell type that produces pancreatic enzymes. These cells constitute spherical secretory units called **acini** (L., grapes) and hence are known as pancreatic **acinar cells.** Each acinus has a central lumen that drains into a duct, but it is rarely sectioned in a plane that discloses the lumen of the acinus. Acinar cells release secretory protein from their luminal (apical) surface, which borders on the lumen (Plates 3-2 and 3-3). The nucleus lies toward the basal surface, and the cytoplasm between the nucleus and the basal border is packed with sufficient rER to render it intensely basophilic (see Plate 3-2). Other protein-secreting cells characterized by an abundance of rER are fibroblasts and osteoblasts, which secrete the organic matrix constituents of connective tissue and bone, and plasma cells, which secrete humoral antibodies.

With the EM, the rER appears as a discrete intracellular compartment bounded by a single unit membrane. Its recognition is easy because 1) most of it typically consists of parallel, flattened sacs called **cisternae**, and 2) its limiting membrane is studded with **ribosomes** (Fig. 3-7). Furthermore, its cisternae are interconnected (see Fig. 2-3) and their luminal content sometimes appears slightly electron-dense. In addition, the outer membrane of the nuclear envelope of all nucleated cells is studded with ribosomes. In all respects, this outer membrane therefore resembles the rER membrane with which it is continuous (see Figs. 2-2, *inset*, and 2-3). The narrow space between the outer and inner membranes of the nuclear envelope is accordingly regarded as an extension of the rER lumen.

The rER is the exclusive site of synthesis of lysosomal hydrolases and secretory proteins. Unlike the cell's cytosolic and nuclear proteins, which are synthesized on free ribosomes, lysosomal enzymes and secretory proteins become segregated within the lumen of the rER in the course of being synthesized. Because lysosomal enzymes are potently hydrolytic, they pose a hazard as soon as they are synthesized. Like secretory proteins, they must be segregated from the rest of the cytoplasm. Moreover, they must be confined by an intracellular membrane until they are used or released by the cell.

The ribosomes that assemble such proteins attach by their large subunit to the outer (cytosolic) surface of the rER membrane. Many of them are organized in polysome configurations. Each polypeptide that they assemble extends down a channel through the ribosome and passes through the rER membrane into the rER lumen (see Fig. 3-7). The details of this process are as follows.

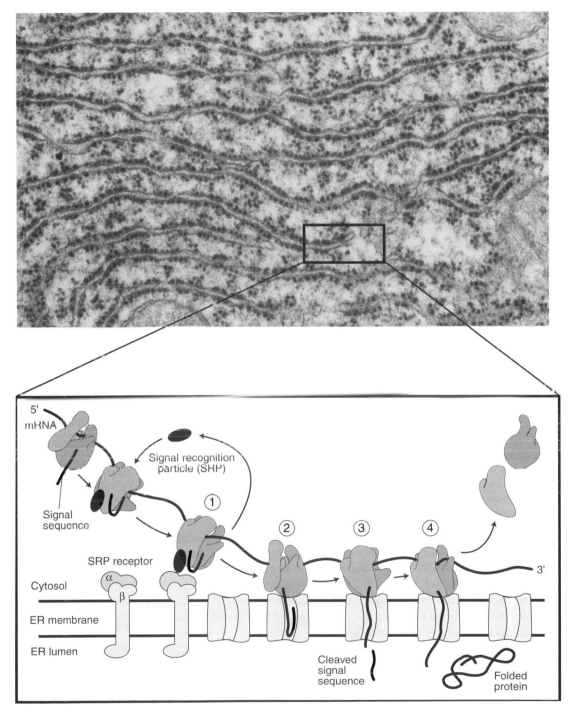

Figure 3-7
Ribosomal binding to the rER membrane and polypeptide assembly with luminal segregation of the synthesized product.
This process is known as the **signal hypothesis**.

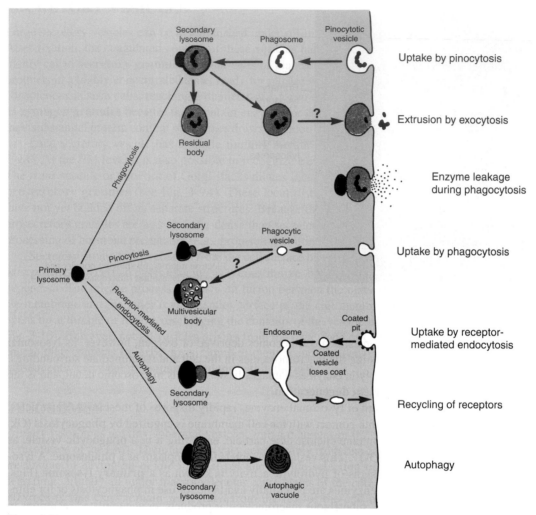

Figure 3-12
The various disposal pathways through which lysosomes eliminate exogenous ingested macromolecules and obsolete cytoplasmic organelles.

CLINICAL IMPLICATIONS

Clinical Importance of Lysosomal Enzymes
Because lysosomal enzymes can degrade a broad range of macromolecular compounds, cells are able to rid the body of most unwanted substances of high molecular weight. In particular, the cell's potent acid hydrolases help to eliminate infectious microbes such as bacteria. Important in this respect are white blood cells known as neutrophils, which are so expert at catching and killing bacteria that they constitute a major defense mechanism against infectious diseases.

When a tissue becomes acutely inflamed (hot, swollen, and tender when pressed), bacterial infection is often the cause. In responding, however, inflammatory cells such as neutrophils may liberate hydrolytic enzymes in sufficient quantities to result in some local tissue destruction. In many instances, this damage is due to premature spilling out of lysosomal hydrolases from forming phagocytic vesicles before these have had time to seal off completely (as shown in Fig. 3-12).

Another problem involving lysosomes is the body's response to chronic inhalation of certain dusts, notably silica particles. Such particles are phagocytosed by macrophages in the lungs, but because the particles are inorganic they resist enzymatic degradation. To make matters worse, the particles can disrupt the intracellular membrane that segregates them from the remainder of the cell. The hydrolytic enzymes leak from the secondary lysosomes into the cytosol and then, through death of the cells, into the surrounding tissues. A similar situation is found in patients with gout whose neutrophils attempt to phagocytose sodium urate crystals deposited in the joint tissues. In this case, the liberated lysosomal enzymes elicit a painful inflammatory reaction that typically is located in the proximal joint of the great toe.

A further example of lysosomal involvement in disease is found in cases where some important enzymatic activity normally present in lysosomes is lacking because of a gene mutation. One consequence of such inherited enzyme deficiency is intracellular accumulation of material that would otherwise be broken down or put to good use by the cell. In the **lysosomal storage diseases,** incompletely degraded cell products accumulate to such an extent that they impair function. If essential cells such as brain neurons are affected, detrimental clinical problems can arise. Patients with **Tay-Sachs disease,** for example, are deficient in the lysosomal enzyme acetylhexosaminidase A, which degrades a neuronal ganglioside. Residual undegraded product, the ganglioside, accumulates in the secondary lysosomes of brain and retinal neurons. This commonly leads to progressive mental impairment, loss of vision, and muscular weakness. It culminates with death in infancy.

Receptor-Mediated Endocytosis Brings in Useful Macromolecules

Endocytosis (Gk. *endon*, within) is a general term for the uptake of macromolecules from the cell's surroundings. A mechanism that normally supplements phagocytosis and pinocytosis is **receptor-mediated endocytosis,** a highly specific form of uptake that is mediated by cell membrane receptors. This important mechanism supplies the cell with some of its required macromolecules. Once such ligands have bound to their receptors on the cell surface, they are rapidly delivered to endosomes (see later). At this site, many of them dissociate from their receptors, which become available for further use. In the case of ligands that do not dissociate from their receptors, however, endocytosis may lower the number of receptors that remain on the cell surface, and this is described as **down-regulation.**

COATED VESICLES

Receptor-mediated endocytosis takes place primarily at sites known as **coated pits.** These are temporary shallow indentations where a protein called **clathrin** coats the cytoplasmic aspect of the cell membrane (see Figs. 3-12 through 3-14). Such pits form and invaginate on a frequent basis. The clathrin coat remains adherent to the cell membrane when the pit invaginates and pinches off to form a **coated vesicle.** The coat on this vesicle is then disassembled by an ATPase and the vesicle fuses with an endosome.

EM sections of the clathrin coat can resemble sparse stubby bristles (see Fig. 3-13A, stage 4). When a coated pit forms, the cytoplasmic surface of the cell membrane becomes coated with clathrin. The same surface remains coated when the pit pinches off to form a coated vesicle. A clathrin-coated vesicle therefore has clathrin on its outer surface and cell coat on its inner surface. The clathrin coat is an enveloping basketwork made up of pinwheel-like subunits that spontaneously assemble into a curved lattice. Such assembly eventually results in formation of a spherical latticework (see Fig. 3-13B) that plays a key role in pinching off and separating coated vesicles from the coated pits in the cell membrane.

In addition, coated vesicles bud from the rER membrane, Golgi saccules, TGN, and secretory vesicles. These coated vesicles are involved in transporting segregated proteins along the cell's separate lysosomal and surface-bound secretory pathways.

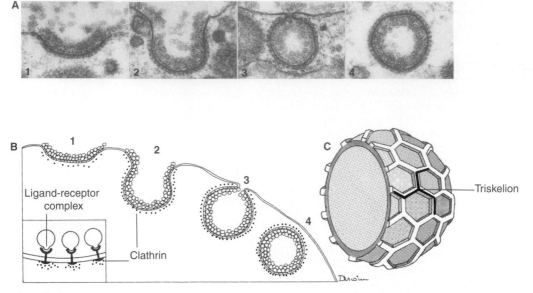

Figure 3-13
(*A*) Electron micrographs showing sequential invagination of a coated pit (*1* and *2*) and formation of a coated vesicle (*3* and *4*) in uptake of lipoprotein particles through receptor-mediated endocytosis (×53,000). (*B*) Interpretive diagram. (*Inset*) A clathrin latticework associates with the lipoprotein receptors. (*C*) This latticework is made up of clathrin-containing subunits termed triskelions.

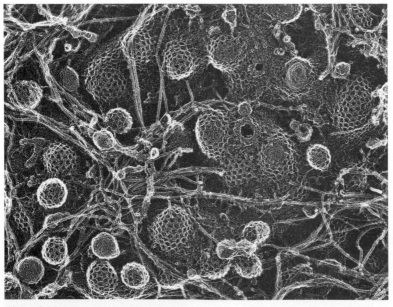

Figure 3-14
Electron micrograph showing coated pits and coated vesicles on the underside of the cell membrane (mouse hepatocyte, deep etched, rotary shadowed replica). The long, straight structures in this region are intermediate filaments representing part of the membrane cytoskeleton.

Coated vesicles constitute a heterogeneous class of transitional vesicular structures that employ either clathrin or coatomer (a complex of seven coat protein subunits) as the basis for budding. Vesicular transport that is *selective* (e.g., receptor-mediated endocytosis, regulated secretion, and routing to lysosomes) is mediated by **clathrin-coated vesicles.** Vesicular transport that is *nonselective* (e.g., bulk progression through Golgi compartments and constitutive secretion) is mediated by **coatomer-coated vesicles.**

ENDOSOMES

Before ingested macromolecules become exposed to the full onslaught of the cell's lysosomal acid hydrolases, they are processed in an intermediate, prelysosomal compartment called an **endosome** (see Figs. 3-10 and 3-12). An endosome is an **endocytic sorting compartment** with an acidic internal pH but only minimal acid hydrolase activity.

Endosomes are categorized as early or late to denote whether there is any delay before the ingested material reaches them following endocytosis. Early endosomes, many of which are tubular, provide an acidic, nondegradative environment in which ligands may *dissociate from their receptors*. In some cases, recovered receptors return to the cell surface for further utilization. Late endosomes lie deeper in the cytoplasm and tend to be larger and more complex in shape. Their pH is slightly lower and they are believed to participate in a comparatively extensive recycling program that involves the TGN as well. Furthermore, endolysosomes (an intermediate compartment that receives lysosomal enzymes from the TGN) represent a late type of endosome. Any ingested macromolecules that are not retrieved from endosomes for further use by the cell are subsequently submitted to the full degradative action of its lysosomal enzymes.

PEROXISOMES

Peroxisomes (known also as **microbodies**) are tiny vesicles, <1 μm in diameter, that are derived from the rER. They are called peroxisomes because oxidase enzymes that they contain are involved in the formation and breakdown of intracellular hydrogen peroxide, which phagocytic cells use to kill phagocytosed bacteria. Hepatocyte peroxisomes have a substantial content of catalase, which can degrade ethyl alcohol, and enzymes that can degrade fatty acids by β-oxidation, indicating that liver peroxisomes play a subsidiary role in the systemic regulation of alcohol, lipid, and cholesterol levels.

The homogeneous content of human peroxisomes is moderately electron-dense and finely granular. In various other species, it is characterized by having a more electron-dense core called a **nucleoid**. This core is considered to be a semicrystalline array of urate oxidase (uricase), an enzyme that degrades urates, because it is absent from the peroxisomes of those species that, like humans, lack this enzyme.

SMOOTH-SURFACED ENDOPLASMIC RETICULUM

In addition to the rER, the cytoplasm contains a **smooth-surfaced endoplasmic reticulum** (sER). Morphologically, this organelle differs from the rER in that 1) its limiting membrane is smooth instead of being studded with ribosomes and 2) it is primarily made up of branched tubules that anastomose in an irregular pattern (Fig. 3-15). Direct continuity nevertheless exists between the two types of endoplasmic reticulum. Furthermore, the integral membrane proteins of the sER are synthesized by the rER, so the sER is derived from the rER. The amount of sER seen varies with the cell type, and in most cells it is inconspicuous.

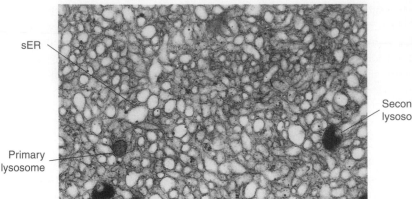

Figure 3-15
Electron micrograph showing tortuous, interconnected tubules of smooth endoplasmic reticulum (sER) in a steroid-synthesizing cell (zona reticularis of human adrenal cortex, ×15,400).

The sER is devoid of ribosomes, so it does not cause cytoplasmic basophilia or synthesize proteins. It does, however, possess most of the enzymes necessary for lipid and steroid synthesis, and in certain cells it has a remarkable capacity for segregating calcium ions. The sER membrane of hepatocytes, which are the metabolically active parenchymal cells of the liver, also contains enzymes that can metabolize, degrade, or detoxify potentially harmful compounds. The details are as follows.

Lipid Synthesis

The sER is the cytoplasmic organelle where lipids and cholesterol-derived compounds are synthesized. It therefore tends to be more conspicuous in cells that secrete lipids, lipoproteins, or steroid hormones. An example of a cell type that synthesizes and also secretes lipids is the common kind of lining cell of the small intestine. Among the many products of digestion that these cells absorb are the breakdown products of fats, which are recombined into lipids in the sER of these cells. The sER is even more extensive in steroid-secreting cells (see Fig. 3-15).

Drug Detoxification

Cytochrome P450 enzymes, the oxidative enzymes present in the sER membrane of hepatocytes, have the capacity to metabolize lipid-soluble drugs (e.g., barbiturates) and other toxic compounds that may be present in the circulation. If blood levels of such drugs or alcohol remain elevated, the sER becomes more extensive, augmenting the liver's detoxification capacity.

Glycogen Metabolism

Much of the glycogen stored in hepatocytes lies in the cytosol present between tubules of the sER (Fig. 3-16). This is probably because glucose-6-phosphatase, which is the enzyme responsible for the last stage of breakdown of glycogen into glucose, and two additional enzymes involved in regulating glycogen metabolism are intimately associated with the sER membrane of these cells.

Calcium Segregation

Whether a muscle cell contracts or relaxes is determined by the concentration of calcium ions reaching its contractile components. The precise intracellular distribution of calcium in skeletal and car-

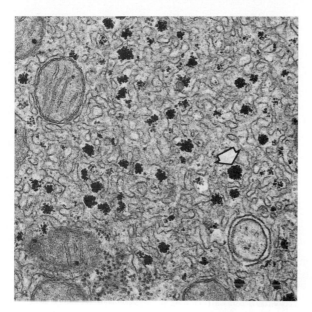

Figure 3-16
Electron micrograph showing glycogen (*arrow*) in proximity to tubules of sER in a hepatocyte.

diac muscle cells is regulated by an elaborate sER that intimately encloses their contractile components (see Chapter 10).

Next, we shall deal with the cytoskeletal components that support the cell, stabilize its limiting membrane, and generate certain forms of cell motility.

MICROTUBULES

Cytoplasmic microtubules are slender, unbranched tubules made of the protein tubulin. They represent the chief structural components of centrioles, mitotic spindles, cilia, and flagella. In interphase, they exist individually as **cytoplasmic microtubules** (Fig. 3-17). At mitosis, cytoplasmic microtubules disappear and spindle microtubules form instead.

With the EM, microtubules appear as long hollow structures of unfixed length with a diameter of 25 nm (Fig. 3-18A). In transverse section, they appear as tiny circles (see Fig. 3-18B). After appropriate staining, it can be discerned that each microtubule is made up of longitudinal rod-like

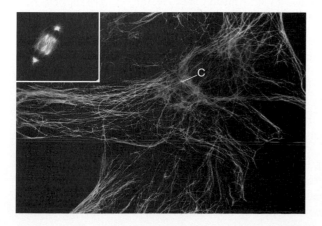

Figure 3-17
Cytoplasmic microtubules of an interphase cell. (*Inset*) Spindle microtubules of an anaphase cell. These are immunofluorescence oil-immersion photomicrographs of mouse embryonic fibroblasts. Near the middle of the interphase cell, centrioles (*c*) appear as a single, intensely fluorescent spot.

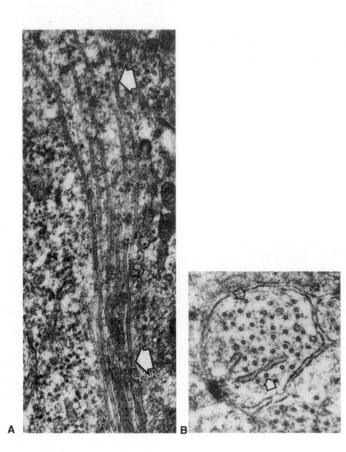

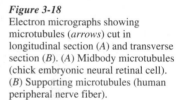

Figure 3-18
Electron micrographs showing
microtubules (*arrows*) cut in
longitudinal section (*A*) and transverse
section (*B*). (*A*) Midbody microtubules
(chick embryonic neural retinal cell).
(*B*) Supporting microtubules (human
peripheral nerve fiber).

elements called **protofilaments** (indicated in Fig. 3-23) assembled from dimeric **tubulin subunits** consisting of α- and β-tubulin. This pattern of organization is evident in the micrograph of a centriole (a structure made up of microtubules) shown in Figure 2-15.

In the cell, tubulin exists both as a soluble protein in the form of free dimeric subunits and in the polymerized state in the form of microtubules. These two forms are in equilibrium with each other. In this connection, the plant alkaloid **colchicine** is extensively employed in experimental studies of the cytoskeleton, chromosome preparation for cytogenetic studies, and investigations relating to mitosis. Its usefulness is due to the fact that it causes existing microtubules to disappear and prevents formation of mitotic spindles, thus blocking cell division. It acts by binding to tubulin subunits, which interferes with microtubule assembly. Also, the disturbed equilibrium between polymerized tubulin and soluble tubulin causes existing cytoplasmic or spindle microtubules to dissociate into free tubulin subunits. Cilia, flagella, and centrioles, however, remain refractory to the action of colchicine and their constituent microtubules stay intact.

As noted in Chapter 2, under Mitosis, microtubules grow mostly at their **plus** end. Their slow-growing, **minus** end lies at the site where their assembly began. **Microtubule-organizing centers**, the initiation sites for microtubule assembly, are most abundant in pericentriolar regions. In general, cytoplasmic microtubules are oriented with their minus end lying toward the middle of the cell and their plus end lying toward the cell periphery. Microtubule assembly is promoted by certain **microtubule-associated proteins** (MAPs). Several MAPs stabilize the assembled microtubules against breakdown; others are able to crosslink them (e.g., to one another, to membranes, or to other organelles). In addition, a small number of microtubule-associated motor proteins have been characterized. Their involvement in microtubule-mediated intracellular transport is considered briefly in the next section.

Microtubules support and provide motility and intracellular transport. Rigid microtubules give cells the necessary internal support. Their role in stabilizing cell shape is most evident in cells with irregular contours (e.g., neurons, the long nerve fibers of which have microtubules extending along them; see Fig. 3-18*B*). Blood platelets have a supporting marginal bundle of microtubules at their periphery that maintains their discoid shape (see Fig. 6-3). In cilia and flagella, mechanical forces generated between adjacent doublet microtubules result in motility (see later).

Microtubules are also involved in intracellular transport. Thus in axons (a type of nerve fiber), microtubules serve as guiding tracks for the transport of organelles and materials from the cell body to the tip of the fiber. There is also evidence that microtubules are involved in certain secretory pathways, e.g., in signal-induced, unidirectional transport of secretory vesicles from the Golgi apparatus to the cell surface, which in some cells appears to be mediated by the **microtubule motor protein, kinesin** (see Chapter 9, under Neurons). **Cytoplasmic dynein** can move vesicles along microtubules in the reverse direction (toward their minus end). Participation of microtubules in the segregation of daughter chromosomes at mitosis was considered in Chapter 2. Corresponding spindle-associated microtubule motor proteins play key roles in the relative movements of spindle microtubules and kinetochores during mitosis.

We shall now consider the cytoplasmic organelles that possess recognizable groups of microtubules. Centrioles, described briefly in Chapter 2, will be reconsidered in connection with basal bodies of cilia.

CILIA AND FLAGELLA

Cilia are hair-like motile processes, 10 μm or so in length and about 0.2 μm in diameter, that extend from the free surface of ciliated cells in the lining of certain internal tubes and cavities. The several hundred cilia on a ciliated cell provides a striking SEM image (Fig. 3-19). Along with **ciliated cells,** respiratory airways are typically provided with **goblet cells** (Fig. 3-20; see also Plate 4-1). These

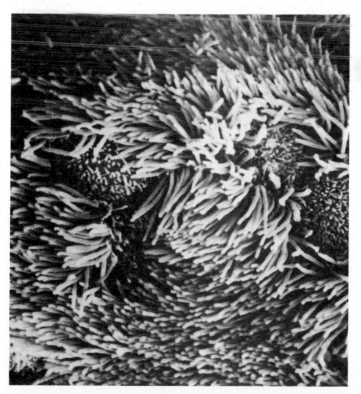

Figure 3-19
Scanning electron micrograph showing cilia on the luminal surface of ciliated luminal lining cells (uterine tube, mouse, ×7000). Three nonciliated cells with microvilli protruding from their luminal surface are also present.

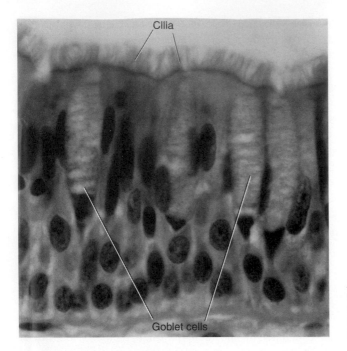

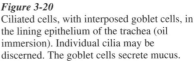

Figure 3-20
Ciliated cells, with interposed goblet cells, in the lining epithelium of the trachea (oil immersion). Individual cilia may be discerned. The goblet cells secrete mucus.

cells become goblet-shaped when they accumulate **mucus**, their glycoprotein secretory product. Mucus is carried along airways as a continuous sheet by the beating of cilia. The traveling mucus blanket not only affords protection but, because it is sticky, traps particles settling out from the inhaled air. With the LM, it is just possible to distinguish individual cilia on such cells, and at the base of the cilium, it is occasionally possible to discern a tiny associated structure called a basal body.

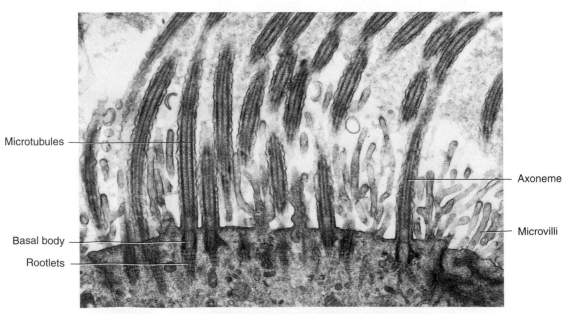

Figure 3-21
Electron micrograph showing ciliated cells of the bronchial lining. Cilia cut in oblique and longitudinal sections may be compared with microvilli cut in corresponding planes.

When viewed with the EM, the **basal body** of a cilium is identical in appearance to a **centriole**, which is a short cylindrical structure, 0.5 μm long and 0.2 μm in diameter, with nine bundles of microtubules in its walls. Each bundle contains three microtubules referred to as **triplet** microtubules (see Fig. 2-15).

In G_1, a typical cell has a pair of closely associated centrioles that is located fairly centrally (*c* in Fig. 3-17). To prepare for ciliation, the cell produces multiple centrioles, one for each cilium. These take up a position just under the free border of the cell and are then called basal bodies. Microtubules grow up from the superficial end of each basal body to produce a cilium, and anchoring **rootlets** subsequently develop from the lower end of the basal body (Figs. 3-21 and 3-22).

In producing a cilium, the microtubules that extend up from a basal body are the two innermost microtubules of each triplet. Hence, the shaft of a cilium, which is termed its **axoneme**, has nine peripheral **doublet** microtubules (see Figs. 3-22 and 3-23). In addition, two **singlet** microtubules

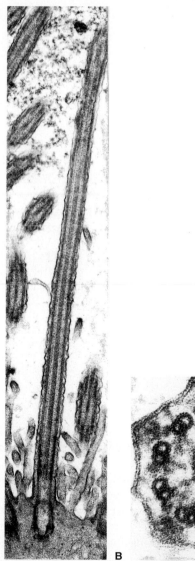

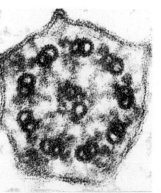

Figure 3-22
Electron micrographs showing cilia cut in longitudinal section (*A*) and transverse section (*B*). These are cilia of human bronchial epithelium.

A   B

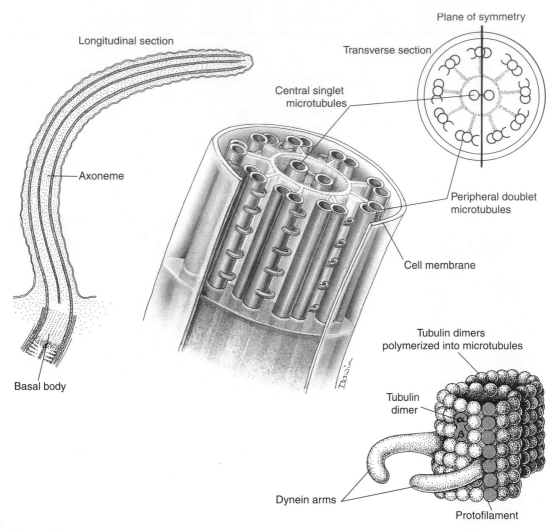

Figure 3-23
Interpretive diagrams of the fine structure of a cilium. In each peripheral doublet, one microtubule possesses dynein arms. It is made up of 13 rod-shaped protofilaments, each assembled from tubulin dimers (*bottom right*). The associated microtubule is made up of 10 or 11 protofilaments; additional protofilaments are shared with the companion microtubule (*bottom right*). Radial spoke linkages connect the peripheral doublet microtubules to an axial tubular sheath that surrounds two central singlet microtubules (*center* and *top right*).

extend along its axis. Thus, a cilium has nine peripheral doublets and two central singlets and is surrounded by cell membrane, whereas its basal body (or a centriole) has nine peripheral triplets and no central singlets, and is surrounded by cytosol.

When cilia execute their strong forward beat (**effective stroke**), they are fairly rigid. When they slip back into their starting position (**recovery stroke**), they are comparatively flexible. The forceful effective stroke can propel a mucus blanket forward. The gentler recovery stroke occurs in the tissue fluid layer that underlies the mucus blanket and does not move the mucus blanket backward. The two strokes are executed in a plane that lies perpendicular to an imaginary line drawn between the two central singlets (see Fig. 3-23, *top right*).

Energy for ciliary motility is obtained from ATP through the enzymatic activity of **dynein**, an ATPase present as tiny hook-like arms on each peripheral doublet of the axoneme (see Figs. 3-22 and 3-23). The forces that bring about ciliary beating are generated by sliding of the peripheral doublets relative to one another. An elaborate interconnecting arrangement between the peripheral doublets and central singlets harnesses forces generated by this sliding action and applies them to bending of the axoneme.

The basic organization of the ciliary axoneme is found also in the tail of the spermatozoon. The sperm tail, however, has additional features and is considerably longer than a cilium (see Chapter 18). Because the sperm tail executes whip-like swimming movements, it is known as a **flagellum** (L., whip) although it resembles a cilium in possessing nine peripheral doublets and two central singlets.

Also of interest is the fact that the *stimulus-sensing region* of certain sensory receptors is a ciliary derivative. Some cells with a modified cilium that serves this purpose are the photoreceptors of the retina and some hair cells of the inner ear (see Chapter 19). Certain other cell types possess a single, unmodified **primary cilium** that is presumed to have a sensory role. The functional significance of this solitary structure remains somewhat speculative.

FILAMENTS

The last nonmembranous organelles that we shall consider are the thread-like cytoplasmic filaments. Three different subclasses of filaments found in cells: 1) **microfilaments**, which are equivalent in function to the **thin filaments** of muscle cells; 2) **thick filaments,** which are found in muscle cells and can exist in a more temporary and much shorter form in other cell types as well; and 3) **intermediate filaments,** a heterogeneous subclass of filaments that are so named because their diameter is intermediate between that of thin and thick filaments. Contractile activity is due to interaction between the microfilament protein **actin** and another contractile protein called **myosin**, an actin-activated ATPase present in thick filaments. The intermediate filaments are not capable of producing contractions.

Contractile Filaments

Seen in the EM, **microfilaments** are slender rods about 7 nm in diameter (Fig. 3-24). They are made up of **actin**, commonly in association with **tropomyosin** and, in muscle cells at least, with proteins that are sensitive to the cytosolic concentration of calcium ions. The role of the calcium ions is to regulate interaction between actin and myosin. The **thick filaments** of muscle cells, composed of myosin, are wider than the thin filaments and more variable in diameter (12 to 16 nm). Nonmuscle cells also contain myosin, but it is seldom in the form of recognizable filaments. Generally, such filaments are assembled in these cells only when needed and, although thick, are too scarce and short to be recognized with confidence.

The thin and thick filaments of skeletal muscle and the heart are distinctively arranged in a pattern (summarized below) that facilitates their interaction in producing contractions. At the periphery of other cells, a basically similar mechanism generates certain forms of cell motility.

Filaments in Skeletal Muscle

The thin and thick filaments are confined to cylindrical structures called myofibrils that extend the full length of the muscle cell. Each myofibril is made up of identical repeated segments termed **sarcomeres**, with conspicuous transverse interconnections called **Z lines.** As shown in Figure 10-3A, equal numbers of thin filaments, attached to each Z line, extend to the middle third of the sarcomere. The thick filaments lie in the middle two thirds of the sarcomere, with the two sets of thin filaments interdigitating between them. When the muscle cell is stimulated to contract, the thin filaments are drawn farther in between the thick ones, while the thick filaments stay in the same position (see Fig. 10-3B). ATP supplies the energy for this process. The

Intermediate filaments

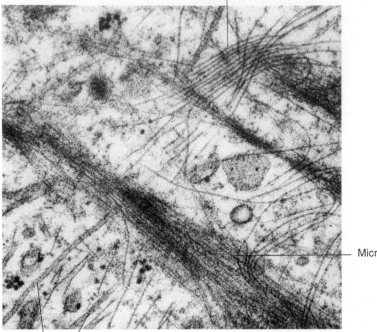

Microfilaments

Microtubules

Figure 3-24
Electron micrograph showing the three main structural components of the cytoskeleton (endothelial cell of pig aorta).
Relative diameters of microtubules, microfilaments, and intermediate filaments may be compared directly in this micrograph.

sliding action pulls the Z lines closer together, and shortening of the myofibrils results in contraction of the cell.
(More details are given under Skeletal Muscle in Chapter 10.)

In almost every kind of cell, the superficial zone of cytoplasm just under the cell membrane is
rich in microfilaments. Many of these microfilaments are probably linked to integral membrane proteins of the cell membrane. In some cells, they are organized into prominent bundles known as **stress
fibers** that occasionally may be discerned in living cells with a phase-contrast microscope (see Fig.
3-4*A*). These bundles are strikingly evident after immunofluorescent staining (Fig. 3-25). Several
different proteins seem to be involved in linking the superficial end of such microfilament bundles
to contact areas where the cell adheres to its substrate.

Contractile activities involving microfilaments and their associated myosin range from alter-
ations in cell shape to cytoplasmic constriction during cell division. At telophase, a band of parallel
microfilaments, known as the **contractile ring,** appears just under the cell membrane and encircles
the cell deep to its developing cleavage furrow. Contractile activity of this ring deepens the cleavage furrow until it splits the cell into two daughter cells.

Crosslinked Microfilaments in Microvilli
On the luminal surface of absorptive cells such as those of the intestinal lining there is a thin layer,
hardly discernible with the LM, of extremely fine perpendicular striations. With the EM, it may be
seen that such a layer, termed a **striated border** or **brush border,** consists of **microvilli** (see Figs.
3-2 and 3-26), which are tiny finger-like processes projecting perpendicularly from the cell surface.

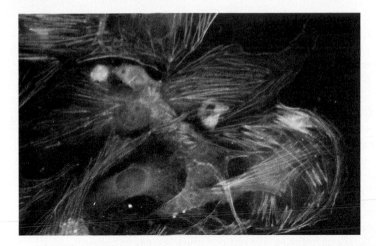

Figure 3-25
Microfilament bundles (mouse
embryonic fibroblast in tissue culture,
oil immersion immunofluorescence
photomicrograph).

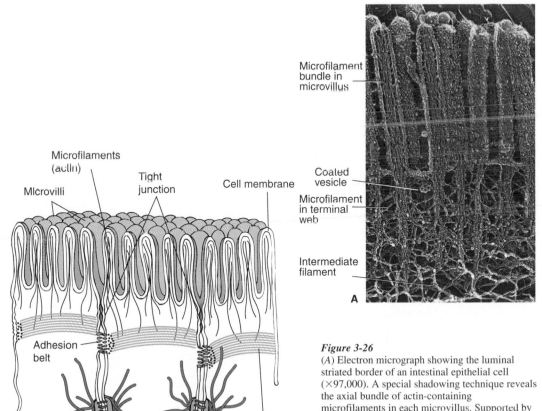

Microfilament
bundle in
microvillus

Coated
vesicle

Microfilament
in terminal
web

Intermediate
filament

A

Microfilaments
(actin)

Tight
junction

Cell membrane

Microvilli

Adhesion
belt

Desmosome

Intermediate
filaments

Marginal band
(microfilaments)

B

Figure 3-26
(*A*) Electron micrograph showing the luminal
striated border of an intestinal epithelial cell
(×97,000). A special shadowing technique reveals
the axial bundle of actin-containing
microfilaments in each microvillus. Supported by
underlying intermediate filaments, these
microfilaments extend up through the terminal
web. A coated vesicle lies near the luminal
surface. (*B*) Microvilli reinforced by axial bundles
of crosslinked microfilaments, the bases of which
are attached to intermediate filaments.

As shown in Figure 3-26, each microvillus is supported by a rigid crosslinked bundle of parallel microfilaments that extends down through the core into the filament-rich superficial zone of cytoplasm. At the tip of the microvillus, the central microfilament bundle is anchored to the cell membrane. Fine myosin-containing crosslinks attach the microfilaments to one another as well as to the overlying region of cell membrane (see Fig. 3-26). The main purpose of this crosslinked arrangement of microfilaments seems to be to provide internal support for the microvillus. The role of the associated myosin is uncertain, but its superficial distribution suggests that it may promote translocation of constituents in the overlying membrane. The chief purpose of the huge number of microvilli extending from this type of border is to expand further the area over which absorption takes place. Other cell types commonly possess a few inconspicuous microvilli.

From electron micrographs such as Figure 3-2, it may be appreciated that microvilli are finger-like projections, not folds. Depending on the plane of section, longitudinal, transverse, oblique, or grazing sections of these structures may be seen. It is important to know how to distinguish between microvilli and cilia, both of which are finger-like extensions of the cell membrane. Remember that microvilli are shorter and narrower (up to 1 μm in length and 90 nm or so in diameter), lack basal bodies, and contain a microfilament bundle instead of the 9 + 2 arrangement of microtubules characterizing cilia (the two structures may be compared directly in Fig. 3-21).

Intermediate Filaments

With a diameter intermediate between the widths of microfilaments and thick filaments, intermediate filaments (see Fig. 3-24) are 8 to 12 nm across and hence are also known as **10-nm filaments.** They constitute a heterogeneous subclass of filaments of diverse protein composition. Table 3-2 lists the main subtypes recognized, together with some cell types in which they are found. The intracellular distribution of intermediate filaments indicates that they play supplemental roles in supporting cells and maintaining asymmetrical shapes. In certain cases these filaments transmit and distribute tensile stresses throughout cells, as for example in smooth muscle cells, where bundles of intermediate filaments transmit the pull of contraction to attachment sites on the cell membrane. Cable-like bundles of **keratin filaments (tonofilaments)** anchored to the cell membrane of epidermal keratinocytes distribute shear stresses, enabling the epidermis to withstand rough treatment. Finally, the nuclear lamina (see Chapter 2) is a fine meshwork of intermediate filaments containing polypeptides called **lamins.** It is held in a more or less central position by intermediate filaments anchored to other parts of the cytoskeleton and also the cell periphery.

Although less information exists about other functions of intermediate filaments, their various subtypes have assisted in malignant tumor identification, particularly in the case of brain tumors, be-

TABLE 3-2

INTERMEDIATE FILAMENTS: MAJOR SUBTYPE PROTEINS AND DISTRIBUTIONS

Constituent Proteins	Cell Types
Keratins (in tonofilaments)	Epithelial cells
Vimentin	Mesenchyme-derived cells
	Neuroectoderm-derived cells
Desmin	Muscle cells
Glial filament (glial fibrillary acidic protein)	Astrocytes and other glial cells
Neurofilament	Neurons
Peripherin	Neurons
Lamins A, B, and C	Nuclear lamina of all nucleated cells

cause the protein composition of the intermediate filaments of tumor cells is a reliable indicator of the cell type from which the tumor originated.

CYTOPLASMIC INCLUSIONS

This category is made up of components that are not always present in the cytoplasm, yet are considered a normal part of the cell.

Stored Foods

Energy sources such as carbohydrates and fat are not stored consistently by every cell. Together with pigments, they are therefore classified as inclusions rather than constituent organelles of the cytoplasm.

Carbohydrate is stored in the cytosol as deposits of the polysaccharide **glycogen**, mostly within hepatocytes and muscle cells. At the EM level, glycogen appears as electron-dense particles that are slightly larger than ribosomes. These particles exist as characteristic aggregates in hepatocytes (see Fig. 3-16).

Fat (lipid) is stored primarily by the fat cells of adipose tissue, but under certain circumstances it accumulates in other cells as well, notably hepatocytes (see Plate 1-3). In all these cells it exists as free droplets in the cytosol that are unsegregated by a limiting membrane.

Cell Pigments

Certain tissues are intrinsically tinted with natural colored compounds termed cell pigments. Exogenous pigments (Gk. *ex*, out) originate outside the body, whereas endogenous pigments (Gk. *endon*, within) are produced by the cell itself.

Exogenous Pigments

Brightly colored lipid soluble food derivatives tend to color fat. Thus body fat is colored yellow if large amounts of **carotene**, the orange pigment in carrots, are ingested and absorbed, and excessive amounts change the color of the skin.

Inhaled colored dusts impart their colors to the lungs, and carbon particles from tobacco smoke blacken the lungs of heavy smokers. Inorganic pigments driven deeply into the skin persist as tattoo marks.

Endogenous Pigments

The red, iron-containing erythrocyte pigment **hemoglobin** has the important function of transporting oxygen around the body. When worn-out erythrocytes are destroyed by macrophages, their hemoglobin is degraded into two other pigments, hemosiderin, which contains iron, and bilirubin, which does not. The iron-containing pigment **hemosiderin**, which is brown, can be conspicuous in macrophages that dispose of worn-out erythrocytes in the spleen. The other pigment, yellowish-brown **bilirubin**, is devoid of iron and superfluous. The liver extracts it from the blood and excretes it as bile.

The brown-to-black pigment that characterizes skin and hair is **melanin**. The skin produces larger amounts of this pigment as a protection against ultraviolet light and it is responsible for the dark skin and hair color of the black race. Melanin light-proofs the eyes and is present in neurons of the substantia nigra of the brain.

Certain long-lived cells, notably heart muscle cells and neurons, produce a brown pigment that is known as **lipofuscin** (L. *fuscus*, brown) or **lipochrome pigment** because of its lipid composition

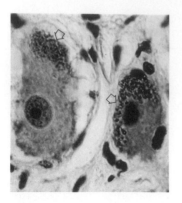

Figure 3-27
Lipofuscin (lipochrome pigment) in the cytoplasm of two neuronal cell bodies (ganglion cells).

and golden brown color. Readily seen in LM sections (Fig.3-27), this pigment represents a normal end-product of wear and tear that resists lysosomal digestion and accumulates in residual bodies (see Fig. 3-12).

SUMMARY

The various cytoplasmic components are listed in Table 3-1. All cytoplasmic membranes appear trilaminar in transverse section at high magnification. The cell membrane is a fluid bilayer of phospholipids and cholesterol that incorporates integral and peripheral membrane proteins. Attached oligosaccharide chains constitute the cell coat. The cell membrane maintains the cell's distinctive internal composition, facilitates exchanges between the cell and its surroundings, and recognizes signals.

Mitochondria are characterized by having a double limiting membrane, the outer one smooth and the inner one invaginated as cristae and studded with enzyme complexes. The mitochondrial matrix contains DNA, RNA, ribosomes, and proteins. Calcium storage granules may also be present in the matrix. Mitochondria generate ATP by oxidative phosphorylation and maintain their population size by asynchronous division.

Basophilic cytoplasm contains numerous ribosomes, including polysomes assembling polypeptides. Ribosomes consist of a large subunit and a small subunit. Assembling secretory, lysosomal, and integral membrane proteins possess an initial signal sequence that ensures the ribosomes assembling them will bind to the rER membrane. The rER, consisting of flat cisternae studded with ribosomes and polysomes, segregates all proteins that are either secretory or lysosomal within its lumen.

From the rER, segregated proteins reach Golgi saccules by way of transfer vesicles. Cells with elaborate Golgi complexes have several stacks of fenestrated saucer-shaped, smooth-walled saccules. Segregated proteins progress through Golgi stacks from their *cis* face to their *trans* face (or TGN), the site where secretory vesicles and lysosomes begin to form. Golgi saccules are the sites where glycoprotein glycosylation is completed and other secretory products are modified. Differential sorting directs secretory products to secretory vesicles and hydrolytic enzymes to lysosomes. The Golgi apparatus also directs and recycles rER-generated integral membrane proteins, replenishing those of the cell membrane.

Lysosomal acid hydrolases are able to dispose of deteriorating organelles and a variety of materials taken up by endocytosis. If liberated from cells, these enzymes can be damaging to tissues. Certain required macromolecules are ingested through receptor-mediated endocytosis. They dissociate from their cell membrane receptors in an endosome compartment. Enzymes for forming and destroying hydrogen peroxide are localized in peroxisomes.

A ramifying tubular system of smooth membrane called the sER is the intracellular site of lipid and steroid synthesis, drug detoxification and glycogen metabolism in hepatocytes, and cytosolic calcium level regulation in muscle.

Microtubules are unbranched tubular assemblies of tubulin subunits. They support the cell, facilitate intracellular transport and mitotic chromosome segregation, and generate the movements of cilia and flagella. Each cilium has a basal body identical to a centriole, with nine peripheral triplet microtubules but no central microtubules. In contrast, the ciliary shaft (axoneme) has nine peripheral doublets with two central singlets and a covering of cell membrane. The axoneme requires ATP for its motility, which is due to sliding between each doublet and the next. In a few special cases, the axoneme has receptor function instead.

Microfilaments contain actin. They are equivalent to the thin filaments that at sarcomeres ends in skeletal muscle are inserted into Z lines. Microfilaments of nonmuscle cells are of similar diameter but are not anchored to Z lines. Myosin, present in the thick filaments of muscle cells, interacts with actin in thin filaments and microfilaments. Thick filaments, however, are not prominent in nonmuscle cells. Interaction between actin and myosin is responsible for muscular contraction and cell separation after mitosis. Actin is also involved in cell motility and adherence. The different subtypes of intermediate (10-nm) filaments have distinctive protein compositions and most, if not all, are thought to have stress-bearing or skeletal roles.

Cytoplasmic inclusions are not consistently present in cells. Examples are the polysaccharide glycogen, which appears as electron-dense particles, and lipid storage droplets. Both lie free in the cytosol, unsegregated by intracellular membranes. Pigments, too, may be present in the cytoplasm. Carotene and carbon are both exogenous, but hemoglobin, hemosiderin (an iron-containing breakdown product of hemoglobin), melanin, and lipofuscin (a superfluous end-product of wear and tear) are endogenous.

Bibliography

Cytoplasmic Organelles (General)

Alberts B, Bray D, Lewis J, et al. Molecular Biology of the Cell, 3rd Ed. New York, Garland Publishing, 1994.

Fawcett DW. The Cell, 2nd Ed. Philadelphia, WB Saunders, 1981.

Goodman SR, ed. Medical Cell Biology, 2nd Ed. Philadelphia, Lippincott-Raven, 1998.

Hollenberg MJ, Cormack DH, Lea PJ. Stereo Atlas of the Cell. Toronto, BC Decker, 1989.

Kessel RG, Kardon RH. Tissues and Organs: A Text-Atlas of Scanning Electron Microscopy. San Francisco, WH Freeman, 1979.

Lodish H, Berk A, Zipursky SL, Matsudaira P, Baltimore D, Darnell J. Molecular Cell Biology, 4th Ed. New York, WH Freeman, 2000.

Tanaka K. Eukaryotes: Scanning electron microscopy of intracellular structures. Int Rev Cytol Suppl 17:89, 1987.

Cell Membrane and Cytosol

Alberts B, Bray D, Lewis J et al. Membrane structure. In: Molecular Biology of the Cell, ed 3. New York, Garland Publishing, 1994, p 478.

Bretscher MS. The molecules of the cell membrane. Sci Am 253(4):100, 1985.

Porter KR, Tucker JB. The ground substance of the living cell. Sci Am 244(3):56, 1981.

Singer SJ. Proteins and membrane topography. Hosp Pract, May 1973.

Singer SJ. The structure and insertion of integral proteins in membranes. Annu Rev Cell Biol 6:247, 1990.

Singer SJ, Nicolson GL. The fluid mosaic model of the structure of cell membranes. Science 175:720, 1972.

Weber K, Osborn M. The molecules of the cell matrix. Sci Am 253(4):110, 1985.

Mitochondria

Attardi G, Schatz G. Biogenesis of mitochondria. Annu Rev Cell Biol 4:289, 1988.

Ernster L, Schatz G. Mitochondria: a historical review. J Cell Biol 91:227S, 1981.

Hinkle PC, McCarty RE. How cells make ATP. Sci Am 238(3):104, 1983.

Kayar SR, Hoppeler H, Mermod L, Weibel ER. Mitochondrial size and shape in equine skeletal muscle: a three-dimensional reconstruction study. Anat Rec 222:333, 1988.

Lea PJ, Hollenberg MJ. Mitochondrial structure revealed by high-resolution scanning electron microscopy. Am J Anat 184:245, 1989.

Mitchell P. Keilin's respiratory chain concept and its chemiosmotic consequences. Science 206:1148, 1979.

Whittaker PA, Danks SM. Mitochondria: Structure, Function, and Assembly. New York, Longman, 1979.

Rough-Surfaced Endoplasmic Reticulum and Ribosomes

Blobel G. Synthesis and segregation of secretory proteins: the signal hypothesis. In Brinkley BR, Porter KR. eds. International Cell Biology 1976—1977. New York, Rockefeller University Press, 1977.

Burgess TL, Kelly RB. Constitutive and regulated secretion of proteins. Annu Rev Cell Biol 3:243, 1987.

Lake JA. The ribosome. Sci Am 245(2):84, 1981.

Lee C, Chen LB. Dynamic behavior of endoplasmic reticulum in living cells. Cell 54:37, 1988.

Siekevitz P, Zamecnik PC. Ribosomes and protein synthesis. J Cell Biol 91:53S, 1981.

Walter P, Blobel G. Translocation of proteins across the endoplasmic reticulum: III. Signal recognition protein (SRP) causes signal sequence-dependent and site-specific arrest of chain elongation that is released by microsomal membranes. J Cell Biol 91:557, 1981.

Endocytosis, Vesicular Transport, and Golgi Apparatus

Alberts B, Bray D, Lewis J et al. Vesicular traffic in the secretory and endocytic pathways. In: Molecular Biology of the Cell, ed 3. New York, Garland Publishing, 1994, p 600.

Brown WJ, Farquhar MG. The mannose-6-phosphate receptor for lysosomal enzymes is concentrated in *cis* Golgi cisternae. Cell 36:295, 1984.

Burgess TL, Kelly RB. Constitutive and regulated secretion of proteins. Annu Rev Cell Biol 3:243, 1987.

Dautry-Varsat A, Lodish HF. How receptors bring proteins and particles into cells. Sci Am 250(5):52, 1984.

Dunphy WG, Rothman JE. Compartmental organization of the Golgi stack. Cell 42:13, 1985.

Farquhar MG. Progress in unraveling pathways of Golgi traffic. Annu Rev Cell Biol 1:447, 1985.

Goldstein JL, Anderson RGW, Brown MS. Receptor-mediated endocytosis and the cellular uptake of low density lipoprotein. In: Membrane Recycling. Ciba Foundation Symposium 92:77, 1982.

Heuser J, Evans L. Three dimensional visualization of coated vesicle formation in fibroblasts. J Cell Biol 84:560, 1980.

Hubbard AL. Endocytosis. Curr Opin Cell Biol 1:675, 1989.

Keen JH. Clathrin and associated assembly and disassembly proteins. Annu Rev Biochem 59:415, 1990.

Morre DJ. The Golgi apparatus. Int Rev Cytol Suppl 17:211, 1987.

Pearse BMF, Robinson MS. Clathrin, adaptors, and sorting. Annu Rev Cell Biol 6:151, 1990.

Rambourg A, Clermont Y, Hermo L. Three-dimensional architecture of the Golgi apparatus in Sertoli cells of the rat. Am J Anat 154:455, 1979.

Rambourg A, Clermont Y, Hermo L. Formation of secretion granules in the Golgi apparatus of pancreatic acinar cells of the rat. Am J Anat 183:187, 1988.

Rodman JS, Mercer RW, Stahl PD. Endocytosis and transcytosis. Curr Opin Cell Biol 2:664, 1990.

Rothman JE. The compartmental organization of the Golgi apparatus. Sci Am 253(3):74, 1985.

Rothman JE, Orci L. Budding vesicles in living cells. Sci Am 274(3):70, 1996.

Schwartz AL. Cell biology of intracellular protein trafficking. Annu Rev Immunol 8:195, 1990.

Shepherd VL. Intracellular pathways and mechanisms of sorting in receptor-mediated endocytosis. Trends Pharmacol Sci 10:458, 1989.

Tanaka K, Mitsushima A, Fukodome H, Kashima Y. Three-dimensional architecture of the Golgi complex observed by high resolution scanning electron microscopy. J Submicros Cytol 18:1, 1986.

Van Deurs B, Petersen OW, Olsnes S, Sandvig K. The ways of endocytosis. Int Rev Cytol 117:131, 1989.

Lysosomes and Peroxisomes

Bainton DF. The discovery of lysosomes. J Cell Biol 91:66S, 1981.

De Duve C. Microbodies in the living cell. Sci Am 248(5):74, 1983.

Hirsch JG. Lysosomes and mental retardation. Q Rev Biol 47:303, 1972.

Kindl H, Lazarow PB, eds. Peroxisomes and glyoxysomes. Ann NY Acad Sci 386:1, 1982.

Kornfeld S, Mellman I. The biogenesis of lysosomes. Annu Rev Cell Biol 5:483, 1989.

Pfeffer SR. Mannose 6-phosphate receptors and their role in targeting proteins to lysosomes. J Membr Biol 103:7, 1988.

Smooth Endoplasmic Reticulum

Cardell RR. Smooth endoplasmic reticulum in rat hepatocytes during glycogen deposition and depletion. Int Rev Cytol 48:221, 1977.

Kappas A, Alvares AP. How the liver metabolizes foreign substances. Sci Am 232(6):22, 1975.

Cytoskeleton, Centrioles, and Cilia

Allen RD. The microtubule as an intracellular engine. Sci Am 256(2):42, 1987.

Bloemendal H, Pieper FR. Intermediate filaments: Known structure, unknown function. Biochim Biophys Acta 1007:245, 1989

Bornens M, Paintrand M, Berges J, Marty MC, Karsenti E. Structural and chemical characterization of isolated centrioles. Cell Motil Cytoskeleton 8:238, 1987.

Brinkley BR. Microtubule organizing centers. Annu Rev Cell Biol 1:145, 1985.

Brokaw CJ, Verdugo P, eds. Mechanism and Control of Ciliary Movement. Progress in Clinical and Biological Research, vol 80. New York, Alan R Liss, 1981.

Dentler WL. Cilia and flagella. Int Rev Cytol Suppl 17:391, 1987.

Drenckhahn D, Dermietzel R. Organization of the actin filament cytoskeleton in the intestinal brush border: a quantitative and qualitative immunoelectron microscope study. J Cell Biol 107:1037, 1988.

Dustin P. Microtubules. Sci Am 243(2):67, 1980

Dustin P. Microtubules, ed 2. New York, Springer Verlag, 1984.

Gelfand VI, Bershadsky AD. Microtubule dynamics: mechanism, regulation, and function. Annu Rev Cell Biol 7:93, 1991.

Groschel-Stewart U, Drenckhahn D. Muscular and cytoplasmic contractile proteins. Coll Relat Res 2:381, 1982.

Hollenbeck PJ. Cell biology: cytoskeleton on the move. Nature 343:408, 1990.

Huxley HE. Sliding filaments and molecular motile systems. J Biol Chem 265:8347, 1990.

Louvard D. The function of the major cytoskeletal components of the brush border. Curr Opin Cell Biol 1:51, 1989.

Mooseker MS. Organization, chemistry, and assembly of the cytoskeletal apparatus of the intestinal brush border. Annu Rev Cell Biol 1:209, 1985.

Mooseker MS, Bonder EM, Conzelman KA et al. Brush border cytoskeleton and integration of cellular functions. J Cell Biol 99:104S, 1984.

Osborn M, Weber K. Intermediate filaments: Cell type-specific markers in differentiation and pathology. Cell 31:303, 1982.

Porter ME, Johnson KA. Dynein structure and function. Annu Rev Cell Biol 5:119, 1989.

Steinert PM, Jones JCR, Goldman RD. Intermediate filaments. J Cell Biol 99:22S, 1984.

Steinert PM, Roop DR. Molecular and cellular biology of intermediate filaments. Annu Rev Biochem 57:593, 1988.

Stewart M. Intermediate filaments: structure, assembly and molecular interactions. Curr Opin Cell Biol 2:91, 1990.

Vale RD. Intracellular transport using microtubule-based motors. Annu Rev Cell Biol 3:347, 1987.

Wheatley DN. The Centriole: A Central Enigma of Cell Biology. New York, Elsevier, 1982.

CHAPTER 4

Epithelial Tissue

OBJECTIVES

This chapter should enable you to do the following:

- Relate the structure of five different types of epithelial membranes to their main functions
- Recognize eight epithelial subtypes
- State two cell renewal mechanisms found in epithelial membranes
- Summarize the structure and function of four different types of cell junctions
- Understand the histological basis on which glands are classified
- Differentiate between serous, mucous, and mixed secretory units in sections
- State three major differences between exocrine and endocrine glands

The exterior of the body and almost all its internal surfaces are covered by continuous cellular sheets called **epithelial membranes** or **epithelia**, which, along with the various **glands** that develop from them, constitute **epithelial tissue.** This simple basic tissue develops from all three embryonic germ layers. The epithelial component of skin, for example, arises from ectoderm. The epithelial lining and glands of the digestive tract are derived from endoderm. The serous linings of the peritoneal, pleural, and pericardial cavities, and also the lining of the circulatory system, are products of mesoderm. Through convention, the membranous lining of the body cavities is called **mesothelium**, whereas that of the heart, blood vessels, and lymphatics is termed **endothelium**. Both linings are nevertheless sheets of contiguous cells and typical epithelial membranes despite their special names.

Epithelial tissue is characterized by intimate cell-to-cell contact of its morphologically polarized cells. Furthermore, epithelia exhibit a broad range of specialization. Epithelia adapted for secretion incorporate secretory cells arranged so that their secretory products reach the free surface. Supplemental secretions come from underlying glands that developed as invaginations and maintained connection with the free surface. In endocrine glands, this continuity is lost and the cells secrete into the bloodstream instead.

EPITHELIAL MEMBRANES

Epithelia are classified on the basis of 1) the number of constituent cell layers and 2) the shape and chief characteristics of their most superficial cells. Some epithelia are only one cell thick, but many are thicker than this. All types of epithelia are nevertheless composed solely of adherent contiguous cells. Furthermore, they contain no capillaries, that is, they are *avascular*. Hence they are dependent on proximity to loose connective tissue for their nutrient and oxygen supplies and byproduct removal (Fig. 4-1). A matrix structure called a **basement membrane** (the composition of which is described in Chapter 5) strongly attaches epithelial cells to the adjacent connective tissue. Some epithelia are unspecialized, whereas others are adapted for absorption, secretion, or protection, as summarized in the following.

Even thin, unspecialized epithelia can impede the passage of macromolecules without restricting the movement of water and ions. Certain epithelia are adapted for selective absorption. Epithelial membranes that are secretory as well as absorptive are able to protect themselves with a coating of mucus. Even more

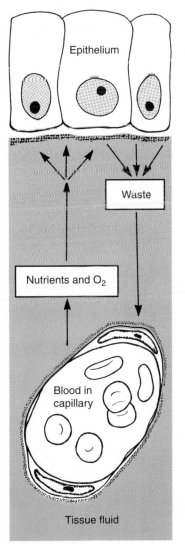

Figure 4-1
Oxygen and nutrients diffuse to cells of epithelial membranes from capillaries in associated connective tissue. Metabolic waste products diffuse in the reverse direction.

protection is afforded if the epithelium is many cells thick. Furthermore, epithelia that are freely exposed to air need to be protected from desiccation. The exterior of the body is accordingly covered with a multilayered epithelium that produces a nonviable layer of keratin instead of having living cells at its surface. Since keratin acts as a resistant barrier that is virtually waterproof, the covering epithelium is tough, highly protective, and renewable. The major airways minimize dehydration by coating their epithelial lining with abundant mucus, which also serves as an excellent dust-catcher for the removal of inhaled particles.

Epithelial membranes are classified according to the number of constituent cell layers and the cell shape at the free surface. A **simple epithelium** is a monolayer of cells (Fig. 4-2A–C). A **stratified epithelium** is at least two cells thick (see Fig. 4-2E–G). A **pseudostratified epithelium** is only one cell thick, but it gives the impression of being stratified because some of its cells are shorter than others and therefore do not reach its free surface (see Fig. 4-2D).

Simple Squamous Epithelium

Squamous means scale-like, so **simple squamous epithelium** consists of a single layer of flat, scale-shaped cells (see Fig. 4-2A) with attenuated cytoplasm that is difficult to see with an LM (Plate 4-1A). Examples of this type of epithelium are the thin-walled tubules in the renal medulla and the endothelial lining of blood vessels. The mesothelial lining of body cavities is a further example of simple squamous epithelium.

Simple Cuboidal Epithelium

Seen face-on, the constituent cells of **simple cuboidal epithelium** have roughly hexagonal perimeters. Through convention, however, this single layer of cells is described as **cuboidal** because in

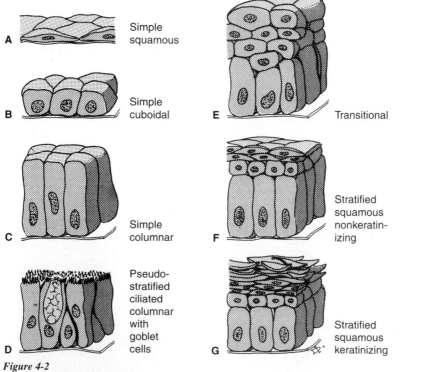

A　Simple squamous

B　Simple cuboidal

C　Simple columnar

D　Pseudostratified ciliated columnar with goblet cells

E　Transitional

F　Stratified squamous nonkeratinizing

G　Stratified squamous keratinizing

Figure 4-2
Principal epithelial membranes.

transverse section the cells appear square (see Fig. 4-2*B*). Simple cuboidal epithelium covers the ovaries, constitutes the lining of the smallest ducts, and lines the narrow renal collecting tubules (see Plate 4-1*B*).

Simple Columnar Epithelium

The single layer of cells in **simple columnar epithelium** are all tall columnar (see Fig. 4-2*C* and Plate 4-1*C*) and fit together in an essentially hexagonal pattern. An unmodified protective form of simple columnar epithelium lines the minor ducts of many exocrine glands. This type of epithelium is commonly adapted for secretion or absorption (or both purposes) as well as protective. Thus, every cell in **simple secretory columnar epithelium** is mucus secreting as well as protective. This type of secretory epithelium lines the stomach and uterine cervix. Its cells are all similar in appearance, and in H&E-stained sections they are pale staining with a frothy appearance due to abundant secretory vesicles (see Plate 4-1*C*). Their glycoprotein secretory product (mucus) may be seen to advantage in sections stained by the PAS procedure (described in Chapter 1).

Simple columnar epithelium also lines the intestine. Here, the membrane is protected from digestion and abrasion by a coating of slippery mucus. Accordingly, interspersed with the absorptive columnar cells are mucus-producing goblet cells, and this epithelium is both absorptive and secretory. A thin refractile layer on the free border of the absorptive columnar cells is known as their **striated (brush) border** (described under Filaments in Chapter 3). Beginners should avoid confusing the word *striated*, as in striated border, with *stratified*, meaning more than one cell thick.

In **simple columnar ciliated epithelium,** cilia cover the free surface of a single layer of columnar cells. Generally, some secretory cells are interspersed with the ciliated cells. This unusual epithelium lines only the uterine tubes and a few regions of the respiratory tract.

Goblet Cells

If individual mucus-producing cells are interspersed with columnar epithelial cells of other kinds in epithelial membranes, they assume the shape of a goblet because the part of the cell in which their secretory vesicles accumulate bulges and compresses the neighboring cells (see Plate 4-1 and Fig. 4-3). Such mucus-producing cells are accordingly known as **goblet cells.** The nucleus lies in the stem-like basal region and the free surface bears a few microvilli (see Fig. 4-3). Synthesis of mucus begins in the rER at the base of the cell. Glycosylation is completed by the cup-shaped Golgi complex lying above the nucleus. Goblet cells appear characteristically pale in H&E-stained sections (see Plate 4-1*D*), but their mucus content stands out vividly in sections stained for glycoprotein using the PAS procedure.

Pseudostratified Columnar Epithelium

In **pseudostratified epithelium**, many but not all of the cells extend up to the free surface of the membrane (see Fig. 4-2*D*). From EM studies, however, it is known that all component cells lie in contact with the basement membrane under the epithelium. Nuclei are visible at more than one level. This gives a false impression that the membrane is more than one cell thick and accounts for its name (see Plate 4-1*D*).

Pseudostratified ciliated columnar epithelium, with liberally scattered **goblet cells,** lines most of the major airways. The ciliated columnar cells and goblet cells that border on its free surface (Fig. 4-2*D* and Plate 4-1*D*) are renewed from a population of unspecialized basal cells. (The ciliated cells in this type of epithelium were described in Chapter 3 under Cilia and Flagella.) Mucus secreted by goblet cells augments that supplied by underlying glands and contributes to a continuous mucus blanket that is propelled toward the pharynx by ciliary action.

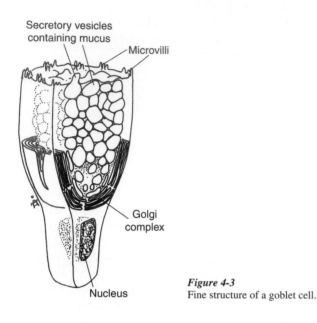

Secretory vesicles
containing mucus
Microvilli

Golgi
complex

Nucleus

Figure 4-3
Fine structure of a goblet cell.

Pseudostratified columnar epithelium is not all mucus secreting and ciliated, however. The pseudostratified columnar epithelium lining the ductus epididymis and certain other parts of the male reproductive tract, for example, possesses neither goblet cells nor cilia.

Stratified Columnar Epithelium

Any membrane that is two or more cells thick is better able to withstand abrasion, but it cannot absorb as efficiently as a simple epithelium. Moreover, it is not suitably adapted for secretion, so any necessary additional secretions have to be produced by accessory glands.

Usually consisting of only two layers of low columnar cells, stratified columnar epithelium lines the larger ducts of skin-derived glands, where it affords marginally more protection than simple columnar epithelium.

Transitional Epithelium

The microscopic appearance of transitional epithelium changes as the membrane stretches. In the unstretched configuration usually seen in sections, the rounded superficial cells bulge out (see Fig. 4-2*E* and Plate 4-1*E*). Under lateral tension, however, these cells are attenuated and squamous. Transitional epithelium lines almost all of the urinary tract and is designed to withstand distention due to the storing and passing of urine. An unexplained feature of the surface cells of the bladder is that many of them are multinucleated and some are polyploid.

Stratified Squamous Nonkeratinizing Epithelium

In the term **stratified squamous nonkeratinizing epithelium,** the word **squamous** describes the superficial cells only. The basal cells are columnar. The cells in the intermediate layers gradually change from a polyhedral (many-sided) shape to a squamous shape as they approach the free surface (see Fig. 4-2*F* and Plate 4-1*F*). This epithelium does not produce keratin, nor is it secretory. Yet it lines wet surfaces submitted to wear and tear, making it necessary for the membrane to be kept moist by fluid or secretions from elsewhere. Sites lined by this epithelium include the inside of the mouth, the esophagus, and the vagina.

Stratified Squamous Keratinizing Epithelium

The cells near the free surface of stratified squamous keratinizing epithelium transform into scales of soft keratin that remain strongly adherent to the underlying layers of living cells (see Fig. 4-2G and Plate 4-1G). Highly suitable for protecting surfaces continuously exposed to air, this epithelium constitutes the epidermal layer of skin. The tough superficial layer of keratin protects against abrasion and microbial infection and resists water loss and uptake. (For further details, see Chapter 12.)

CELL JUNCTIONS

A distinctive though not exclusive feature of the contiguous cells of epithelial tissue is their local adjoining and interconnecting specializations of the cell membrane. Known as **cell junctions,** the specialized sites are of three main types, each with specific functions. Yet only one kind of junction is exclusive to epithelial tissue. Known as a **tight** or **occluding** junction, its role relates to the partitioning function of epithelial linings of separate body compartments. At tight junctions, cell membranes of contiguous cells are in intimate contact with each other along systems of anastomosing ridges. Because they occlude the intercellular space, these ridges produce a selective seal that obstructs the paracellular route between cells. Cell junctions of the second main type are classified as **adhering** or **anchoring junctions** because they are sites of strong adhesion between the contiguous cells and also between the cells and their substrate. Moreover, they are sites where cytoskeletal components are anchored strongly to the cell membrane. Not restricted to epithelial cells, such junctions also maintain adhesion between heart muscle cells. In the third type of cell junction, the **gap junction,** a characteristic narrow gap exists between the cell membranes of the contiguous cells. However, this gap is traversed by minute tubular passageways that enable ions and other small molecules to pass directly from the interior of one cell to that of the other without involving the intercellular space. Gap junctions, again not unique to epithelial tissue, facilitate direct cell-to-cell communication. The elaborate terminology used for cell junctions includes three expressions that denote the shapes of junctions, irrespective of their type. A cell junction that circumscribes the entire cell perimeter and is shaped like a belt is termed a **zonula** (see Figs. 4-4A and 4-6, *left*). If instead of entirely surrounding the cell, the junction constitutes only a strip or patch on the cell surface, it is called a **fascia**. Finally, if the junction is small, circular, and spot-like, it is called a **macula**. Hence the *shape* is generally specified along with the *type* of junction.

Tight Junctions

In some locations, it is necessary to prevent certain molecules from passing unimpeded across an epithelium by way of the narrow paracellular (Gk. *para*, beside) spaces that exist between the lateral borders of the epithelial cells. These borders are fused together along a system of anastomosing ridges (Figs. 4-4 through 4-6). Commonly, the ridges extend around the entire perimeter of each cell close to its free or luminal border (see Figs. 4-4A and 4-6, *left*). The continuous belt-like junction they constitute is termed a **continuous tight** (or **occluding**) **junction**, known also as a **zonula occludens** (L. *zonula,* belt). The matching ridges on the adjacent cells are made up of aligned transmembrane integral proteins of each cell membrane that interlock across the intercellular space and constitute sealing strands that occlude the intercellular space (see Fig. 4-4B). The number of sealing strands in a tight junction varies with location but is not a reliably consistent indicator of sealing efficiency. The multistranded junctions between intestinal epithelial cells (see Fig. 4-5) keep macromolecules that are present in the intestinal lumen from gaining access to intercellular spaces by the paracellular route. They also prevent loss into the lumen as a result of passage in the opposite direction. Depending on their site, tight junctions vary in permeability to ions and water-soluble molecules of low molecular weight. Tight junctional permeability is also dependent on the

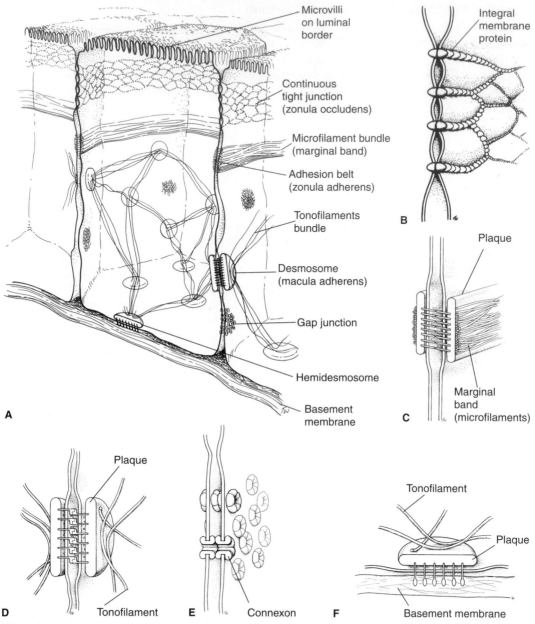

Figure 4-4
Cell junctions in epithelia. (*A*) General distribution of junctions over the epithelial cell surface. (*B*) Continuous tight (occluding) zonular junction. (*C*) Adhesion belt (zonula adherens). (*D*) Desmosome (macula adherens). (*E*) Gap junction. (*F*) Hemidesmosome.

molecule's charge and shape. Thus to some extent all tight junctions are selectively leaky, and the degree of tight junctional permeability can probably be regulated by the cell.

Because a tight junction consists of multiple anastomosing sealing strands, it accommodates and conforms to most variation in cell shape by stretching in some dimension. Even if a few of its sealing strands become breached, enough of them remain intact to maintain selectivity of the seal.

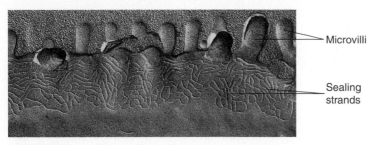

Figure 4-5
Electron micrograph showing part of a continuous tight (zonular occluding or zonula occludens) junction on a lateral border of an intestinal lining epithelial cell (freeze-fracture replica, ×50,000).

In morphologically polarized cells, a second important role of the zonular tight junction is to delineate and hence separate markedly different domains of the cell membrane. Integral membrane proteins of the apical domain are prevented from intermixing with those of the basolateral domain (and vice versa), which otherwise would occur due to random free diffusion of these proteins in the plane of the membrane. Hence the zonular tight junction can act as a selective diffusion barrier for integral cell membrane proteins as well as for extracellular macromolecules.

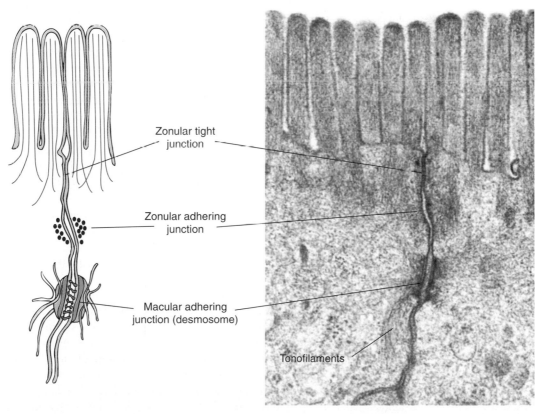

Figure 4-6
The three component cell junctions of a junctional complex, showing their positions relative to the luminal surface of intestinal epithelial lining cells. The level of the terminal web is also indicated in the micrograph.

The **fascia occludens** (L. *fascia*, band) is a similar but discontinuous tight junction that is strip- or band-shaped instead of extending around the whole cell as a belt. This interrupted type of junction is present between endothelial cells of blood vessels. Since it does not occupy the entire cell perimeter, the selective seal between lateral borders of such cells is incomplete.

Adhering (Anchoring) Junctions

Epithelial cells are held together by strong adhering (anchoring) junctions that are of two distinct types. The first type, present for example between intestinal epithelial cells, extends around the entire perimeter of each cell like a belt and is therefore called an **adhesion belt** or **zonula adherens.** It lies near the free (luminal) border of the cell, at a level just deep to the zonular occluding junction on the lateral borders (see Figs. 4-4*A* and 4-6, *left*). Below these two parallel belt-like junctions lies a horizontal discontinuous row of spot-like (macular) adhering junctions (the second type of adhering junction, see later). This distinctive combination of the three different cell junctions is known as a **junctional complex** (see Fig. 4-6).

The relatively wide intercellular gap at an adhesion belt (see Figs. 4-4*C* and 4-6) contains a slightly electron-dense material representing adhesion domains of cell membrane glycoproteins (chiefly **E-cadherin**). Strong cell-to-cell adhesion is mediated at this site by calcium-dependent, zipper-like, homophilic interaction between antiparallel terminal extracellular adhesion domains of the transmembrane linker glycoproteins.

A key feature of an adhesion belt is that it represents a major site of attachment of **microfilaments** to the cell membrane. It counteracts the tendency for cell separation to occur as a result of contractile activities involving microfilaments, many of which are arranged circumferentially around the cell as a **marginal band.** The marginal band of microfilaments extends along the adhesion belt (see Figs. 3-24 and 4-4*C*) and is attached to it by several intracellular attachment proteins. Because strong cell-to-cell adhesion occurs along the adhesion belt, contraction of the marginal bands causes a decrease in the total surface area of the epithelium. This mechanism of reducing the surface area is believed to play a key role in the morphogenesis of epithelial and neuroepithelial derivatives such as tubes and ducts, and also expedites epithelial repair.

The **focal contact (adhesion plaque)** is essentially similar to the adhesion belt, except that it is found on the basal surface of the cell and is a localized kind of junction instead of extending as a belt around the entire cell perimeter. It is a site where intracellular attachment proteins anchor a microfilament bundle to a contact site between the cell membrane and the substrate, and it plays a role in cellular adhesion to the extracellular matrix.

The second major type of adhering (anchoring) junction is termed a **desmosome**. It is also known as a **spot desmosome** or **macula adherens** because it is circular or spot-like in outline (L. *macula*, spot), not belt- or band-shaped. Besides being present in junctional complexes, desmosomes are present elsewhere on contiguous cell surfaces (see Figs. 4-4*A*, and 4-6, *left*). In epithelial desmosomes, bundles of keratin-containing intermediate filaments (**tonofilaments**) are anchored in electron-dense, disk-like **plaques** containing **plakoglobin** and **desmoplakins**. The plaques are attached to the cytoplasmic surfaces of the apposed areas of cell membrane (see Figs. 4-4*D* and 4-7). Also, a fine electron-dense line may be seen extending along the midline of the comparatively wide intercellular gap (see Fig. 4-7). The current interpretation of this line is that it, too, represents the site where adhesion ectodomains of transmembrane linker glycoproteins (e.g., **desmogleins** and **desmocollins**, which are cadherin proteins) extend across the intercellular gap, securing the apposed regions of cell membrane to each other (see Fig. 4-4*D*). Desmosomes are particularly abundant in epithelia that need to withstand abrasion. Deep in the epidermis, for example, the keratinocytes have a distinctive LM appearance that earned them the name **prickle cells.** Their characteristic prickly out-

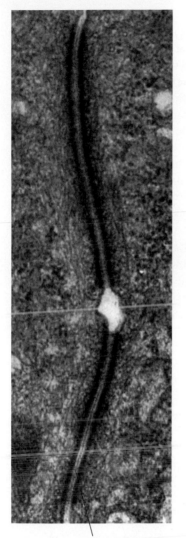

Figure 4-7
Electron micrograph of desmosomes (epithelial lining cells of chick trachea). A thin electron-dense line extends along the midline of the thin, electron-lucent intercellular region. Electron-dense plaque material lies on both sides of the junction, and tonofilaments are discernible lateral to the plaque.

Electron-dense line

line discloses sites where desmosomes prevented cell separation during fixation. The essential role of desmosomes is maintenance of strong cell-to-cell adhesion. The membrane-anchored intermediate filament bundles transmit and distribute tension and shear stresses through the cell, and the desmosomal transmembrane linker glycoproteins resist cell separation as a result of these stresses. Desmosome-like junctions are not exclusive to epithelial tissue. Junctions with similar morphology are present between cardiac muscle cells, but the intermediate filaments anchored in their plaques are made of desmin, not keratin.

A **hemidesmosome** (see Fig. 4-4*F*) is a second type of spot-like adhering junction that in EM sections looks like half a desmosome (Gk. *hemi*, half). Here, intermediate filament bundles are attached to the cell membrane along the basal surface of the cell, and the role of the junction is to anchor these keratin-containing filaments (tonofilaments) strongly to the underlying basement membrane through an integrin, which is a transmembrane linker protein (see Fig. 4-4*A* and *F*).

Gap Junctions

Gap junctions are spot-like (i.e., macular) in outline (see Fig. 4-4A). Their most obvious morphological feature is a narrow gap that lies between the apposed areas of cell membrane. However, it is an array of tubular aqueous **channels** traversing the gap rather than the gap itself that is significant. The cylindrical walls of these tiny interconnecting channels (**connexons**) are constructed from six aligned transmembrane protein subunits (**connexins**) that project from both membranes and interlock halfway across the narrow gap (see Fig. 4-4E). The central channels of the numerous connexons link the interiors of adjacent cells, allowing ions and small molecules to diffuse freely between the cells without entering the intercellular space. Gap junctions not only enable amino acids, sugars, and nucleotides to pass directly from one cell to another but also ensure widespread dispersal of ions or small molecules that can act as intracellular signals. Besides maintaining direct communication between epithelial cells, gap junctions enable waves of electrical excitation to spread unimpeded throughout the heart and visceral smooth muscle. They also transmit nerve impulses at certain synapses (but not the usual kind).

The permeability of gap junctions is regulated by the intracellular concentration of calcium ions. Normally, the cell keeps its cytosolic calcium level below the extracellular calcium level. At such low calcium concentrations, connexons remain in the open configuration. A massive influx of extracellular calcium, however, will close these channels. This is a self-sealing mechanism that preserves the integrity of living cells if an epithelium or epithelial organ is damaged. Connexons also close when the cytosolic pH decreases.

Terminal Web

Just deep to the striated border of an intestinal absorptive cell, at the level where the adhesion belt encircles the cell, lies a narrow superficial zone of cytoplasm that is reinforced by a dense meshwork of intermediate filaments. The abundant filaments that pervade this region give it a web-like texture, hence it is known as the **terminal web** (see Figs. 3-26 and 4-6, *right*). Many of the intermediate filaments in this zone are keratin filaments (tonofilaments) anchored to desmosomes of junctional complexes (see Fig. 4-6). Furthermore, the microvilli constituting the striated border contain crosslinked bundles of microfilaments, and these bundles extend down as far as the terminal web and are supported by it (see Fig. 3-26). In addition, other kinds of crosslinks are present on the superficial side of the terminal web. Lastly, it should be recalled that the marginal band of microfilaments is situated along the adhesion belt at the periphery of the terminal web, where they are attached to the cell membrane (see Figs. 3-26 and 4-4A and C).

EPITHELIAL CELL RENEWAL

Two separate arrangements exist for epithelial cell renewal. In the simplest case, which is found in simple squamous, simple cuboidal, and simple unmodified columnar epithelium, specialization is not extreme, and all the cells retain the capacity to divide. In those epithelia with nondividing, specialized cells that need to be replaced, however, stem cells are involved (see Chapter 2 under Cell Renewal). The stem cells of simple columnar epithelium that is adapted for absorption and secretion lie below the luminal surface of the epithelium, protected in small invaginations called **crypts**. In pseudostratified epithelium, the stem cells are distributed basally among taller, nondividing cells. In stratified epithelium, the stem cells are situated in the basal layer, and the differentiating progeny cells displaced toward the free surface are nondividing.

Atypical Histologic Appearances of Epithelia

Chronic exposure to certain detrimental environmental conditions can lead to replacement of particular areas of a given type of epithelium by patches of different epithelium. Termed **metaplasia** (Gk. *meta*, after; *plasia*, shaping), focal or extensive transformation of one epithelial cell type to another is widely viewed as an adaptive response to persisting abnormal environmental conditions. An acquired reversible change, such replacement is evidence that gene re-expression has been induced on a scale that is sufficient to redirect the epithelial cell's course of differentiation. Fairly common examples of epithelial metaplasia are 1) the replacement of stratified squamous nonkeratinizing epithelium by mucus-secreting, simple columnar epithelium in the distal part of the esophagus in patients with chronic gastric acid reflux (**Barrett's esophagus**), 2) the replacement of bronchial pseudostratified ciliated columnar cells and goblet cells by stratified squamous nonkeratinizing epithelium as an epithelial response to repeated heavy exposure to tobacco smoke, and 3) the widespread squamous replacement of several different epithelia as a consequence of prolonged deficiency of vitamin A.

Histologic evidence of genetic damage in epithelia resulting from long-term exposure to detrimental conditions also includes microscopically detectable inconsistencies of cell organization and position within the epithelial membrane. Described as **dysplasia** (Gk. *dys*, bad), these atypical histological features are a manifestation of induced disorderly cell division and incomplete maturation. Although reversible and benign, observed disruption of a normal epithelial growth pattern implies dysregulation of proliferation and maturation. Of clinical importance is the fact that associated with dysplasia is an increased risk of malignant change. A familiar example of dysplasia is the **actinic keratosis**, a lesion developing at epidermal sites damaged by overexposure to sunshine.

Excessive, dysregulated proliferation of epithelial cells can give rise to a noninvasive epithelial tumor. Localized benign tumors conventionally bear the suffix *-oma* (Gk. *-oma*, tumor), but tumor terminology is not consistent. Examples of benign epithelial growths are projecting **polyps**, finger-like or frond-like **papillomas**, and hollow, cyst-like **cystadenomas** (Gk. *adenos*, gland). In contrast, invasive cancers derived from epithelial cells are termed **carcinomas** ((Gk. *karkinos*, cancer or crab). Cancers arising from glandular epithelial cells are known as **adenocarcinomas** even if a gland-like organization is lacking. When carcinoma cells penetrate the underlying basement membrane of an epithelium, they can gain access to lymphatics or blood vessels and thereby spread to distal sites, forming secondary malignant tumors.

EPITHELIAL GLANDS

Epithelial glands constitute the other major subdivision of epithelial tissue. They are subdivided further into 1) **exocrine glands**, which develop as downgrowths of an epithelial membrane and secrete onto its surface through their **ducts** (Fig. 4-8), and 2) **endocrine glands**, many of which develop in a similar way but *lack ducts* because they lose their connection with the surface epithelium (Fig. 4-8, *bottom*). Instead of channeling their secretions through a duct onto an epithelial surface, endocrine glands release their secretory products close to the external surface of thin-walled blood vessels, with the result that these products enter the bloodstream.

Goblet cells are sometimes classified as mucus-secreting, unicellular exocrine *glands* instead of being considered an intrinsic component of epithelial *membranes*.

Exocrine Glands

Exocrine glands are constructed from secretory units, ducts, and, in all but the simplest glands, the connective tissue that supports these components. A **secretory unit** is a group of secretory epithelial cells that release their secretion into a lumen, whereas a **duct** is an epithelially lined tube that

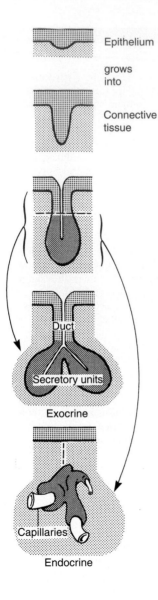

Epithelium

grows
into

Connective
tissue

Duct

Secretory units

Exocrine

Capillaries

Endocrine

Figure 4-8
Epithelial glands develop by downgrowth of an epithelial membrane.

conveys the secretion from a secretory unit to an epithelially lined surface. Ducts can also alter the concentration or composition of the secretion that passes along them.

Four different ways of classifying exocrine glands are in general use (Table 4-1). A major distinction that is made is whether the duct system is branched or not. Thus, a gland with a single *unbranched* duct is called a **simple gland** (Fig. 4-9*A* and *B*), whereas a gland with a *branched*, tree-like duct system that drains a number of secretory units is called a **compound gland** (Fig. 4-9*C*). A sweat gland of the skin is an example of a simple gland, and the pancreas is an example of a compound gland.

Exocrine glands are also categorized according to the overall shape of their secretory units. Thus, tubular secretory units characterize **tubular glands** (see Fig. 4-9*A*), whereas spherical or flask-like secretory units characterize **acinar** (L. *acinus*, grape) or **alveolar** (L. *alveolus*, small hollow sac) glands (see Fig. 4-9*B*). All such spherical or flask-shaped secretory units are often referred

TABLE 4-1

CRITERIA USED FOR CLASSIFYING EXOCRINE GLANDS

Duct Arrangement

Unbranched in simple glands

Branched in compound glands

Shape of Secretory Units

Tubular

Alveolar or acinar

Type of Secretion

Serous

Mucous

Mixed

Secretory Mechanism

Merocrine

Holocrine

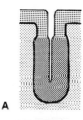

Tubular

A

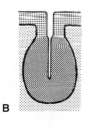

Acinar
or
Alveolar

B

Figure 4-9
Basic histologic types of exocrine glands. (*A* and *B*) Simple glands, in which the duct does not branch. (*C*) A compound gland, in which the duct system branches. Exocrine glands possess tubular secretory units (*A*), acinar or alveolar secretory units (*B*), or secretory units of both kinds (*C*).

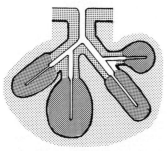

C Tubuloalveolar

to as *alveoli*, except that in the case of the pancreas they are conventionally called *acini*. Glands with a mixture of tubular and alveolar secretory units are termed **tubuloalveolar glands** (see Fig. 4-9*C*). The third system of classification is based on the secretory product of exocrine glands. **Serous glands** produce watery secretions that in many cases contain enzymes, and **mucous glands** secrete the viscid glycoprotein mucus. **Mixed glands** produce both kinds of secretion in a regulated manner. Serous units, mucous units, and mixed secretory units made up of serous and mucous cells both in the same unit are distinguishable from one another in H&E-stained sections.

The secretory cells in secretory units typically appear triangular in outline. In the case of **serous secretory units**, the wide basal part of the cell is intensely basophilic due to abundant rER, and it contains a large spherical nucleus (Plate 4-2). In serous secretory units of some enzyme-secreting glands, acidophilic zymogen granules may also be seen in the apical part of the cell. These granules represent secretory vesicles containing enzymes or their precursors.

In contrast to brightly stained serous secretory units, **mucous secretory units** appear pale (Plate 4-3). The nucleus of the constituent mucus-secreting cells is relatively small and generally lies flattened against the basal cell border. The whole cell looks pale because it is packed with mucus-containing secretory vesicles. The mucus content of these vesicles may be demonstrated by the PAS procedure, which stains glycoproteins.

Mixed glands, with serous and mucous units, produce **seromucous** (i.e., mixed) secretions. Some of them also have **mixed secretory units** with mucous and serous cells secreting into the same lumen. Mixed secretory units are composed primarily of mucous cells, but serous cells constitute a cap on one side of the unit. In transverse section, the cap of serous cells is suggestive of a crescent moon, hence it is known as a **serous demilune** (see Plate 4-3).

Enveloping each secretory unit of an exocrine gland, and in some cases the ducts too, are epithelial cells of a third type that lie at the border between the secretory cells and the basement membrane around the unit. The long branched cytoplasmic processes of these cells wrap around the secretory unit in the form of a loose basket, but they are not evident without use of special staining techniques. Their function is to contract and squeeze the secretion out of the secretory unit and along the duct system. Because such cells are contractile yet epithelial in origin, they are known as **myoepithelial cells**.

The fourth major distinction is based on the way secretory cells of different kinds of exocrine glands produce a secretion. The secretory cells of **merocrine glands** release their secretion by exocytosis, that is, through fusion of the limiting membrane of secretory vesicles with the cell membrane (see Plate 3-3). This is the way the secretory cells of most exocrine glands (eg, pancreatic acinar cells) release their secretory products. In the flask-shaped sebaceous glands associated with hair follicles, however, the secretory product is formed in a different manner. In this case, entire cells are sacrificed in producing the secretion, so this type of gland is described as **holocrine** (Gk. *holos*, all). As cells derived from the epithelial lining layer become displaced toward the interior of the gland, they accumulate lipid and take on a pale, vacuolated appearance (Fig. 4-10). Subsequently, they die and disintegrate. In this manner, entire secretory cells become sebum, the oily secretion that preserves the suppleness of hair and skin.

Apocrine glands were formerly regarded as an additional category of exocrine gland. From LM studies, it appeared that the secretory cells of glands such as apocrine sweat glands lost portions of their apical cytoplasm and cell membrane in the process of releasing their secretions. In most cases, however, EM studies failed to substantiate this notion. The only exception is milk fat secretion by the simple columnar alveolar secretory cells of the breast, where some depletion of the luminal region of the cell membrane and occasional loss of traces of superficial cytosol are thought to occur. Secretion of proteins by the same cells, however, is merocrine. The remainder of the glands formerly described as apocrine are now regarded as merocrine. Apocrine sweat glands have nevertheless retained their original name, primarily to distinguish them from eccrine sweat glands, which differ from them in certain respects (see Chapter 12).

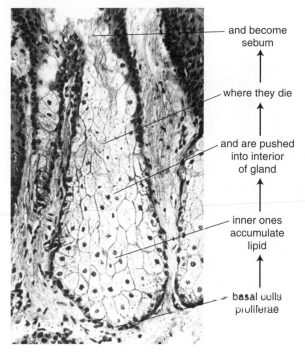

and become
sebum

↑

where they die

↑

and are pushed
into interior
of gland

↑

inner ones
accumulate
lipid

↑

basal cells
proliferae

Figure 4-10
Process of holocrine secretion (sebaceous gland, thin skin).

Compound Exocrine Glands: General Organization

The design of all **compound exocrine glands** is based on the same general plan. The epithelial component (i.e., secretory units and ducts) constitutes the **parenchyma**, whereas the supporting connective tissue (together with blood vessels and nerve fibers) constitutes the **stroma**. The gland is enclosed by a fibrous connective tissue **capsule**. Internally, it is supported by fibrous **septa**, which are sheet-like partitions extending inward from the capsule that subdivide the parenchyma. The substantial parenchymal segments of some large compound glands constitute anatomically separate **lobes**. Parenchymal segments existing only at the LM level are called **lobules**. Hence, the fibrous partitions that separate lobes are **interlobar septa**, and those separating lobules are **interlobular septa** (Fig. 4-11 and Plate 4-4). Septa support major branches of the duct system and, like the ducts, converge toward the site where the main duct leaves the gland. **Interlobular ducts** extending along interlobular septa are generally large enough to be evident in sections. Furthermore, they are embedded in the fibrous connective tissue characterizing septa. **Intralobular ducts** lie *within* lobules and have a smaller lumen. Also, they are surrounded by relatively little connective tissue because they lie outside septa (the two kinds of ducts may be compared in Plate 4-4). Lastly, the simple columnar epithelium of intralobular ducts is low or essentially cuboidal (Fig. 4-12), whereas that of interlobular ducts is typically somewhat taller. The remainder of the stroma, namely the delicate connective tissue between the secretory units, is supplied with numerous capillaries that provide nutrients and oxygen for the secretory cells.

Regulation of Exocrine Secretory Activity

Exocrine glands release secretions in response to efferent autonomic nerve impulses and certain hormones. This autonomic response is involuntary (see Chapter 9).

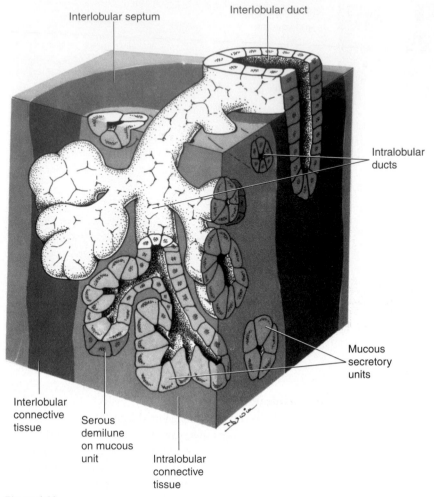

Figure 4-11
Basic histologic organization of a compound gland lobule.

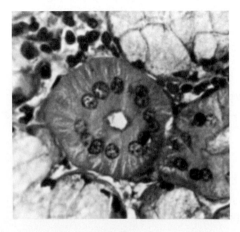

Figure 4-12
Intralobular duct of a mucus-secreting gland. Its lining epithelium is
essentially cuboidal or low columnar.

Endocrine Glands

Endocrine glands have a simpler organization. Instead of releasing their secretions into ducts, they discharge them into the bloodstream. Typically, their secretory cells are grouped around wide fenestrated capillaries (see Fig. 4-8, *bottom*). Extensions of the strong connective tissue **capsule** that encloses the gland ramify inward, conveying blood vessels. Known as **trabeculae** (L. for small beams), these fibrous extensions provide internal support and in certain cases give the gland a lobular appearance in sections.

Secretions of endocrine glands are known as **hormones** (Gk. *hormaein*, to set in motion, spur on) because they elicit functional changes in target cells that they reach by way of the bloodstream. However, cells of endocrine glands are not the only cells that synthesize hormones. The gastrointestinal tract, for example, produces a variety of peptide hormones, but this was discovered many years after the classic endocrine organs were recognized. The pancreas is considered both exocrine and endocrine because its serous secretory units release pancreatic digestive enzymes into its duct system and small groups of endocrine islet cells release pancreatic hormones into its capillaries.

Endocrine glands commonly *store* the secretions that they synthesize. In most cases, the hormone accumulates intracellularly within secretory vesicles and is discharged intermittently by exocytosis. The thyroid is somewhat different, however, because it stores its hormone extracellularly in the form of an inactive macromolecular precursor. The thyroid consists of spherical storage units with walls composed of secretory cells and a central lumen containing the precursor.

Many endocrine glands contain hormone-secreting cells of more than one type. Regulation of secretory activity, a complex matter, generally depends on *negative feedback*. The feedback arrangements counteract deviations in rates of specific cellular activities without overcompensation. An example of such an arrangement is protection from substantial drops in blood calcium. In response to the declining calcium concentration, certain endocrine cells release their stored hormone. The circulating hormone facilitates several compensatory mechanisms for bringing blood calcium back to the normal range. The rising blood calcium then begins to have a negative feedback effect, inhibiting further hormonal release. As a result, the blood calcium level reaches an equilibrium level.

SUMMARY

Epithelial tissue, derived from each of the embryonic germ layers, includes both epithelial membranes and glands. A simple epithelium has one layer of cells, whereas a stratified epithelium has more than one layer. Epithelia are made up of contiguous cells possessing cell junctions. Since they are avascular, they are nourished from adjoining connective tissue. Whereas the cells of simple squamous, simple cuboidal, and unmodified simple columnar epithelium are capable of mitosis, the principal cells of specialized epithelia are renewed from stem cells. For example, stem cells are present in the simple columnar linings of the stomach (mucus-secreting), the intestine (absorptive and mucus-secreting), and the uterine tubes (ciliated). Solitary mucus-secreting cells have the distinctive shape of goblet cells. Mucus-secreting, pseudostratified ciliated epithelium is one cell thick, but it includes a basal cell population that contains stem cells. Protective stratified columnar epithelium lines certain ducts. Urinary transitional epithelium withstands distention. Stratified epithelia nevertheless do not secrete. Stratified squamous epithelium is highly protective. Where freely exposed to air, it keratinizes, minimizing dehydration and providing a resistant barrier to the outside world. Stratified epithelia contain stem cells in their basal layer.

Cell junctions are highly specialized regions of the cell membrane. Tight junctions selectively regulate paracellular diffusion between epithelial cells. Adhering (anchoring) junctions hold cells in place. Gap junctions provide a basis for cell-to-cell communication. Adhering and gap junctions are also found in other tissues, eg, cardiac muscle. Zonular junctions extend around cell perimeters like belts. Fascia junctions are discontinuous strips or patches. Macular junctions are spot-shaped.

At zonular tight junctions, integral membrane proteins interlock across the narrow intercellular space as occluding strands These junctions constrain paracellular passage of macromolecules between lateral borders of contiguous epithelial cells and lateral mixing (through diffusion) of integral membrane proteins characterizing different domains of the cell membrane. Occluding fascia junctions, present between the endothelial cells at most sites, provide comparable seals that are only partial because the junctions are discontinuous.

The adhesion belt or zonula adherens (an adhering junction) lies just deep to the zonular tight junction in junctional complexes. At adhesion belts, transmembrane linker glycoproteins strongly attach the contiguous cell membranes and marginal microfilament bands are anchored to the membranes. Crosslinked bundles of microfilaments supporting microvilli of the striated border on absorptive cells of the intestinal epithelium are anchored to a dense terminal web of intermediate filaments. The spot-like desmosome (the other main type of adhering junction) is found in junctional complexes and scattered along contiguous cell surfaces. Transmembrane linker glycoproteins also strongly attach cell membranes at desmosomes. Tonofilaments anchored in desmosome plaques distribute tensile stresses. Hemidesmosomes and focal contacts play a role in anchoring epithelial cells to their underlying basement membrane. Gap junctions, which are spot-like, are sites where transmembrane proteins constitute tiny tubular channels that permit ions and small molecules to pass directly from cell to cell.

Glands with ducts opening onto epithelial surfaces are termed exocrine glands, and those with branched duct systems are classified as compound. Glandular secretory units are tubular, alveolar, or a combination. Secretions are serous, mucous, or a combination. Serous cells are basophilic and may have acidophilic secretory granules. Mucus-secreting cells are characteristically pale-staining in H&E-stained sections. Serous demilunes are present in mixed secretory units. Exocrine secretory units and certain ducts are enveloped by contractile myoepithelial cells. Most glands release secretions by exocytosis (merocrine secretion), but entire disintegrating cells become the secretion of sebaceous glands (holocrine secretion). The parenchyma of compound exocrine glands is enclosed by a capsule and subdivided into lobes and lobules by septa. The connective tissue component of glands constitutes their stroma. Ducts may be intralobular or interlobular in position. Exocrine secretory activity is regulated by autonomic nerve impulses and certain hormones.

Endocrine glands possess no ducts and secrete hormones into the bloodstream. They are highly vascular, and although provided with a connective tissue capsule and trabeculae, most are relatively simple in organization. Most hormones or their precursors are stored intracellularly, but the precursor of thyroid hormone is stored extracellularly. Hormone release is generally subject to negative feedback regulation.

Bibliography

Epithelial Tissue (General)

Gumbiner B. Generation and maintenance of epithelial cell polarity. Curr Opin Cell Biol 2:881, 1990.
Jost SP, Gosling JA, Dixon JS. The morphology of normal human bladder urothelium. J Anat 167:103, 1989.
Slater NJ, Raftery AT, Cope GH. The ultrastructure of human abdominal mesothelium. J Anat 167:47, 1989.

Cell Junctions

Boyer B, Thiery JP. Epithelial cell adhesion mechanisms. J Membr Biol 112:97, 1989.
Burridge K, Fath K. Focal contacts: transmembrane links between the extracellular matrix and the cytoskeleton. BioEssays 10:104, 1989.
Cereijido M, ed. Tight junctions. Boca Raton, FL, CRC Press, 1992.

Cereijido M, Ponce A, Gonzalez-Mariscal L. Tight junctions and apical/basolateral polarity. J Membr Biol 110:1, 1989.

Geiger B, Avnur Z, Volberg T, Volk T. Molecular domains of adherens junctions. In: Edelman GM, Thiery J-P, eds. The Cell in Contact: Adhesions and Junctions as Morphogenetic Determinants. New York, John Wiley & Sons, 1985, p 461.

Grove BD, Vogl AW. Sertoli cell ectoplasmic specializations: a type of actin-associated adhesion junction. J Cell Sci 93:309, 1989.

Hertzberg EL, Lawrence TS, Gilula NB. Gap junctional communication. Annu Rev Physiol 43:479, 1981.

Hull BE, Staehelin LA. Functional significance of the variations in the geometrical organization of tight junction networks. J Cell Biol 68:688, 1976.

Pappas GD. Junctions between cells. Hosp Pract 8(8):39, 1973.

Schneeberger EE, Lynch RD. Tight junctions: their structure, composition, and function. Circ Res 55:723, 1984.

Schneeberger EE, Lynch RD. Structure, function, and regulation of cellular tight junctions. Am J Physiol 262:L647, 1992.

Schwarz MA, Owaribe K, Kartenbeck J, Franke WW. Desmosomes and hemidesmosomes: constitutive molecular components. Annu Rev Cell Biol 6:461, 1990.

Staehelin LA. Structure and function of intercellular junctions. Int Rev Cytol 39:191, 1974.

Staehelin LA, Hull BE. Junctions between living cells. Sci Am 238(5):140, 1978.

Stauffer KA, Unwin N. Structure of gap junction channels. Semin Cell Biol 3:17, 1992.

Stevenson BR, Anderson JM, Bullivant S. The epithelial tight junction: structure, function and preliminary biochemical characterization. Mol Cell Biochem 83:129, 1988.

Weinstein RS, McNutt NS. Cell junctions. N Engl J Med 286:521, 1972.

Brush Border and Terminal Web

Drenckhahn D, Dermietzel R. Organization of the actin filament cytoskeleton in the intestinal brush border: a quantitative and qualitative immunoelectron microscope study. J Cell Biol 107:1037, 1988.

Heintzelman MB, Mooseker MS. Assembly of the intestinal brush border cytoskeleton. Curr Top Dev Biol 26:93, 1992.

Hirokawa N, Tilney LG, Fujiwara K, Heuser JE. Organization of actin, myosin, and intermediate filaments in the brush border of intestinal epithelial cells. J Cell Biol 94:425, 1982.

Louvard D. The function of the major cytoskeletal components of the brush border. Curr Opin Cell Biol 1:51, 1989.

Mooseker MS. Organization, chemistry, and assembly of the cytoskeletal apparatus of the intestinal brush border. Annu Rev Cell Biol 1:209, 1985.

CHAPTER 5

Loose Connective Tissue and Adipose Tissue

OBJECTIVES

After you have read this chapter, you should be able to do the following:

- Summarize the main structural similarities and differences between collagen and elastin
- Explain the histologic changes associated with edema
- State what is meant by a basement membrane and discuss its distinctive composition
- Differentiate between six different cell types present in loose connective tissue
- Outline how the structure of plasma cells reflects their chief function
- Discuss the functional significance of four mast cell-derived inflammatory mediators

Loose connective tissue, known also as **areolar tissue,** belongs to a large family of diverse connective tissues that develop from the embryonic connective tissue, **mesenchyme** (Table 5-1). The fundamental roles of loose connective tissue are to support, interconnect, and nourish the other tissues, for which purposes it produces substantial quantities of extracellular matrix. The extracellular matrix is organized in several different ways. In loose connective tissue, the **interstitial matrix** is an elaborately structured complex of intercellular macromolecular matrix constituents of two main kinds—**fibrous proteins** that constitute strong intercellular fibers, and the so-called amorphous **ground substance,** a soft and shapeless yet molecularly organized gel (Gk. *a*, without; *morphē*, form). Fibers made of **collagen** are extremely resistant to stretch, whereas fibers made of **elastin** yield to stretch but then recoil like stretched elastic bands. Another type of collagen is the main constituent of **basement membranes,** which are comparatively organized sheets made of various matrix macromolecules that lie along the interface between loose connective tissue and adjoining tissues (e.g., epithelial tissue). Basement membranes have a distinctive composition and their macromolecular constituents are not all derived from connective tissue cells. In dense connective tissue (see Chapter 8), collagen fibers predominate and the ground substance, cells, and blood vessels represent relatively minor components.

The amorphous ground substance of the interstitial matrix occupies the intercellular space between cells and capillaries. It serves as more than a filler because tissue fluid held by extensive aque-

TABLE 5-1

MAJOR SUBTYPES OF CONNECTIVE TISSUE	
Ordinary	**Special**
Loose connective tissue (areolar tissue)	Adipose tissue (fat)
	Blood cells
Dense ordinary connective tissue (fibrous tissue):	Blood cell-forming tissues: Myeloid tissue Lymphoid tissue
Regular Irregular	Cartilage
	Bone

ous channels in its elaborate gel structure facilitates (1) diffusion of nutrients and oxygen from capillaries and (2) diffusion of waste products in the reverse direction (see Fig. 4-1). Thus, loose connective tissue has a substantial content of intercellular matrix constituents and tissue fluid, and its cells are separated fairly widely by these constituents.

CONNECTIVE TISSUE FIBERS

Loose connective tissue (e.g., from superficial fascia) may be stretched out as a flat spread for observation with the LM (Plate 5-1). Figure 5-1 is a composite drawing of the fibers and cells in such preparations. **Collagen fibers** appear unbranched, wide, and wavy and stain pink with eosin. Longitudinal bundles of fibrils are sometimes discernible in collagen fibers (see Plate 5-1). **Elastic fibers** are comparatively straight and narrow, and they branch. They have affinity for certain stains (e.g., they stain reddish-brown with orcein) but in H&E-stained sections they are not readily distinguishable. In contrast, the elastic laminae represented in certain kinds of blood vessels are moderately acidophilic.

Other special stains reveal delicate, finely branching fibers called **reticular fibers** (Fig. 5-2) that constitute supporting networks (L. *rete*, net). These additional fibers, however, are not prominent enough to be discernible in connective tissue spreads. They represent narrow bundles of *collagen fibrils*, coated with associated glycoproteins and proteoglycans that account for their special staining properties. Their branching is due to the fact that collagen bundles can split longitudinally. Reticular fibers provide intimate support for capillaries, nerves, and muscle cells, and are intimately associated with basement membranes (see later). Also, they constitute the main supporting elements of blood-forming tissues and the liver. Although indistinguishable in H&E-stained sections, their presence is demonstrable by silver impregnation, which stains them black (see Fig. 5-2). Furthermore, reticular fibers are PAS-positive, mainly because of their associated glycoproteins. The collagen in reticular fibers is **type III collagen** (Table 5-2). The chief source of this collagen is fibroblasts, with supplemental production by reticular cells in the case of blood-forming tissues.

Before considering assembly and the fine structure of collagen fibers and elastic fibers, we briefly describe the principal forms of collagen.

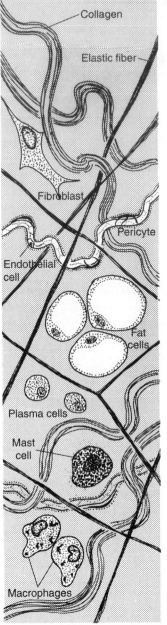

Figure 5-1
Fibers and cells of loose connective tissue.

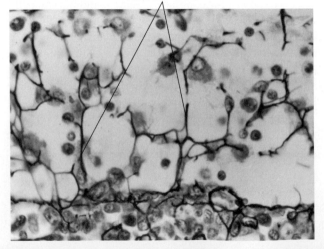

Reticular fibers

Figure 5-2
Reticular fibers of a lymph node (PA-silver stain).

TABLE 5-2

SUMMARY OF TYPE I—V COLLAGEN DISTRIBUTION WITH CELLULAR SOURCES		
Collagen Type	**Major Distribution**	**Major Sources**
I	Loose and dense ordinary connective tissue (collagen fibers)	Fibroblasts, reticular cells, and smooth muscle cells
	Fibrocartilage	
	Bone	Osteoblasts
	Dentin	Odontoblasts
II	Hyaline and elastic cartilage	Chondrocytes
	Vitreous body of eye	Retinal cells
III	Papillary layer of dermis and loose connective tissue (reticular fibers)	Fibroblasts and reticular cells
	Blood vessels	Smooth muscle cells and endothelial cells
IV	Basement membranes	Epithelial and endothelial cells, muscle cells, Schwann cells
	Lens capsule of eye	Lens fibers
V	Fetal membranes; placenta	Fibroblasts
	Basement membranes	
	Bone	
	Smooth muscle	Smooth muscle cells

COLLAGEN

Collagen is the most abundant connective tissue protein. Each molecule consists of three polypeptide subunits (**α chains**) wound together in the form of a triple helix. Covalent crosslinking within and between the constituent α chains confers great tensile strength on the molecule. A number of different collagen types representing distinctive combinations of α chains have been isolated. Table 5-2 summarizes the respective tissue distributions and main sources of five prevalent forms of collagen.

Type I collagen, the most widely represented type, accounts for approximately 90% of total body collagen. Types I, II, and III collagen assemble into **collagen fibrils,** and type I collagen fibrils aggregate into **collagen fibers.** Type II collagen fibrils, however, remain widely dispersed. Type IV collagen is the only form of collagen known to assemble into a layer of meshwork instead of fibrils.

Procollagen Secretion

Collagen is extracellularly derived and assembled in the intercellular space from a secreted larger precursor called **procollagen.** The only difference between procollagen (which is made up of three pro-α chains) and collagen is that the procollagen polypeptide subunits are slightly longer. Both ends of the constituent pro-α chains are elongated by propeptide **extension sequences.** The pro-α chains are synthesized by the rER, which is accordingly extensive in procollagen-secreting cells. Transfer vesicles deliver the constituent precursor polypeptide subunits, assembled as procollagen triple helices, to the Golgi apparatus. Secretory vesicles then carry this precursor to surfaces where it is released by exocytosis. When types I, II, or III procollagen enter the intercellular space, extracellular peptidases cleave off both propeptide extension sequences. The collagen molecules thus produced assemble into collagen fibrils. In the case of type IV collagen, however, the extension sequences stay attached, and their extracellular interaction results in assembly of a sheet-like meshwork instead of fibrils.

Collagen Assembly: Axial Periodicity of Collagen Fibrils

Extracellular assembly of collagen fibrils produces the unique staggered molecular arrangement represented in Figure 5-3*A*, in which collagen molecules are depicted as *arrows*. Each collagen molecule incorporated into the parallel array extends beyond its neighbor by one fourth of its length. Furthermore, a short gap region persists at each intermolecular position along the fibril (see Fig. 5-3*A*). Transverse alignment of these gap regions is evident following negative staining because the intermolecular spaces become permeated by EM stain (compare Fig. 5-3*A* with Fig. 5-3*B*, which shows a fibril with the gap regions filled after negative staining). After negative staining, the gap-containing regions appear *more* electron-dense. Also, a repeating unit **(period)** consisting of one dark segment plus a light one becomes evident. Conventional EM staining produces a comparable underlying pattern (periodicity) of dark and light segments, but their positions are reversed because the gap-containing regions contain less collagen to stain and therefore appear *less* electron-dense (compare Fig. 5-3*B* with Fig. 5-3*C*, which shows a fibril stained in the conventional manner). Superimposed on the underlying periodicity, however, is a bar code-resembling pattern of narrow lines reflecting the transverse alignment of charged amino acids (see Figs. 5-3*C* and 5-4).

In summary, collagen fibrils are readily recognized at the EM level by their interstitial distribution and distinctive **axial periodicity,** that is, a repeating basic pattern of dark and light segments every 64 nm along their length. This characteristic periodicity arises from their staggered pattern of molecular assembly.

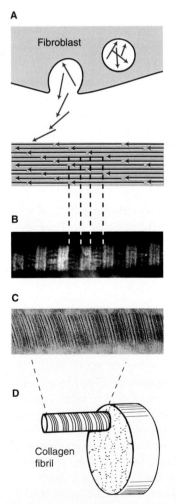

Figure 5-3
Collagen fibrils of loose connective tissue, showing the molecular basis of their axial periodicity. Collagen molecules (*arrows*) are derived from procollagen molecules secreted by fibroblasts (*A*). They assemble into collagen fibrils in the interstitial space (*D*). Electron micrographs show a collagen fibril after negative staining (*B*) and after conventional staining (*C*).

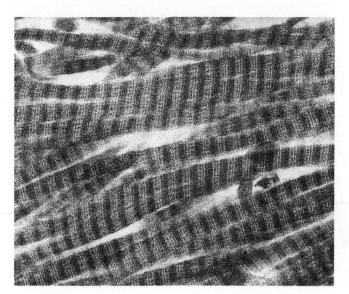

Figure 5-4
Electron micrograph showing the
characteristic axial periodicity of collagen
fibrils (×37,000).

ELASTIN

Elastin is an interstitial *amorphous* protein that unless molded into fibers forms fenestrated sheets called **elastic laminae,** an important role of which is to supplement elastic recoil of elastic fibers in the walls of certain blood vessels.

Elastic Fiber Assembly

Elastin assembly from its soluble precursor, **tropoelastin,** takes place near the extracellular surface of the cell membrane. Unlike collagen fibers, **elastic fibers** are not homogeneous structures made of multiple, identical extracellular fibrils, nor does their assembly process produce axial periodicity. Elastic fiber assembly requires ancillary formation of fibrils of another type, termed **microfibrils** (Fig. 5-5). For secreted tropoelastin to become incorporated into fibers, a roughly cylindrical scaffolding of microfibril bundles is required. As a result, at least two different sorts of proteins, namely elastin and microfibrillar glycoproteins called **fibrillins,** are present in elastic fibers. The generally pale-staining interior of an elastic fiber represents the amorphous protein elastin. Surrounding and embedded in the elastin are the thin microfibrils that originally served as its scaffolding. They stain more darkly than the elastin and therefore outline the perimeter of the fiber. In addition to their role in shaping elastin as it forms, these microfibrils contain proteins that are believed to bind to tropoelastin and crosslink it into a network-like polymer.

The functional importance of fibrillin is evident in patients with **Marfan syndrome,** an autosomal recessive disease that is partly characterized by predispositions to aortic aneurysms, dissection (splitting) of the aortic wall, and bilateral dislocation of the ocular lenses. In Marfan syndrome, the elastic recoil of elastin and the zonular attachments of the lenses are compromised by a gene mutation that results in defective fibrillin 1.

The original broad classification of interstitial matrix into fibrous and amorphous constituents is complicated by the findings that collagen is not exclusively fibrous and, as just explained, elastin is itself an essentially amorphous protein. Also, calling the ground substance amorphous when at the molecular level it is elaborately structured rather loses sight of its key functions. In descriptions of connective tissue, the term **ground substance** is still widely used in a generic sense to denote the macromolecular constituents of interstitial matrix other than collagen and elastin. The finding that certain matrix constituents are functionally indistinguishable from cell surface molecules makes the task of defining the borderline between the cell coat and the adjacent extracellular matrix a somewhat contentious issue.

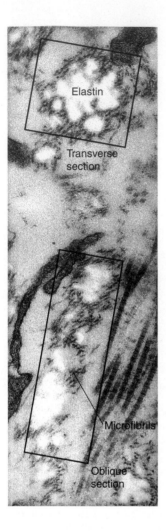

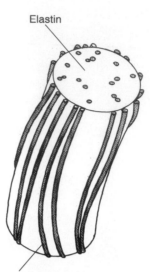

Figure 5-5
Electron micrograph showing elastic fibers in
transverse and oblique section. Elastic fibers
consist of pale-staining elastin with a
microfibril scaffolding. Collagen fibrils are
also included (lower right, outside boxed-in
area).

GROUND SUBSTANCE (AMORPHOUS COMPONENT OF INTERSTITIAL MATRIX)

The nonfibrous supporting component (i.e., **ground substance**) of connective tissue has the typical properties of an extensively hydrated semisolid gel. Its macromolecular organic content is so minimal that it scarcely stains at all, hence its existence is rarely noticed in H&E-stained sections. It contains **glycosaminoglycans,** most of which are sulfated and complexed with proteins as **proteoglycans,** along with some **glycoproteins** (e.g., fibronectin). Hyaluronic acid, the chief glycosaminoglycan, constitutes a particularly voluminous hydrated gel that holds vast amounts of tissue fluid in the numerous interstices of a mesh-like arrangement. The source and ultimate destination of this all-important fluid are as follows.

Interstitial Fluid and Lymphatic Drainage

At most sites in the body, the lateral margins of squamous endothelial lining cells of blood capillaries are interconnected by tight junctions of the **fascia occludens** type (described in Chapter 4 under Cell Junctions). Because these junctions extend only partway around cell perimeters, slit-like intercellular spaces positioned between the junctions remain unsealed. Under normal conditions, the narrow unsealed spaces permit only small molecules and ions to slip between the lateral margins of endothelial cells, passing either from the vessel's lumen into the interstitial space or in the opposite direction. Normally, proteins and other plasma macromolecules are restricted from taking this paracellular route.

In considering why tissue fluid is produced, it will be appreciated that the narrow luminal diameter of blood capillaries offers considerable resistance to viscous blood flow, with resulting fall of the blood pressure within them. The already reduced hydrostatic pressure of blood reaching capillaries from arterioles (the smallest arterial branches) therefore continues to drop along the course of open capillaries. This pressure drives a certain amount of the fluid component of blood, depleted of macromolecules, through the narrow slits between endothelial cells. The blood dialysate that forms in this manner is termed **tissue fluid.**

The macromolecules retained by blood plasma (i.e., the fluid component of blood) exert an osmotic pressure that opposes hydrostatic pressure, bringing tissue fluid back into the lumen. When capillaries are open (Fig. 5-6A), the luminal hydrostatic pressure exceeds the osmotic pressure, hence open capillaries *produce* tissue fluid (plasma minus most of its protein). When increased tonus of the precapillary sphincters shuts down capillary blood flow, however, the luminal hydrostatic pressure remains below the osmotic pressure, and as a result, closed capillaries *resorb* tissue fluid (Fig. 5-6B). Surplus interstitial fluid collects in **lymphatic capillaries,** a separate system of thin-walled vessels resembling blood capillaries. **Lymph** (L. *lympha*, clear water), the clear watery fluid that collects in them, is essentially surplus tissue fluid with a significant accumulated content of interstitial protein. From lymphatic capillaries, lymph passes through lymphatic vessels into lymphatic ducts that empty into large veins at the root of the neck, and here lymph joins the blood.

Continuous production and resorption of tissue fluid promotes interstitial fluid circulation through minute internal aqueous channels in the gel structure of the ground substance. If, at any site, tissue fluid is being produced in larger volumes than the combined volume being resorbed by closed blood capillaries and collected by open lymphatic capillaries, the imbalance leads to swelling of the ground substance, i.e., **edema.** A familiar example of edema is connective tissue swelling at a site of acute inflammation (described under Neutrophils in Chapter 6).

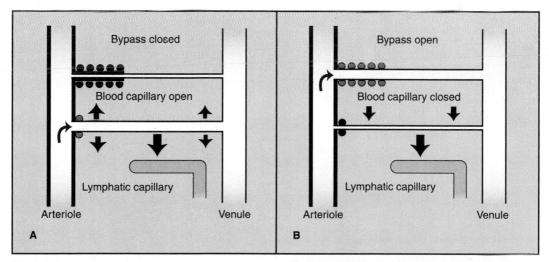

Figure 5-6
Tissue fluid production, resorption, and drainage in loose connective tissue. Under conditions of capillary blood flow, while precapillary sphincters are relaxed and the bypass channels remain constricted, most of the interstitial fluid being produced (*colored arrows*) passes into lymphatic capillaries (*A*). While precapillary sphincters are contracted and the bypass channels are open, part of the interstitial fluid enters closed capillaries and the remainder passes into lymphatic capillaries (*B*).

BASEMENT MEMBRANE

Extending along the extensive interface between connective tissue and the other basic tissues (epithelial, nervous, and muscle tissue) is a thin sheet of specialized extracellular matrix known as a **basement membrane.** At the LM level, basement membranes are seen as homogeneous extracellular layers that are PAS-positive because of their substantial glycoprotein content (Plate 5-2). In electron micrographs taken at high enough magnification, an inconspicuous fuzzy line of low or moderate electron density may be seen approximately 60 nm from the cell membrane, extending parallel to the cell surface (Fig. 5-7). This structure is sometimes referred to as a **basal lamina.** The constituent layers and molecular composition of basement membranes are summarized in Table 5-3.

The electron-dense layer of a basement membrane is called its **lamina densa.** An indistinct electron-lucent layer lies on each side of the lamina densa. The almost unstained layer on the cellular side is termed the **lamina lucida.** The lightly stained indistinct layer on the interstitial side is known as the **lamina fibroreticularis** because in some instances it is associated with reticular fibers of the underlying connective tissue. At certain sites, additional **anchoring filaments (fibrils)** containing type VII collagen are attached to this interstitial border of the basement membrane.

As shown in Figure 5-8, the lamina densa contains a delicate meshwork of **type IV collagen** associated with a glycoprotein called **laminin,** both produced by the cell or cells on the lamina lucida side of the basement membrane. Type IV collagen is a unique nonfibrillar collagen that is distinct from the types I, II, and III fibrillar collagen characteristic of loose connective tissue. (The five major types of collagen, characterized by slightly different combinations of α chains, are distributed as indicated in Table 5-2.) Other collagens, too, are associated with the interstitial side of the basement

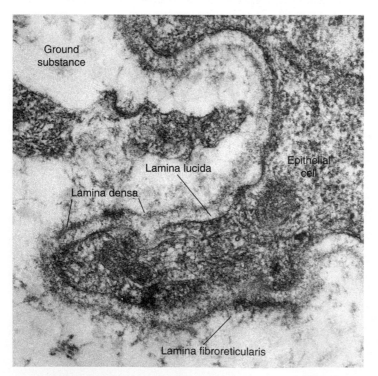

Figure 5-7
Electron micrograph showing the basement membrane associated with the basal surface of an epithelial cell (tracheal epithelial lining). The three component layers of the basement membrane are discernible.

TABLE 5-3

BASEMENT MEMBRANES: COMPONENT LAYERS AND CONSTITUENT MACROMOLECULES

Component Layers

Lamina lucida

Lamina densa

Lamina fibroreticularis

Constituent Macromolecules

Exclusive to Basement Membranes

Type IV collagen

Laminin

Heparan sulfate proteoglycans

Entactin (nidogen)

Not exclusive to Basement Membranes

Fibronectin

Type III collagen

Type VII collagen

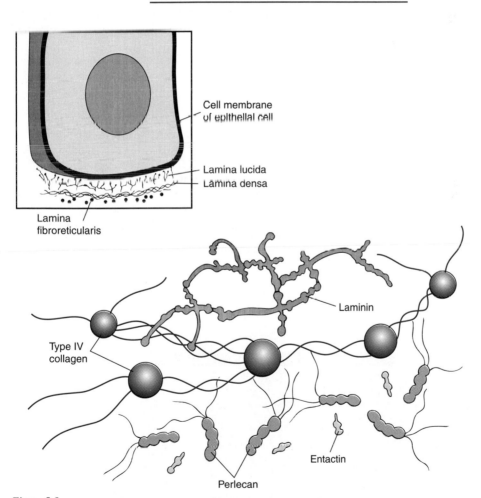

Figure 5-8
Essential macromolecular organization in a basement membrane.

membrane. Sparse, wispy strands of type IV collagen and associated laminin also extend between the lamina densa and the cell membrane (see Fig. 5-8).

Besides possessing cell-binding domains, the adhesive glycoprotein **laminin** has strong affinities for type IV collagen and heparan sulfate in proteoglycans. **Fibronectin,** a cell-binding glycoprotein that is present in the interstitial matrix as well as basement membranes, has affinities for a wide variety of extracellular macromolecules. Another basement membrane glycoprotein named **entactin (nidogen)** has affinity domains for the cell membrane, type IV collagen, and laminin. Also present are **heparan sulfate proteoglycans,** e.g., **perlecan,** with multiple affinity domains. Complex macromolecular associations such as these impart to basement membranes the distinctive properties that we next describe.

Basement membranes are situated under epithelial membranes (including endothelium), around epithelial glands, around fat cells, and along boundaries between loose connective tissue and (1) muscle fibers or (2) Schwann cells (the cells that invest peripheral nerve fibers). They attach such cells strongly to the adjacent connective tissue, providing them with flexible support. Although basement membranes are freely permeable to small molecules, they impede the passage of macromolecules. This differential retention property gives them functional importance in the kidneys, where their combined capacity for selective filtration minimizes loss of plasma proteins into the urine. Basement membranes are the first-formed organized extracellular matrix components of the embryo. They play key roles in promoting and maintaining the fully differentiated state, morphological polarization of cells, and cell migrations during morphogenesis, tissue repair, and regeneration. They also bind certain growth factors and enzymes (e.g., acetylcholinesterase at motor end plates).

LOOSE CONNECTIVE TISSUE CELLS

Connective tissue cells arise from **mesenchyme,** an embryonic connective tissue consisting of relatively widely spaced, pale-staining cells with slender cytoplasmic processes, embedded in a gelatinous ground substance with extremely fine intercellular fibers. Mesenchymal cells are directly or indirectly ancestral to the loose connective tissue cells listed in Table 5-4.

Key functions of the various cells in loose connective tissue include the production of interstitial matrix constituents and defense roles associated with inflammatory and immune responses. Figure 5-1 depicts the cell types found in loose connective tissue. It is a composite drawing based on various kinds of preparations, however, and not all these cell types would be seen in a single field. Furthermore, some of them develop in the tissue itself, and others are immigrant cells arising elsewhere in the body that reach loose connective tissue by way of the bloodstream.

TABLE 5-4

CELLS IN LOOSE CONNECTIVE TISSUE

Fibroblasts

Endothelial cells

Pericytes

Fat cells (adipocytes)

Plasma cells

Mast cells

Macrophages

FIBROBLASTS

The macromolecular constituents that constitute the interstitial matrix of ordinary connective tissues are produced by cells called **fibroblasts** (L. *fibra*, fiber; Gk. *blastos*, germ). Actively secreting fibroblasts are spindle-shaped or have wide cytoplasmic processes (see Fig. 5-1). Their ample cytoplasm is basophilic and their nucleoli are prominent, indications that they are actively engaged in protein synthesis. Less active, nondividing fibroblasts predominate in adult life. Often referred to as **fibrocytes,** their nuclear chromatin is much more condensed and their scant cytoplasm is pale staining or only slightly basophilic (see Plate 5-1). Although fibrocytes can still secrete matrix constituents in diminished amounts, major connective tissue repair involves the formation of new fibroblasts, many of which are derived from pericytes (see later).

All regions of the fibroblast surface can release matrix constituents, which include procollagen, tropoelastin, proteoglycans, and fibrillin (the microfibrillar glycoprotein in elastic fibers). Fibroblasts also produce collagenase for their own internal use in breaking down interstitial collagen that they ingest by phagocytosis.

In **wound healing,** certain growth factors (e.g., basic fibroblast factor, platelet-derived growth factor) bind to their respective receptors in the fibroblast cell membrane. **Activated fibroblasts** resulting from the ensuing activation cascade show increased levels of chemotactic cell motility, cellular proliferation, and collagen synthesis. Contractile fibroblasts called **myofibroblasts** commonly also are generated. Representing a contractile phenotype of the secretory fibroblast, these cells are involved in **wound contraction** (reduction is size of scars).

ENDOTHELIAL CELLS

Endothelial cells constitute the simple squamous endothelium lining the circulatory system and hence are epithelial cells. Developmentally and functionally, however, they are a component of loose connective tissue. Besides playing a key role in tissue fluid formation and necessary exchanges across capillary walls, endothelial cells produce interstitial matrix macromolecules, e.g., type III collagen and proteoglycans. Furthermore, endothelial cells are derived from mesenchyme, and the tumors that arise from them are considered to be of connective tissue origin. Hence, in several respects endothelial cells resemble connective tissue cells as well as being epithelial cells.

Few features of endothelial cells are discernible in LM sections other than their nucleus, but the EM discloses that these squamous cells wrap around a vessel lumen as depicted in Figure 5-9. The endothelial cells of capillaries and other small blood vessels have **tight junctions** between their lateral cell borders. Typically, such junctions are strip shaped, with narrow interposed intercellular slits through which tissue fluid can pass. At sites where maximal capillary permeability is required, the endothelial cells are provided with round window-like areas called **fenestrae** (L. for windows). A distinction is therefore made between **fenestrated capillaries** (see Fig. 5-9*B*) and unfenestrated or **continuous capillaries** (see Fig. 5-9*A*). Generally, fenestrations are closed by thin, selectively permeable **diaphragms** that are rarely evident in EM sections. The fenestrated capillaries that produce urinary filtrate in the kidneys are an exception because they are provided with open pores that lack diaphragms. Capillaries of both types are enclosed by basement membranes that anchor the endothelial cells to surrounding interstitial matrix. Endothelial cells actively engage in endocytosis. They are also able to divide. **Factor VIII-related antigen,** one of the many proteins that endothelial cells secrete, serves a marker by which these cells may be reliably identified (factor VIII is one of the blood coagulation factors). **Endothelium-derived relaxing factor (nitric oxide radical),** another endothelial cell product, brings about the relaxation of vascular smooth muscle cells, ie, has vasodilator activity. **Endothelin 1,** a potent vasoconstrictor that is also produced by endothelial cells, has the antagonistic action. In acutely inflamed tissues, venular endothelial cells express cell

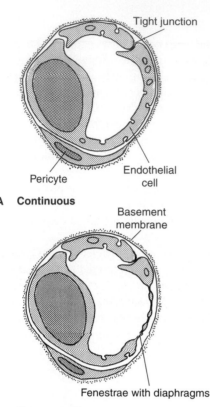

A   Continuous

B   Fenestrated

Figure 5-9
Basic structure of a continuous capillary (*A*) and a fenestrated
capillary (*B*).

adhesion molecules that mediate leukocyte adhesion and spreading (see under Neutrophils in
Chapter 6).

PERICYTES

Pericytes (perivascular cells) are inconspicuous, pale-staining cells that remain intimately associated with the endothelium of 1) blood capillaries and 2) small venules into which capillaries drain.
Hard to discern even in EM sections, and fairly widely separated along the vessel, pericytes lie
wrapped around the endothelium (Gk. *peri*, around) on the luminal side of the basement membrane
(see Fig. 5-9). Their narrow, pale-staining cytoplasmic processes ramify around the vessel.

A distinctive characteristic of pericytes is that they remain incompletely differentiated and capable of division. Pericytes represent a continuing potential source of new fibroblasts and smooth
muscle cells. Persisting partial differentiation and broad potentiality, along with characteristic pale
staining and a stellate shape, suggest that rather than representing essentially contractile cells (a
property that remains incompletely substantiated in undifferentiated pericytes), pericytes represent
residual mesenchymal cells. A key role played by pericytes is their availability for producing fibroblasts and smooth muscle cells if connective tissues or blood vessels become damaged and need
to be repaired. In addition, pericytes can secrete basement membrane and interstitial matrix constituents and several regulatory functions have been ascribed to them.

FAT CELLS OF ADIPOSE TISSUE

In certain regions of the body, **fat cells** (alternatively known as **adipocytes**) are relatively common in loose connective tissue. Tissue sites where adipocytes constitute the vast majority of the connective tissue cells are generally referred to as deposits of **adipose (fat) tissue.** Specialized for fat storage, adipose tissue is the body's chief depot of long-term energy reserves. Also, it reduces heat loss, fills in crevices, and softly cushions some parts of the body. Mature fat cells that are laden with lipid do not divide but they are comparatively long lived, hence those with overabundant fat cells risk becoming obese if they overeat. Furthermore, additional fat cells arise postnatally from adipocyte precursors that persist in adipose tissue.

Although lipids become extracted from paraffin sections, they are readily demonstrable in frozen sections if a fat stain is used (see Plate 1-3). In the common type of fat cell, the accumulating fat droplets coalesce and form a large central droplet surrounded by an extremely thin rim of cytoplasm (see Figs. 5-1 and 5-10). Thus mature, lipid-laden fat cells are characterized by having a signet-ring appearance. The flattened nucleus resembles the signet, and the pale-staining thin rim of peripheral cytoplasm resembles the ring (see Fig. 5-1). Another helpful analogy for recognizing groups of fat cells or adipose tissue in H&E-stained sections is their superficial resemblance to chicken wire. This similarity is due to the large empty space formerly filled with lipid that is left in each fat cell (see Fig. 5-10). EM sections of fat cells show that most of the organelles lie in proximity to the nucleus. Abundant mitochondria provide enough energy to sustain a high level of metabolic activity. The lipid droplets lie freely suspended in the cytosol, without a limiting membrane. Adipose tissue is richly supplied with capillaries and postganglionic adrenergic nerve fibers belonging to the sympathetic division of the autonomic nervous system (see Chapter 9).

White and Brown Adipose Tissue

Two distinct subtypes of adipose tissue are known as white fat and brown fat. The more widely distributed subtype is **white fat,** which usually appears yellow because of its content of the lipid soluble pigment, carotene. Its microscopic appearance is as just described, and it constitutes the primary site of lipid storage and metabolism in the body. **Brown fat** is comparatively scant in distribution. Its cells are smaller than those of

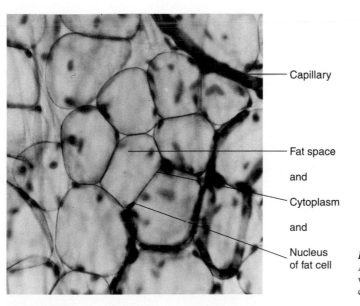

Capillary

Fat space

and

Cytoplasm

and

Nucleus
of fat cell

Figure 5-10
Adipose tissue (white fat) prepared as a whole mount to show its adipocytes and capillaries.

white fat, and its lipid is stored as multiple droplets, not as a single large central droplet. Also, its mitochondria are larger, have shelf-like cristae, and are more numerous. The tissue appears brown due to its extensive capillary blood supply and because of the colored enzymes (cytochromes) in its abundant mitochondria. The main role of brown fat is to provide body heat, critical for newborn babies and for mammals that are emerging from hibernation.

PLASMA CELLS

Plasma cells were originally classified as connective tissue cells because they are commonly present in the loose connective tissue associated with certain wet epithelia. However, since they arise from the B cells of secondary lymphoid organs and mucosal connective tissue, they are more appropriately regarded as a component of lymphoid tissue. Hence, plasma cells are often described as belonging to both loose connective tissue and lymphoid tissue.

A characteristic association of LM features facilitates the recognition of plasma cells. Except where crowded or compressed, plasma cells are typically rounded (Plate 5-3). Also, their spherical or ovoid nucleus commonly lies eccentrically in the cell. A large nucleolus may be discernible. The condensed peripheral chromatin may resemble the numerals on a dial, giving the nucleus a distinctive "clockface" appearance. Other features of plasma cells are that their cytoplasm is markedly basophilic, and sometimes they exhibit a negative Golgi image, additional indicators of active protein secretion.

Seen at the EM level, plasma cells have abundant ribosomes and an extensive rER, the dilated cisternae of which contain the cell's secretory product, **immunoglobulin** (Fig. 5-11). Secretory vesicles rapidly convey this secretory protein from the prominent Golgi complex to all parts of the cell surface.

The functional importance of plasma cells and their immediate precursors (**plasmablasts**) is that they are the source of **circulating antibodies (immunoglobulins),** the significance of which is discussed in the following section.

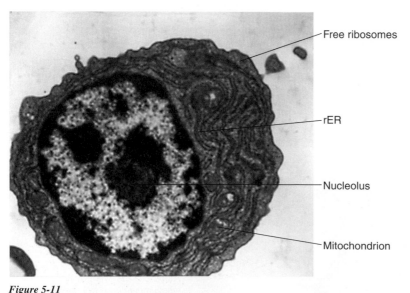

Free ribosomes

rER

Nucleolus

Mitochondrion

Figure 5-11
Electron micrograph of a plasma cell.

Plasma Cells Are Key Immune Effector Cells
To develop **immunity** means to become safe or exempt from reinfection. The usual kind of immunity develops when immunologically responsive cells respond to foreign macromolecules and produce specific **immune responses** directed against them. A macromolecule capable of eliciting specific immune responses is termed an **antigen** (Gk. *anti*, against; *gennan* to produce). The secretory protein, produced by a plasma cell, that interacts specifically with an antigen is called an antibody. **Antibodies**, known more precisely as **immunoglobulins**, are carried in the blood plasma and constitute a class of **γ-globulins.**

Patients who catch infectious diseases generally ward off reinfection by producing antibodies that recognize specific antigenic determinants on the disease-causing microorganisms. Compounds that elicit antibody formation are generally macromolecules (or their derivatives) that are foreign to the body. The plasma cells formed during immune responses to antigens synthesize and liberate antibody molecules capable of specifically recognizing and interacting with these antigens. Since such antibodies circulate to all parts of the body in the plasma, they are widely known as **humoral antibodies** (L. *humor*, liquid).

The plasma cells found in loose connective tissue under wet epithelia are derived from immigrant B cell progeny generated in immune responses to foreign antigens. For further information, see Chapter 7.

MAST CELLS

Mast cells may generally be found along the course of small blood vessels in loose connective tissue spreads (see Plate 5-1). In most cases, the numerous membrane-bounded secretory granules in these relatively large cells obscure the central spherical or ovoid nucleus (see Plate 5-1 and Fig. 5-1). A distinctive staining feature of mast cells is **metachromasia** of their large secretory granules (Gk. *meta*, after; *chroma*, color), meaning that certain basic stains impart to these granules a color other than that of the dye itself (e.g., toluidine blue imparts a purple color instead of blue). The metachromasia is due chiefly to the sulfated glycosaminoglycan heparin, present in human mast cell granules as **heparin proteoglycan.** Unlike exogenous heparin, the form of heparin found in human mast cells is only weakly anticoagulant. The tiny amount of heparin released when these cells degranulate has little effect other than enhancing lipid clearance from blood plasma through a facilitating action on lipoprotein lipase, for which enzyme heparin acts as cofactor. Heparin proteoglycan, along with a minor amount of chondroitin sulfate B proteoglycan in mucosal mast cells, constitutes the granule matrix. The chief role of the negatively charged matrix macromolecules is ionic binding of a variety of positively charged mediator molecules. Seen in the EM, secretory granules of mast cells present in most connective tissue sites exhibit distinctive lattice or grating-like internal patterns. The granules of mucosal mast cells, however, exhibit scroll-like internal patterns. The different patterns may reflect a variety of mediator–matrix associations.

Another major preformed constituent of mast cell granules is the amine **histamine,** a potent inflammatory mediator. In some species, but not humans, serotonin is present as well. An important action of the histamine released in degranulation is the induction of contraction in endothelial cells of venules. Their cell perimeters separate to a certain extent at the sites where the cell membranes are not tightly apposed in forming discontinuous tight junctions. Widening of endothelial intercellular slits results in local paracellular leakage of immunoglobulins and other plasma proteins from venules, an important stage of the acute inflammatory reaction (described in Chap. 6). Other functional consequences of significant histamine release are bronchoconstriction and vasodilatation.

The secretory granules of mast cells contain a number of additional inflammatory mediators and cytokines (i.e., cell-to-cell signaling molecules), including **eosinophil chemotactic factors of anaphylaxis** (ECF-A),

neutrophil chemotactic factor (NCF), several interleukins, and lysosomal **hydrolases.** Mast cells are also able to generate several other inflammatory mediators with great rapidity and liberate them along with the preformed mediators. **Leukotriene 3** (formerly known as the **slow-reacting substance of anaphylaxis,** SRS-A), **platelet activating factor** (PAF), and **prostaglandins** are produced in this manner at the time of degranulation.

Whereas NCF is specifically chemotactic to neutrophils, ECF-A attracts both neutrophils and eosinophils. Enzymes produced by the typical connective tissue mast cells include chymase, tryptase, and carboxypeptidase (neutral proteases). Mucosal mast cells produce tryptase and leukotriene C_4, but not chymase or carboxypeptidase. Leukotriene 3 effects are similar to those of histamine but are more prolonged. PAF causes platelets to aggregate and stimulates them to undergo their release reaction (see Chapter 6). Histaminase and aryl sulfatase produced by eosinophils can degrade two of the liberated mast cell-derived mediators, dampening their action.

CLINICAL IMPLICATIONS

Mast Cells Play a Key Role in Allergy Development

Mast cells degranulate and liberate their mediators 1) if a specific **antigen–antibody interaction** occurs at their cell surface or 2) in response to *direct trauma* to these cells. The immunological basis of degranulation is as follows. The cell membrane of mast cells possesses receptors for antibodies belonging to the **immunoglobulin E** (IgE) class. Irrespective of antigenic specificity, antibodies of this relatively minor class of γ-globulins bind to the cell surface, not only in *mast cells* but also in *basophils,* the rarest type of white blood cell. Some persons are predisposed genetically to producing antibodies of the IgE class in response to pollens, dusts, or fungal spores, when such particles (or their antigens) gain access to their body through tiny breaks in the epithelial lining of the respiratory tract. Other persons tend to respond in a similar way to allergens that they absorb from their gastrointestinal tract. Any IgE thus formed, irrespective of its antigenic specificity, can bind to the high affinity IgE receptors on mast cells or basophils with its antigen-recognition site exposed at the microenvironmental interface. Thus, if a particular antigen has elicited production of an IgE antibody, mast cells and basophils carrying that antibody on their surface will respond to the same antigen when it re-enters the body. Specific interaction between the antigen and surface-bound IgE on mast cells or basophils causes crosslinking of the bound IgE (Fig. 5-12). This leads to immediate discharge of se-

(continued)

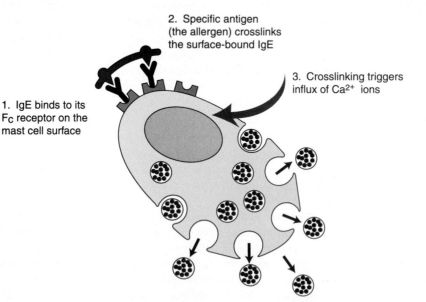

2. Specific antigen (the allergen) crosslinks the surface-bound IgE

3. Crosslinking triggers influx of Ca^{2+} ions

1. IgE binds to its F_C receptor on the mast cell surface

4. Granules containing preformed mediators discharge by exocytosis

Figure 5-12
Stages involved in IgE-mediated mast cell degranulation.

cretory granules, with accompanying liberation of the cell's impressive battery of inflammatory mediators. Moderate local responses involving only mast cells bring on the signs and symptoms of **allergies (immediate hypersensitivity reactions).** Ragweed pollen, for example, is notorious for causing sufferers of **hay fever** to develop **rhinorrhea** (Gk. *rhis*, nose; *rhoia*, flow; i.e., a runny nose), itchy eyes, and bouts of sneezing, all mediated by the histamine released by mast cells. A significant risk also exists that there will be a more profound adverse reaction to an allergen. Immediate hypersensitivity reactions of greater severity can occur in persons who produce substantial amounts of IgE in response to wasp stings, antibiotics derived from penicillin, or other antigenic sources that lead to patient sensitization. Further exposure to the sensitizing allergen triggers massive systemic release of histamine and other mediators from basophils as well as mast cells. Widespread release of these mediators has the potential to cause **systemic anaphylaxis,** a profound adverse reaction that is potentially fatal because it can lead to cardiovascular collapse.

Mast cells closely resemble blood basophils. The main differences are their respective nuclear shapes and the tissues in which these cells are found. Immunological release of their mediators occurs under essentially similar conditions, and both cell types arise from myeloid progenitors. Hence, mast cells of loose connective tissue are essentially immigrant cells derived from bone marrow. Two phenotypes, often referred to as **typical connective tissue mast cells** and **mucosal mast cells,** result from the influence of different cytokines acting in slightly different microenvironments.

MACROPHAGES

Macrophages (histiocytes) are considered a normal component of loose connective tissue and hence are classified as connective tissue cells. They are also found in certain other tissues, notably the blood cell-forming tissues and liver. As suggested by their name, they are voracious eaters with a big appetite for the particulate material that they ingest and then try to destroy. They are typically round or oval in outline, with an eccentric nucleus that has the shape of an indented oval or kidney bean (Plate 5-4). Their nucleus, however, may be obscured by particles that they have phagocytosed. The presence of substantial particles in a fairly large cell often indicates that this cell is a macrophage of some kind. Engulfed particles are taken into the cytoplasm in phagosomes that subsequently fuse with primary lysosomes. Ingested macromolecular organic compounds are then submitted to enzymatic degradation by the lysosomal hydrolases. At the EM level, macrophages are characterized by having abundant ingested material in phagosomes and secondary lysosomes. Typically, they also contain residual bodies with indigestible remains.

The various distinctive functions of macrophages include the phagocytosis and elimination of infectious microorganisms, removal of cell debris, and clearance of inhaled particulate matter from the lungs. Also, macrophages secrete complement proteins and a number of important growth factors (see Table 7-2). The macrophages in the spleen dispose of worn-out blood cells. Various kinds of macrophage-like cells are capable of antigen processing, an essential preliminary stage of most immune responses.

The various kinds of macrophages are derived from white blood cells known as **monocytes** that migrate from small blood vessels into loose connective tissue and transform directly into macrophages. Hence, macrophages represent immigrant cells derived from myeloid tissue. Macrophages are able to divide. In addition, macrophages and their precursors (monocytes) have the capacity to fuse together, resulting in huge multinucleated cells known as **foreign body giant cells** that are capable of walling off relatively large masses of foreign material from the remainder of the body.

SUMMARY

Loose connective tissue, derived from mesenchyme, consists of cells, fibers, and an amorphous matrix component with the consistency of a soft gel. Collagen fibers are made up of parallel narrow fibrils that resist stretch. Elastic fibers branch, recoil if stretched, and are not made up of identical fibrils. Reticular fibers branch, constituting fine supporting networks. They represent fine bundles of collagen fibrils with closely associated matrix glycoproteins and proteoglycans. The ground substance of connective tissue is rich in protein-complexed glycosaminoglycans. Its abundant tissue fluid content facilitates the diffusion of nutrients and waste products. The tissue fluid (blood plasma depleted of plasma proteins) produced by open capillaries is partly resorbed by closed capillaries in which hydrostatic pressure is lower than osmotic pressure. Much of the surplus tissue fluid, containing accumulated interstitial protein, enters lymphatic capillaries as lymph. Edema results if tissue fluid production exceeds fluid removal through lymphatic drainage and capillary resorption.

Basement membranes are sheets of distinctively organized interstitial matrix with a characteristic electron-dense lamina densa and commonly with associated reticular fibers. Produced by epithelial, endothelial, fat, muscle, and Schwann cells, basement membranes contain type IV collagen, adhesive glycoproteins, and proteoglycans. Besides providing flexible support, they constitute the main selective filter in the kidneys.

Fibroblasts are secretory cells that produce the matrix constituents of ordinary connective tissue. Most types of collagen are produced through enzymatic processing of fibroblast procollagens followed by extracellular assembly into collagen fibrils, but type IV collagen is an exception. Because of their distinctive assembly, collagen fibrils possess a unique axial periodicity manifested as a "bar-code" pattern. Fibroblasts also produce tropoelastin and form fibrillin-containing microfibrils that mold forming elastin into elastic fibers.

Intercellular slits between the discontinuous tight junctions of capillary endothelial cells permit the passage of tissue fluid. In most fenestrated capillaries, diaphragms close the endothelial fenestrations. Endothelial cells secrete endothelium-derived relaxing factor (nitric oxide radical) and endothelin 1, two important vasoactive products. In acute inflammation, their cell adhesion molecules become upregulated. The walls of capillaries and small venules also contain pericytes, which are incompletely differentiated cells that can produce new fibroblasts and smooth muscle cells.

Fat cells, the predominant cell type of adipose tissue, have abundant mitochondria and are metabolically active. Their lipid is unsegregated by an intracellular membrane. In white fat, the body's chief energy reserve, each fat cell contains a single fat droplet. In brown fat, which produces body heat and is scant, each fat cell contains multiple fat droplets. Plasma cells are characteristically round, with an eccentric clockface nucleus, basophilic cytoplasm, and a negative Golgi image. They secrete specific humoral antibodies (immunoglobulins) capable of recognizing specific antigens.

Mast cells have a conspicuous content of metachromatic granules that contain preformed histamine and heparin proteoglycan. Histamine released through degranulation permits immunoglobulins and other plasma proteins to escape from venules. Other potent inflammatory mediators are generated just prior to degranulation. In mast cells and basophils, degranulation is triggered by interaction between antigen and surface-bound IgE. It also results from direct damage. Allergies are manifestations of local IgE-mediated mast cell responses to foreign antigens. Anaphylaxis can occur if there is systemic involvement of basophils as well.

Because macrophages are actively phagocytic, they commonly contain exogenous constituents. In addition, they secrete complement proteins and certain growth factors and can process antigens. Macrophages, derived from blood monocytes, have the potential to fuse to form foreign body giant cells.

Bibliography

Fibroblasts, Interstitial Matrix, and Tissue Fluid

Buck CA, Horwitz AF. Cell surface receptors for extracellular matrix molecules. Annu Rev Cell Biol 3:179, 1987.

Gabbiani G, Rungger-Brándle E. The fibroblast. In: Glynn LE, ed. Tissue Repair and Regeneration: Handbook of Inflammation, vol 3. Amsterdam, Elsevier/North Holland Biomedical Press, 1981, p 1.

Gallagher JT. The extended family of proteoglycans: social residents of the pericellular zone. Curr Opin Cell Biol 1:1201, 1989.

Gotte L. Molecular morphology of elastin. In Robert AM, Robert L, eds. Biology and Pathology of Elastic Tissues: Frontiers of Matrix Biology, vol 8. Basel, S Karger, 1980, p 33.

Hay ED, ed. Cell Biology of the Extracellular Matrix. New York, Plenum Press, 1981.

Imayama S, Braverman IM. Scanning electron microscope study of elastic fibers of the loose connective tissue (superficial fascia) in the rat. Anat Rec 222:115, 1988.

Intaglietta M, Endrich BA. Experimental and quantitative analysis of microcirculatory water exchange. Acta Physiol Scand Suppl 463:59, 1979.

Montes GS, Bezerra MSF, Junqueira LCU. Collagen distribution in tissues. In Ruggeri A, Motta PM, eds. Ultrastructure of the Connective Tissue Matrix. Boston, Martinus Nijhoff, 1984, p 65.

Piez KA, Reddi AH (eds). Extracellular Matrix Biochemistry. New York, Elsevier, 1984.

Reddi AH, ed. Extracellular Matrix Structure and Function. UCLA Symposia on Molecular and Cellular Biology, New Series, vol 25. New York, Alan R Liss, 1985.

Ross R, Bornstein P. Elastic fibers in the body. Sci Am 224(6):44, 1971.

Basement Membranes

Eady RAJ. The basement membrane: interface between the epithelium and the dermis: structural features. Arch Dermatol 124:709, 1988.

Inoué S. Ultrastructure of basement membranes. Int Rev Cytol 117:57, 1989.

Inoué S, Leblond CP. Three-dimensional network of cords: the main component of basement membranes. Am J Anat 181:341, 1988.

Laurie GW, Leblond CP, Inoué S et al. Fine structure of the glomerular basement membrane and immunolocalization of five basement membrane components to the lamina densa (basal lamina) and its extensions in both glomeruli and tubules of the rat kidney. Am J Anat 169:463, 1984.

Martin GR, Timpl R. Laminin and other basement membrane components. Annu Rev Cell Biol 3:57, 1987.

Schittney JC, Yurchenco PD. Basement membranes: molecular organization and function in development and disease. Curr Opin Cell Biol 1:983, 1989.

Macrophages and Endothelial Cells

Auger MJ, Ross JA. The biology of the macrophage. In: Lewis CE, McGee J, eds. The Macrophage: The Natural Immune System. Oxford, IRL Press, 1992.

Bearer EL, Orci L, Sors P. Endothelial fenestral diaphragms: a quick-freeze, deep-etch study. Cell Biol 100:418, 1985.

Carr I. The Macrophage. A Review of Ultrastructure and Function. New York, Academic Press, 1973.

Carr I. The biology of macrophages. Clin Invest Med 1:59, 1978.

Fuller RW. Macrophages. Br Med Bull 48:65, 1992.

Page RC. The macrophage as a secretory cell. Int Rev Cytol 52:119, 1978.

Mast Cells

Austen KF. Biological implications of the structural and functional characteristics of the chemical mediators of immediate-type hypersensitivity. In: The Harvey Lectures, series 73. New York, Academic Press, 1979, p 93.

Beaven MA. Histamine, pt 1. N Engl J Med 294:30, 1976.

Erb KJ, Holloway JW, Le Gros G. Innate Immunity: mast cells in the front line. Curr Biol 6:941, 1996.

Galli SJ. New concepts about the mast cell. N Engl J Med 328:257, 1993.

Gordon JR, Burd PR, Galli SJ. Mast cells as a source of multifunctional cytokines. Immunol Today 11:458, 1990.

Holgate ST, ed. Mast Cells, Mediators and Disease. Boston, Kluwer Academic, 1988.

Holgate ST, Church MK. The mast cell. Br Med Bull 48:40, 1992.

Stevens RL, Austen KF. Recent advances in the cellular and molecular biology of mast cells. Immunol Today 10:381, 1989.

Adipocytes and Adipose Tissue

Angel A, Hollenberg CH, Roncari DAK, eds. The Adipocyte and Obesity: Cellular and Molecular Mechanisms. New York, Raven Press, 1983.

Julien P, Despres J-P, Angel A. Scanning electron microscopy of very small fat cells and mature fat cells in human obesity. J Lipid Res 30:293, 1989.

Poissonnet CM, Lavelle M, Burdi AR. Growth and development of adipose tissue. J Pediatr 113:1, 1988.

Roncari DAK. Pre-adipose cell replication and differentiation. Trends Biochem Sci 9:486, 1984.

Thompson JF, Habeck DA, Nance SL, Beetham KL. Ultrastructural and biochemical changes in brown fat in cold exposed rats. J Cell Biol 41:312, 1969.

CHAPTER 6

Blood Cells

OBJECTIVES

On completion of this chapter, you should be able to do the following:

- Examine and evaluate blood films
- Recognize erythrocytes, the various leukocytes, and platelets
- Discuss the significance of reticulocytes and reticulocyte counts
- Explain what happens if intravascular platelets encounter vessel wall damage
- List five types of leukocytes present in peripheral blood and state their respective cell counts
- Summarize the similarities and chief differences between the five types of leukocytes, specifying key functions in each case
- Name two types of leukocytes playing major roles in acute inflammation

Blood contains red blood cells or **erythrocytes** (Gk. *erythros*, red), white blood cells or **leukocytes** (Gk. *leukos*, white), and cytoplasmic fragments known as blood **platelets.** These components are freely suspended in **plasma,** the fluid portion of blood. Blood is considered a special connective tissue not because its cells produce intercellular matrix constituents but because they develop from mesenchyme (see Table 5-1).

Erythrocytes contain **hemoglobin,** a distinctive red protein that has the necessary properties to bring about efficient oxygen transport from the lungs to the tissues. The same blood cells also facilitate transfer of carbon dioxide from the tissues to the lungs. A unique feature of erythroid maturation is that each forming erythrocyte extrudes its nucleus before entering the circulation. Nuclei are also lacking in blood platelets since they are membrane-covered fragments of cytoplasm. Platelets play a key role in arresting bleeding from damaged blood vessels.

Leukocytes are so named because after bulk sedimentation they look almost white. They are largely protective in function, defending the body from the ravages of infection in a variety of ways. Most types of leukocytes carry out major extravascular activities in loose connective tissue. Five different types of leukocytes are recognized, each with varied functions and distinctive microscopic features. The fact that leukocytes are greatly outnumbered by erythrocytes is obvious when blood films are observed. These films are prepared by drawing out small drops of peripheral blood on slides to make thin films (Fig. 6-1A) and staining them with a blood stain (a mixture of red acid stains

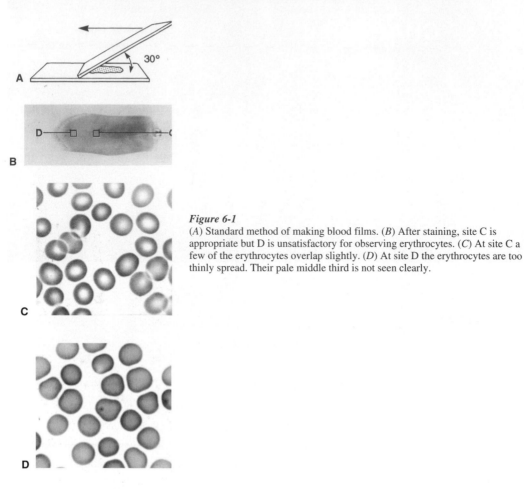

Figure 6-1
(*A*) Standard method of making blood films. (*B*) After staining, site C is appropriate but D is unsatisfactory for observing erythrocytes. (*C*) At site C a few of the erythrocytes overlap slightly. (*D*) At site D the erythrocytes are too thinly spread. Their pale middle third is not seen clearly.

and blue basic stains) such as Wright's stain, which gives the colors described in this chapter and Chapter 7. Blood films are thicker where the drops first spread out, and the appearance of erythrocytes varies according to the area chosen for observation. The best area to select for examining erythrocytes is a region where some of them just overlap, as in Figure 6-1*C*. Part *D* of the same illustration shows their appearance at a site where they are too thinly spread. Erythrocytes should appear as pink circles with a central pale area representing about one third of their diameter (see Plate 6-1*B*). Leukocytes stand out in contrast mainly because they possess a nucleus, and in general they are larger than erythrocytes. They are not as numerous, however, and some types of leukocytes can be tracked down only with diligent searching. Platelets are relatively easy to recognize, especially if they have aggregated, as sometimes happens in preparing fresh blood films (see Plate 6-1*C*).

ERYTHROCYTES

Each liter of normal adult peripheral blood contains almost 5×10^{12} erythrocytes (i.e., 4.3×10^{12} in females, 4.8×10^{12} in males). The erythrocyte is a biconcave disk, 7 to 8 μm in diameter (Fig. 6-2), with a finite life span of about *4 months*. Erythrocytes sometimes stick together temporarily, forming columns called **rouleaux** that resemble stacks of coins. The role of the erythrocytic protein

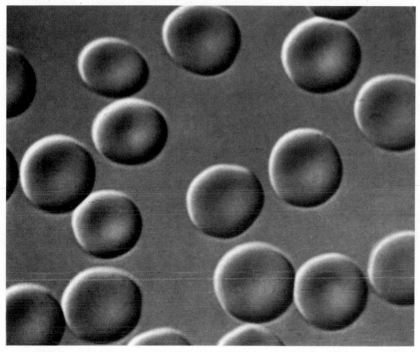

Figure 6-2
Erythrocytes (fresh preparation, interference microscope).

hemoglobin, which consists of iron-containing **heme** groups conjugated to the protein **globin,** is to transport oxygen. **Oxyhemoglobin,** the red oxygenated form of this protein, turns darker and slightly blue as it yields its oxygen to the tissues. Erythrocytes also contain the enzyme carbonic anhydrase, which facilitates uptake of carbon dioxide from the tissues and its discharge from the lungs.

CLINICAL IMPLICATIONS

Anemias
Any significant lowering of the blood concentration of hemoglobin, due either to reduction in the total number of circulating erythrocytes or to decrease in their individual hemoglobin content, is described as an **anemia** (Gk., without blood). Anemic patients generally appear pale and may be chronically tired and listless due to impaired oxygen delivery to their tissues. If their peripheral blood films are examined with an LM, the erythrocytes may appear undercolored **(hypochromic)** because of hemoglobin insufficiency, as in an iron-deficiency anemia, or they may be larger than normal but reduced in number, as in a vitamin B_{12}—deficiency anemia. In the case of a genetically transmitted condition called **sickle cell anemia,** erythrocytes become deformed into elongated crescents (sickles) in the process of yielding their oxygen. A single amino acid substitution in hemoglobin causes this protein to polymerize and crystallize as it gives up its oxygen. The damage that this physical change inflicts on the erythrocyte membrane leads to premature erythrocyte destruction. Normally, erythrocytes circulate for 100 to 120 days and then are phagocytosed, mostly by macrophages in the spleen. If erythrocytes are destroyed prematurely, or if erythrocyte production fails to keep up with daily requirements, anemias result. The daily rate of erythrocyte production can be assessed from the proportion of newly formed erythrocytes. These recently formed cells can be recognized and counted in blood films, as explained in the next section.

Reticulocytes

Most erythrocytes seen in routinely stained blood films appear pink because of acidophilic staining of their hemoglobin (Plate 6-1*B*). A small proportion of erythrocytes, however, are slightly larger and tinged with blue (see Plate 6-1*A*). Known as **polychromatophilic erythrocytes** (meaning red cells that love many colors), these are immature erythrocytes with enough residual RNA from prior hemoglobin synthesis to add a trace of basophilic staining to their otherwise acidophilic staining properties. These cells are easier to recognize if they are stained with new methylene blue or cresyl blue, which shows up their cytoplasmic RNA as a distinctive blue wreath-like network (Plate 6-2). Red cells that exhibit such a network are referred to as **reticulocytes** (L. *rete*, net). Reticulocytes, which represent erythrocytes that are still immature and polychromatophilic, are comparatively easy to distinguish from mature erythrocytes. They lose their polychromatophilic and reticulocyte staining properties 2 days or so after entering the circulation. Conditions that stimulate erythrocyte production cause newly formed erythrocytes to enter the circulation in greater numbers. Hence, a rise in the reticulocyte count (i.e., an increase in the proportion of erythrocytes that are reticulocytes) indicates that erythrocyte production has increased. Under normal conditions, only 1 to 2.5% of peripheral blood erythrocytes are reticulocytes.

PLATELETS

Each liter of normal adult peripheral blood contains between 150×10^9 and 350×10^9 small platelike structures, 2 μm to 3 μm in diameter, called **blood platelets** or **thrombocytes.** These potentially secretory circulating structures are produced by **megakaryocytes,** giant cells of red bone marrow. Platelets represent entirely cytoplasmic fragments, covered by cell membrane and lacking a nuclear component because they are produced through fragmentation of subdivided megakaryocyte cytoplasm. They tend to aggregate in drawn blood, so platelet clumps may be found as well as individual platelets in blood films (see Plate 6-1*C*). The central region of a platelet contains purple-staining granules, whereas the nongranular periphery stains a transparent pale blue.

Electron micrographs indicate that the platelet's biconvex discoid shape is maintained by a supporting ring of marginal microtubules (Figs. 6-3 and 6-4). Platelets take up the potent vasoconstric-

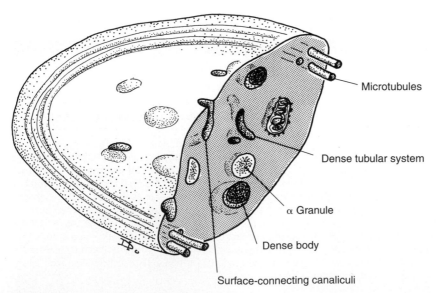

Microtubules

Dense tubular system

α Granule

Dense body

Surface-connecting canaliculi

Figure 6-3
Internal details of a platelet discernible at the EM level.

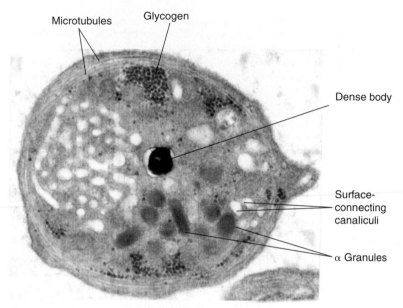

Figure 6-4
Electron micrograph of a blood platelet (×30,000).

tor **serotonin** from the blood and store it in electron-dense granules termed **dense granules** or **dense bodies.** Also important is **platelet-derived growth factor,** a major proliferation promoter in fibroblasts, smooth muscle cells, and a few other cells. This potent growth factor is localized, along with certain constituents involved in blood coagulation, in a different population of platelet granules called *α*-granules. Platelets can discharge their granular contents by exocytosis, and they have the potential for active phagocytosis. Some of their granular discharge occurs by way of surface-connecting canaliculi that are tubular invaginations of the surface membrane. Platelets also possess a second tubular system, known as the **dense tubular system,** the functional significance of which remains inconclusively evaluated.

At any given moment, one third of the body's total complement of platelets is temporarily out of circulation. Noncirculating platelets sequestered in the red pulp of the spleen are nevertheless able to exchange freely with the platelets circulating in the peripheral blood. The maximum circulation time for platelets is about 10 days, after which they are phagocytosed by macrophages, primarily those of the spleen.

CLINICAL IMPLICATIONS

A Key Role of Platelets Is to Terminate Hemorrhage
Damage to the endothelial lining of a blood vessel can expose collagen and other normally hidden components of the vessel wall directly to the blood. When circulating platelets come into contact with some of these vascular components they adhere to them. Furthermore, direct contact with collagen is also one of the stimuli that causes platelets to release their secretory granules, a key response known as the **release reaction.** The serotonin thus released elicits contraction of the circular layer of smooth muscle cells present in most blood vessel walls, and this action reduces loss of blood from damaged vessels.

Platelets rapidly accumulate on the luminal surface of a bleeding vessel as increasing numbers of them adhere to those already attached (**platelet aggregation**). This is largely an effect of ADP liberated during the release reaction. The temporary seal or **platelet plug** that they constitute grows large enough to stem

(continued)

further blood loss from the vessel. Another consequence of the release reaction is that **fibrin** is produced from its soluble precursor **fibrinogen** through the complex process of **blood coagulation.** The outcome is a fibrin mass (a blood clot or **thrombus**) that is stronger and more substantial than the platelet plug it replaces. Platelets therefore have a dual role in the arrest of bleeding (**hemostasis**). By aggregating they temporarily seal off bleeding vessels. Then by initiating local coagulation they provide a more permanent seal, namely a blood clot.

Platelets show a similar tendency to adhere to certain components of the vessel wall if these become exposed as a result of degenerative or pathological changes. Ensuing **thrombosis** (formation of a blood clot) can have critical consequences if it occludes the arterial supply to some part of the brain or heart, leading either to a stroke or a heart attack.

Finally, spontaneous bruising, tiny cutaneous hemorrhages on the arms or thighs, or undue bleeding of the gums can indicate a platelet deficiency (**thrombocytopenia**).

LEUKOCYTES

A liter of normal adult peripheral blood contains a total of 4.5×10^9 to 11×10^9 leukocytes. These motile cells are subdivided into five types according to their staining characteristics and respective functional activities within and outside the bloodstream.

Leukocytes are also broadly categorized as 1) granule-containing **granular leukocytes** and 2) **nongranular leukocytes** that lack conspicuous granules. A few tiny granules may nevertheless be present in nongranular leukocytes. The three types of granular leukocytes are (1) **eosinophils** with specific granules that stain with acid dyes such as eosin (see Plate 6-1*F*); (2) **basophils** with specific granules that are markedly basophilic (see Plate 6-1*G*); and (3) **neutrophils** with specific granules that are not markedly acidophilic or basophilic at neutral pH (see Plate 6-1*D* and *E*). Neutrophils are also known as **polymorphonuclear leukocytes (polymorphs** for short) because their nucleus can have from two to five lobes. The two types of nongranular leukocytes are (1) **lymphocytes** (see Plate 6-1*J* and *K*), which are found in lymph as well as blood, and (2) **monocytes**, the large circulating cells that are the precursors of macrophages (see Plate 6-1*H*).

Identifying Leukocytes in Peripheral Blood Films

By systematically searching under low or scanning power, it is possible to find each type of leukocyte in a blood film. However, leukocytes do not stain well in the thicker part of the film where the drop first spreads out. It is advisable to look for them in the thinner part of the film even though they are less numerous there. Also, the middle of the film is more useful than the edges, where leukocytes tend to be distorted and poorly stained. Sometimes it is necessary to observe more than one blood film to see everything. The following pitfalls should be avoided.

Degenerating and Damaged Leukocytes

Degenerating and disintegrating leukocytes are commonly also present. Endeavouring to identify them is a waste of time. For reference purposes, a degenerating neutrophil is shown in Plate 6-1*I*.

Platelet Aggregates

Beginners may misinterpret the purple-staining granular material in platelets (see Plate 6-1*C*) as a nucleus, and this can lead them to confuse platelets or platelet aggregates with leukocytes.

"Difficult" and Poorly Stained Leukocytes

Those who are inexperienced in identifying leukocytes should search for fairly obvious examples of each type and avoid agonizing over cells that are hard or impossible to identify.

NEUTROPHILS (POLYMORPHS)

Most leukocytes present in a blood film are mature neutrophils. These cells represent 50% to 70% of the total leukocyte count of adult peripheral blood. The nucleus of the mature neutrophil is segmented, with two to five lobes interconnected by fine strands and chromatin that is condensed and dark staining (see Plate 6-1*E*). In persons having two X chromosomes per cell (e.g., karyotypically normal females), one X chromosome (the sex chromatin, described in Chap. 2) has the form of a distinctive nuclear lobe called a **drumstick appendage** (Fig. 6-5). Neutrophils contain abundant fine neutrophilic granules, referred to as **specific granules** (i.e., specific to this type of leukocyte), that impart a mauve (lavender) color to the cytoplasm. In addition, they have a few larger granules that stain a reddish purple (see Plate 6-1*E*). Termed **azurophilic granules** because of their affinity for one of the dyes in blood stains (methylene azure), these larger granules correspond to lysosomes.

Neutrophils circulate in the blood for 6 to 10 hours. They then enter the tissues as motile cells and continue their important phagocytic activities for another 2 or 3 days. Their prime target is bacteria, which they engulf and promptly destroy using hydrogen peroxide and other bactericidal molecules, together with many different enzymes from their membrane-bounded granules. Most of the molecules employed for this purpose come from their lysosomal (azurophilic) granules, but lactoferrin is supplied by the specific granules, and the hydrogen peroxide-producing enzymes are located in their peroxisomes.

The neutrophils seen in a peripheral blood film generally include up to 5% that are slightly immature. The immature forms are recognizable by the fact that their nucleus remains band-shaped, sometimes resembling a horseshoe, hence they are termed **band neutrophils** (see Plate 6-1*D*).

CLINICAL IMPLICATIONS

Neutrophils Play a Key Role in Acute Inflammation

The acute inflammatory reaction is typically a localized, acute tissue response elicited by some sort of local injury. It often succeeds in eliminating its cause or reversing the adverse effects of the injury, and it patches up the resulting damage. This reaction occurs in loose connective tissue and involves not only neutrophils but also monocytes, mast cells, and the endothelial cells of venules. The classic signs of acute inflammation can become noticeable, for example, after the skin has been pierced by a dirty sliver (Fig. 6-6*A*). They are redness, hotness, and swelling of the underlying connective tissue, usually with some pain and tenderness. The first two changes are due to augmented blood flow (**hyperemia**), and in sections of the inflamed region the venules and capillaries appear dilated and congested (see Fig. 6-6*B*). The swelling (**edema**) is a

(continued)

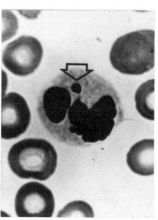

Figure 6-5
Mature neutrophil (peripheral blood). Arrow indicates the drumstick appendage (sex chromatin) found in neutrophils of persons with two X chromosomes.

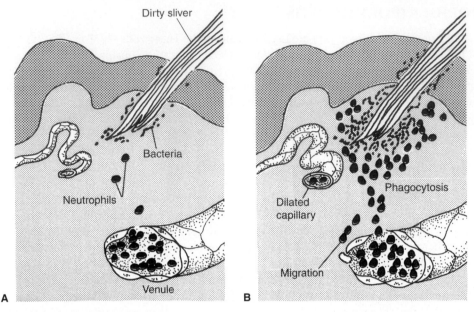

Figure 6-6
Neutrophil emigration in acute inflammatory reactions. Neutrophils that migrate from dilated venules (*A*) track down bacteria introduced during injury and engulf them by phagocytosis (*B*).

manifestation of plasma leakage from affected venules. It should be recalled from Chapter 5 that histamine released from mast cells induces limited separation of the margins of the endothelial cells of venules. This partial separation provides an escape route for fibrinogen, immunoglobulins, complement proteins, and other plasma proteins. Infecting microorganisms introduced with the sliver therefore come into direct contact with any immunoglobulins that may be present as a result of previous exposure to the same organisms or their antigens. The excess fluid that accumulates in the ground substance as a consequence of the permeability increase results in edema and also in tenderness owing to increased pressure on sensory nerve endings. In addition, certain inflammatory mediators elicit pain directly by stimulating pain-sensitive nerve endings.

Early in the acute inflammatory reaction, **neutrophils** start adhering to the endothelial cells of affected venules and escape by squeezing between these cells, as illustrated in Figure 6-7. They then become attracted chemotactically toward bacteria, which they phagocytose and destroy. Local accumulation of neutrophils is a consistent indication that an acute inflammatory reaction is underway. The migrating neutrophils are accompanied by **monocytes** that escape from venules in a similar manner and rapidly transform into **macrophages** as they enter the tissues. Macrophages actively phagocytose some strains of bacteria and dispose of residual debris as inflammation subsides. In addition, macrophages are a source of a number of important cytokines, including chemotactic factors, inflammatory mediators (notably **interleukin 1** and **tumor necrosis factor**), and several growth factors, that collectively promote tissue repair. In the terminal phase of tissue repair, which is often referred to as **fibrosis** or **fibroplasia**, fibroblasts actively secrete procollagen. Also, a capillary blood supply becomes reestablished, primarily as a result of sprouting from undamaged vessels at the periphery of the inflammatory focus. A distinctively contractile phenotype of the fibroblast, termed the **myofibroblast**, subsequently emerges and supersedes the collagen-producing variety. Its contractile activity reduces the overall dimensions of the newly formed repair tissue and hence the size of the residual scar.

An elevated peripheral neutrophil count, termed a **neutrophilia**, can represent an acute response to bacterial infection. Furthermore, immature cells of the neutrophil series (band neutrophils and earlier forms) enter the peripheral blood in greater numbers when there is an increased demand for neutrophils, for example, in combatting a severe bacterial infection. Progressive increase in the number of immature forms leaving the bone marrow, indicating progression of bacterial infection, is known as a **shift to the left.**

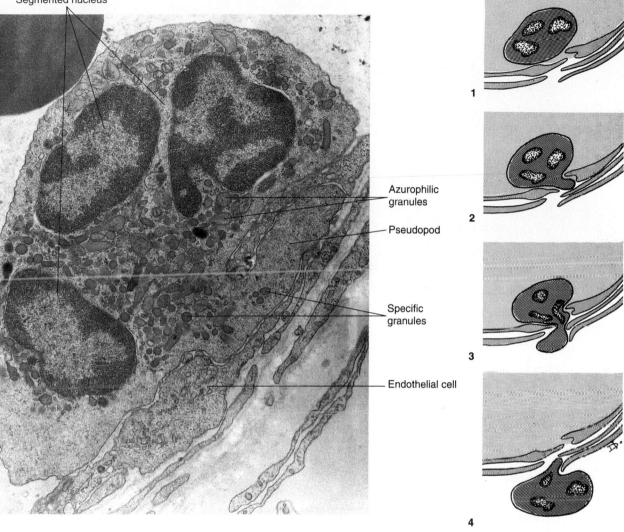

Segmented nucleus

Azurophilic granules

Pseudopod

Specific granules

Endothelial cell

Figure 6-7
Electron micrograph and interpretive diagram of neutrophil migration from a venule in an acute inflammatory reaction.
This neutrophil corresponds to stage 2 of the series.

EOSINOPHILS

Only 1% to 4% of the leukocytes in adult peripheral blood are eosinophils. These granulocytes are slightly larger than neutrophils, and their nucleus consists of only two lobes. Their most striking feature, however, is their large acidophilic specific granules, which stain bright red or reddish-purple (see Plate 6-1*F*). With the EM, the specific granules appear ovoid with a lattice-structured crystalloid core and a limiting membrane (Fig. 6-8). The enzyme complement of these granules indicates that in the case of eosinophils, the specific granules are derived from lysosomes.

Four cationic (basic) proteins present in the eosinophil's specific granules have substantial destructive potential: **major basic protein,** a crystalloid core constituent that is toxic to certain parasites, bacteria, and epithelial cells; **eosinophil cationic protein,** which is toxic to some parasites, bacteria, and neurons; **eosinophil-derived neurotoxin,** a ribonuclease that is toxic to neurons and mildly toxic to parasites; and **eosinophil peroxidase,** which destroys microorganisms and certain parasites and is toxic to mast cells and some epithelial and tumor cells.

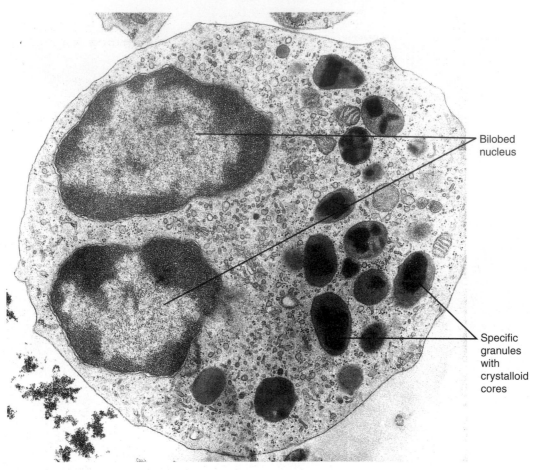

Bilobed
nucleus

Specific
granules
with
crystalloid
cores

Figure 6-8
Electron micrograph showing the characteristic structure of an eosinophil. Its large lysosomal specific granules have a
distinctive appearance, and its nucleus is bilobed.

In addition, eosinophils produce O_2^- (the superoxide radical ion) and two lipid-derived mediators: platelet-activating factor (which exerts a chemotactic and activating action on eosinophils) and leukotriene C_4. Eosinophils release this varied complement of mediators when their surface-bound IgA, IgG, or IgE becomes bridged by antigen.

Eosinophils circulate for 1 to 10 hours in the peripheral blood and then enter loose connective tissue (e.g., the gastrointestinal lamina propria) and remain there for up to 10 days.

CLINICAL IMPLICATIONS

Eosinophils Regulate Allergic Inflammation and Kill Certain Parasites

Eosinophils migrate from the peripheral blood into the mucosal connective tissue adjacent to wet epithelia (e.g., in the respiratory and gastrointestinal tracts). Eosinophils that accumulate at sites of local allergic responses phagocytose antigen–antibody complexes. In addition, eosinophils produce **histaminase** and **aryl sulfatase B,** enzymes capable of inactivating two inflammatory mediators from mast cells. Hence eosinophils have the capacity to subdue and regulate local inflammatory reactions of allergic origin. A high peripheral blood eosinophil count (**eosinophilia**) may therefore indicate an **allergic reaction.** In addition, eosinophils play a key role in killing parasitic helminth worms at the larval stage, so eosinophilia is equally consistent with certain forms of **parasitic infestation.**

BASOPHILS

Basophils are a rare type of leukocyte representing 0.5% to 1% of the total peripheral blood leukocytes, so to find even a single basophil in a blood film is a real challenge. Almost as large as neutrophils, basophils possess a nucleus that generally has two lobes but may have more. When observed in blood films, however, the nucleus of a basophil may be largely or entirely obscured by a moderate number of substantial blue-staining specific granules (see Plate 6-1*G*) that contain **histamine** in ionic association with a matrix of **sulfated glycosaminoglycans** (chiefly chondroitin and dermatan sulfates), stain metachromatically, and essentially resemble large mast cell granules. These specific granules have a limiting membrane and represent the secretory granules of the cell.

Basophils are only mildly phagocytic. Of greater functional significance is their direct involvement in bodywide **(systemic) allergic responses.** Antigen–IgE antibody interactions occurring at their surface trigger release of histamine and other inflammatory mediators, as explained in Chapter 5 under Mast Cells. This release may be sufficiently massive to result in **fatal systemic anaphylaxis.** In addition, basophils participate in **cutaneous basophilic hypersensitivity,** a delayed hypersensitivity reaction with signs and symptoms that resemble those of allergic contact dermatitis.

LYMPHOCYTES

Lymphocytes comprise 20% to 40% of peripheral blood leukocytes. These highly motile nongranular leukocytes are relatively easy to find in blood films. Besides being present in blood, they enter the tissues and also are present in lymph (hence their name). Peripheral blood lymphocytes are of two sizes. Most of them are **small lymphocytes** with a diameter of 6 to 9 μm (see Plate 6-1*K*). The remainder (<10%) are **large lymphocytes** (known also as **medium-sized lymphocytes**) with an average diameter of 12 μm (see Plate 6-1*J*). Lymphocytes are classified as *nongranular* leukocytes because they lack specific granules. In approximately 10% of them, however, there are fine purple-staining (azurophilic) granules representing lysosomes.

Small lymphocytes possess a small, spherical or slightly indented nucleus with abundant dark-staining condensed chromatin (see Plate 6-1*K*). Only a thin external rim of slightly basophilic cytoplasm is visible in blood films. The cytoplasm is scarcely discernible in LM sections. Ribosomes are numerous but other cytoplasmic organelles are scant. When small lymphocytes having this poorly differentiated appearance become activated by antigen, they proliferate, and among the cells they produce are differentiated effector cells capable of mediating immune responses. Furthermore, the small lymphocyte population represents two different types of antigen-responsive cells—**B lymphocytes** and **T lymphocytes.** Whereas B lymphocyte differentiation occurs entirely in the bone marrow, certain critical stages of T lymphocyte differentiation take place in the thymus. The two kinds of lymphocytes nevertheless have identical morphological appearances and special techniques are necessary to distinguish between them. B and T lymphocytes, more commonly known as **B cells** and **T cells**, and an overview of their respective roles in immune responses are described in Chapter 7. In addition to B and T cells, peripheral blood contains a population of **null cells.** Although these cells look like small lymphocytes, they lack the specific markers that would characterize them as B or T cells.

Large lymphocytes possess a nucleus that is slightly larger and darker staining, though also spherical or slightly indented (see Plate 6-1*J*). The cytoplasm is slightly more copious than that of small lymphocytes and equally or more basophilic (compare *J* and *K* in Plate 6-1). Large lymphocytes possess more free ribosomes and mitochondria, with a more extensive rER and Golgi apparatus. Some large lymphocytes present in blood films may initially be confused with monocytes. The nucleus in large lymphocytes, however, is not indented enough to be kidney-shaped, and large lymphocytes are smaller than most monocytes. Large lymphocytes represent a heterogeneous population that may include antigen-activated lymphocytes and even reactive lymphoid cells.

MONOCYTES

Monocytes are nongranular leukocytes that constitute 2% to 6% of the total blood leukocytes. Because they represent the largest type of leukocyte they are relatively easy to find in blood films. Beginners nevertheless sometimes confuse monocytes with large lymphocytes (compare *H* with *J* in Plate 6-1). The nucleus of monocytes varies from being deeply indented or roughly kidney-shaped to having the form of a wide horseshoe (see Plate 6-1*H*). It may even become twisted over as an artifact of preparation. The chromatin of monocytes is less condensed and lighter staining than that of lymphocytes (compare *H* with *J* and *K* in Plate 6-1). The cytoplasm of monocytes is abundant and stains a distinctive pale blue or light blue-gray (see Plate 6-3*H*). Specific granules are lacking, but a few fine purple-staining (azurophilic) granules may be present in the cytoplasm. In EM sections, free ribosomes, a Golgi region, some rER, and scattered lysosomes corresponding to azurophilic granules are discernible in the cytoplasm.

Circulating monocytes, with only a limited capacity for phagocytosis, represent the immediate precursors of tissue macrophages that are actively phagocytic. After circulating in the blood for 1 to 3 days, monocytes enter body tissues and transform directly into macrophages. Substantial numbers of monocytes and neutrophils escape from the venules of acutely inflamed tissues. Monocytes represent a major source of certain cytokines (see Table 7-6). They have the potential for fusing with each other, producing foreign body giant cells and osteoclasts.

Summary

The main features of erythrocytes and platelets are summarized in Table 6-1. Among the circulating erythrocytes are 1% to 2% that are still slightly polychromatophilic and immature. With special staining they appear as reticulocytes. Erythrocytes have a finite life span of 100 to 120 days. Platelets are actively phagocytic during their 9 to 10 day period of circulation. By undergoing their release re-

TABLE 6-1

ERYTHROCYTES AND PLATELETS

	Erythrocytes	Platelets
Morphology and Staining in Blood Films[*]		
Cytoplasm	Mature: pink Immature: bluish pink	Pale blue, with purple granules
Nucleus	No nucleus	No nucleus
Diameter (mean)	7 μm	3 μm
Functions	Transport oxygen and carbon dioxide	Arrest bleeding
Blood Counts		
Total number per liter blood	4.3×10^{12} (women) 4.8×10^{12} (men)	150×10^9–350×10^9
Proportion of total number	Mature 97.5%–99% Immature 1%–2.5%	

[*] Wright's blood stain.

action, they elicit local blood coagulation and liberate the vasoconstrictor serotonin. At sites of blood vessel damage, platelet adhesion and aggregation curtails extravasation of blood.

The main features of leukocytes are summarized in Table 6-2. Distinction between the three types of granular leukocytes is based on differential staining of their specific granules. Neutrophils, and also lymphocytes and monocytes, contain additional lysosomal azurophilic granules. In eosinophils, however, the lysosomal granules correspond to the acidophilic specific granules.

Up to 5% of circulating neutrophils are band neutrophils. Mature neutrophils (polymorphs), efficient at phagocytosing bacteria, are a hallmark of acute inflammation. Eosinophils can regulate local allergic reactions, phagocytose antigen–antibody complexes, and destroy helminth parasites. Basophils, which closely resemble mast cells, respond to antigens by liberating histamine and other inflammatory mediators, occasionally in massive amounts affecting the entire body. Small lymphocytes are uniform in microscopic appearance but include both B and T cells, which collaborate in producing immune responses to antigens. Monocytes represent a moderately phagocytic precursor stage of macrophages. They can also give rise to giant cells and osteoclasts.

TABLE 6-2

LEUKOCYTES

	Granular Leukocytes			Nongranular Leukocytes	
	Neutrophils (Polymorphs)	**Eosinophils**	**Basophils**	**Lymphocytes**	**Monocytes**
*Morphology and Staining in Blood Films**					
Cytoplasm	Small mauve granules	Large red-to-purple granules	Large dark blue granules	Blue, without conspicuous granules	Pale blue, without conspicuous granules
Nucleus	Segmented (2–5 lobes)	2 lobes	2 lobes or segmented	Round or slightly indented	Indented oval or kidney shaped
Diameter (mean or range)	13 μm	15 μm	11 μm	Small: 6–9 μm Large: 9–15 μm	12–20 μm
Functions	Phagocytose bacteria	Counteract local allergic responses and mediate antiparasitic responses	Mediate systemic allergic responses	Mediate immune responses	Phagocytic precursor stage of macrophages, giant cells, and osteoclasts
Blood Counts					
Total number per liter blood (total leukocyte count, all types included) = 4.5×10^9–11×10^9					
Proportion of total number (= differential WBC count)	50%–70%	1%–4%	0.5%–1%	20%–40%	2%–6%

* Wright's blood stain.

Bibliography

Comprehensive

Beck WS, ed. Hematology, ed 5. Cambridge, Mass., MIT Press, 1991.

Bessis M. Living Blood Cells and Their Ultrastructure. New York, Springer-Verlag, 1973.

Cline MJ. The White Cell. Cambridge, MA, Harvard University Press, 1975.

Hoffbrand AV, Pettit JE. Color Atlas of Clinical Hematology, ed 2. London, Mosby-Wolfe, 1994.

Erythrocytes and Platelets

Bearer EL. Platelet membrane skeleton revealed by quick-freeze deep-etch. Anat Rec 227:1, 1990.

Bessis M. Corpuscles. In: Atlas of Red Blood Cell Shapes. Berlin, Springer-Verlag, 1974.

Mustard JF, Packham MA. The reaction of the blood to injury. In Mozat HZ, ed. Inflammation, Immunity and Hypersensitivity. Molecular and Cellular Mechanisms, ed 2. Hagerstown, Harper & Row, 1979, p 558.

Roth GJ. Platelets and blood vessels. The adhesion event. Immunol Today 13:100, 1992.

Surgenor D. The Red Blood Cell, ed 2, vols 1 and 2. New York, Academic Press, 1974.

Weiss JH. Platelet physiology and abnormalities of platelet function. N Engl J Med 293:531, 1975.

White JG. The secretory process in platelets. In Cantin M, ed. Cell Biology of the Secretory Process. Basel, S Karger, 1984, p 546.

White JG. Views of the platelet cytoskeleton at rest and at work. Ann NY Acad Sci 509:156, 1987.

Zucker MB. The functioning of blood platelets. Sci Am 242(6):86, 1980.

Leukocytes* and Their Roles in Inflammation

Abramson JS, Wheeler JG, eds. The Neutrophil. Oxford, IRL Press at Oxford University Press, 1993.

Bass DA. The functions of eosinophils. Ann Intern Med 91:120, 1979.

Bevilacqua MP, Nelson RM, Mannori G, Cecconi O. Endothelial-leukocyte adhesion molecules in human disease. Annu Rev Med 45:361, 1994.

Brines R, ed. Adhesion molecules. Immunol Today, Immune Receptor Suppl:17, 1996.

Dvorak AM. Ultrastructural morphology of basophils and mast cells. In: Blood Cell Biochemistry, vol 4, Basophil and Mast Cell Degranulation and Recovery. New York, Plenum Press, 1991, p 67.

Gleich GJ. Current understanding of eosinophil function. Hosp Pract 23:137, 1988.

Gleich GJ, Adolphonson CR, Leiferman KM. The biology of the eosinophilic leukocyte. Annu Rev Med 44:85, 1993.

Hastie R. Methods in laboratory investigation: Ultrastructure of human basophil leukocytes studied after spray freezing and freeze-substitution. Lab Invest 62:119, 1990.

Kay AB. The role of the eosinophil in physiological and pathological processes. In Thompson RA, ed. Recent Advances in Clinical Immunology, no 2. Edinburgh, Churchill Livingstone, 1980, p 113.

Kay AB, Corrigan CJ. Eosinophils and neutrophils. Br Med Bull 48:51, 1992.

Klebanoff SJ, Clark RA. The Neutrophil: Function and Clinical Disorders. New York, Elsevier/North Holland Biomedical Press, 1978.

Movat HZ. The Inflammatory Reaction. Amsterdam, Elsevier, 1985.

Parwaresch MR. The Human Basophil: Morphology, Origin, Kinetics, Function and Pathology. Berlin, Springer-Verlag, 1976.

Spry CJF, Kay AB, Gleich GJ. Eosinophils 1992. Immunol Today 13:384, 1992.

Weissmann G, ed. The cell biology of inflammation. In: Handbook of Inflammation, vol 2. Amsterdam, Elsevier/North Holland Biomedical Press, 1980.

*For references on Lymphocytes, see Chapter 7; see also Chapter 5, under Mast Cells.

CHAPTER 7

Myeloid Tissue, Lymphoid Tissue, and Immune System

OBJECTIVES

The information found in this chapter should enable you to do the following:

- Outline the basic functional organization of myeloid tissue
- Specify four distinctive characteristics of hematopoietic stem cells
- Name five hematopoietic progenitor cells present in myeloid tissue
- Distinguish morphologically between the erythroid and the granulocytic precursors in bone marrow films
- Compare the functional roles and distinguishing features of two important subclasses of small lymphocytes
- State key differences between cell-mediated and humoral immune responses
- Compare the basic histological organization and main functions of four different forms of lymphoid tissue

When blood cells terminate their useful life span, they must be renewed. Highly differentiated blood cells, however, do not divide. A continuing supply of new blood cells is nevertheless provided by the **hematopoietic (hemopoietic) tissues** (Gk. *hemato*, blood; *poiein*, to make), which are two of the special connective tissues derived from mesenchyme (see Table 5-1). An additional important function of hematopoietic tissues is elimination of old or worn-out blood cells. **Myeloid tissue,** alternatively known as **red bone marrow** (Gk. *myelos*, marrow), is the body's essential source of most kinds of blood cells. **Lymphoid (lymphatic) tissue,** the other hematopoietic tissue, is characterized by an evident abundance of lymphocytes. It is chiefly involved with the body's immune defenses. Whereas T lymphocytes differentiate in the thymus (one of the lymphoid organs), B cells arise in myeloid tissue, hence lymphocytes are not exclusively a product of lymphoid tissue, as was once generally assumed.

MYELOID TISSUE

Red bone marrow (myeloid tissue) is largely confined to the medullary cavity of certain flat bones. For marrow transplants, it may be taken from the **iliac crest** or **sternum** under local anesthesia. The **yellow marrow** typical of adult long bones stores fat instead of producing blood cells.

The histological organization of myeloid tissue is hard to discern in LM sections (Figs. 7-1 and 7-2). Basically, myeloid tissue consists of 1) a highly vascular **stroma,** made up of connective tissue cells with a supporting network of delicate reticular fibers, and 2) a heterogeneous population of **forming blood cells** at their various stages of differentiation and maturation.

Myeloid Sinusoids and Stromal Cells

Numerous wide venous channels known as **sinusoids** provide the escape route for the newly formed blood cells to enter the circulation from the stromal interstices. Blood flow is predominantly radially inward, from the cortical bone at the periphery of the medullary cavity to a wide central sinusoid. The stromal interstices are so tightly packed with blood-forming cells that the sinusoids are often difficult to recognize in sections of myeloid tissue (see Fig. 7-1). They become more evident, however, if hematopoiesis is temporarily inhibited (see Fig. 7-2). The fenestrated endothelial lining of their thin walls is supported by a discontinuous basement membrane and reticular fibers. Maturing blood cells are able to make transient **migration pores** through the attenuated endothelial cells margins, and squeeze through these pores to enter the lumen of the sinusoid. Imperfect new blood cells, residual cell fragments, and any blood-borne particles in the lumen are avidly phagocytosed by sinusoid-associated stromal macrophages.

In addition to sinusoid **endothelial cells** and the resident population of **macrophages**, myeloid stroma contains numerous **fibroblasts**. Collagen fibers produced by these cells reinforce the walls of the medullary blood vessels and provide strong internal support for the tissue. Some myeloid fibroblasts have *osteogenic* potential, meaning that they can produce bone-forming cells. A related but less well characterized type of stromal cell is the myeloid **reticular cell.** It should be noted that the word *reticular* is used to describe either 1) cells with long cytoplasmic processes, interconnecting with those of similar cells, that constitute a network (L. *rete*, net) or 2) cells that lay down networks of reticular fibers. Myeloid reticular cells originate from mesenchyme and produce networks of delicate **reticular fibers.** In H&E-stained sections, they appear comparatively large and pale staining.

Care should be taken to distinguish between the terms *reticular cell* and *reticulocyte* (an erythrocyte at the polychromatophilic stage).

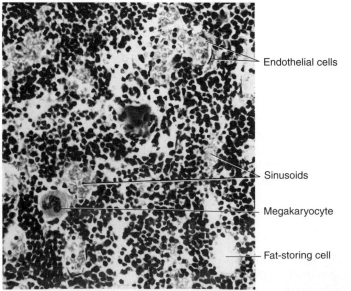

Endothelial cells

Sinusoids

Megakaryocyte

Fat-storing cell

Figure 7-1
Section of red bone marrow (low power).

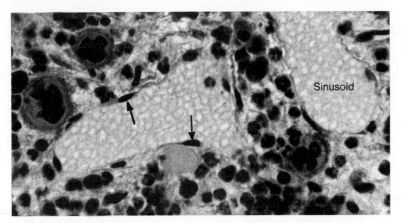

Figure 7-2
Sinusoids of myeloid tissue (mouse) following induced depletion of its hematopoietic cells. Arrows indicate nuclei of the fenestrated endothelial cells that constitute the sinusoidal lining.

Fat-storing cells, too, are plentiful in myeloid tissue. The same cells predominate in yellow marrow. The round empty spaces left when their fat is extracted (see Fig. 7-1) are often distinguishable from sinusoids by the fact that they contain no blood cells. Stromal fat-storing cells and some of the myeloid fibroblasts seem to originate from stromal reticular cells.

Myeloid stromal cells produce several **hematopoietic growth factors** that regulate myeloid cell production by acting primarily at early stages of differentiation. Hematopoietic growth factors are cell-to-cell signaling proteins (cytokines) that stimulate or inhibit specific hematopoietic functions. Stromal substrate-adherent fibroblast-like reticular cells, endothelial cells, and macrophages represent major sources of such factors (see Table 7-2).

We shall next consider the succession of cells and various differentiation pathways through which blood cells are renewed.

Myeloid Differentiation and Maturation

Myeloid tissue contains a diverse population of hematopoietic cells representing innumerable stages of blood cell differentiation and maturation. The earlier, poorly differentiated stages are rather uniform in microscopic appearance, but the subsequent stages may be recognized morphologically.

The blood cell-forming population of myeloid tissue is made up of 1) **self-renewing stem cells,** 2) **differentiating progenitors** that become progressively committed to specific cell lineages as differentiation advances, and 3) **functional blood cells** and derivatives such as platelets (Table 7-1).

The various types of blood cells are derived from **pluripotential hematopoietic stem cells,** small undifferentiated reserve cells with an extensive potential for proliferation and self-renewal that represent an enduring uncommitted hematopoietic compartment. Each of these pluripotential reserve cells can be life-saving because it has the capacity to regenerate the full hierarchy of hematopoietic cells in each blood cell lineage. Bearing some resemblance to small lymphocytes, pluripotential hematopoietic stem cells arise from mesenchymal cells of the embryonic **yolk sac.** Traveling by way of the bloodstream, they settle first in the **liver** and then the **spleen,** after which they seed the fetal **bone marrow.** In adult life they are present mostly in red marrow, which persists in the pelvis, sternum, ribs, vertebrae, skull, short bones, and proximal ends of the femora and humeri. Experimental studies indicate that the hematopoietic stem cell population is actually a composite of various successions of multipotential and pluripotential self-renewing cells, so

TABLE 7-1

HEMATOPOIETIC DIFFERENTIATION: (A) LYMPHOID AND (B) MYELOID LINEAGES

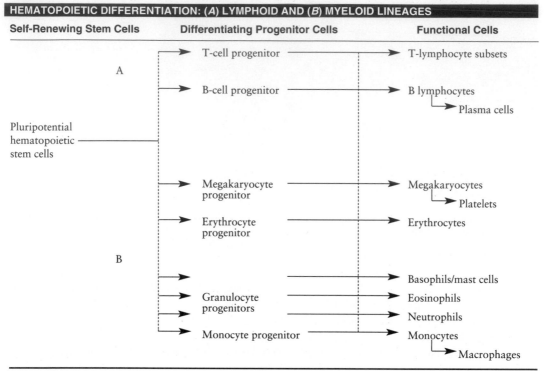

Self-Renewing Stem Cells	Differentiating Progenitor Cells	Functional Cells

hematopoietic stem cells should not be considered a single cell type. Postnatally, these stem cells remain quiescent (i.e., in G_0) unless they are triggered into cell cycle by a myeloid growth factor.

Not included in Table 7-1 is a putative further succession of stem cells with diminishing potentiality and diminishing self-renewal capacity. The progeny become increasingly restricted to **lymphoid** or **myeloid** lines of differentiation. Lymphoid lineages produce lymphocytes and plasma cells, whereas myeloid lineages produce the other blood cells and platelets (see Table 7-1).

Bone marrow transplantation succeeds if the recipient's marrow becomes permanently repopulated by pluripotential hematopoietic stem cells, also known as **myeloid repopulating cells.** These uncommitted stem cells seldom proliferate except to compensate for a substantial decline in the restricted stem cells and progenitor cells arising from them. Blood cell renewal on a day-to-day basis is primarily the result of proliferation and differentiation of progenitor cells, the cells that follow in the hierarchy.

Hematopoietic progenitor cells arise from the more restricted hematopoietic stem cells. Although capable of further differentiation, they have negligible capacity for self-renewal and hence are unable to replace themselves effectively. Furthermore, they become increasingly committed to specific cell lineages. Although progenitor cells are capable of producing microscopically recognizable differentiated progeny cells, until they do so they remain inconspicuous and unrecognizable from their individual microscopic appearances. The existence and respective potentialities of these cells has been deduced from the various kinds of cells present in the colonies that they produce in vitro.

Proliferation and differentiation of myeloid progenitors are precisely regulated by later-acting **myeloid growth factors** with various lineage specificities (Table 7-2). Erythrocyte production, for example, is stimulated by the glycoprotein hormone **erythropoietin**, which acts in the following

TABLE 7-2

MYELOID GROWTH FACTORS

	Factor*	Chief Sources**	Principal Responding Myeloid and Lymphoid Cells
Regulators of Early Myeloid Differentiation	IL-1	Macrophages, keratinocytes	Pluripotential stem cells, myeloid and lymphoid stem cells
	IL-3	T cells, macrophages	Pluripotential stem cells, early and intermediate myeloid progenitors
	IL-4	T cells	Pluripotential stem cells, lymphoid stem cells
	IL-6	T cells, macrophages, fibroblasts, endothelial cells	Early megakaryocyte and neutrophil progenitors, B cell progenitors
	SCF (MGF)	Myeloid stromal cells	Pluripotential stem cells, early myeloid progenitors, mast cell progenitors
	GM-CSF	T cells, fibroblasts, endothelial cells	Early, intermediate, and late myeloid progenitors
Later-Acting Regulators	EPO	Kidney peritubular interstitial cells***, liver	Intermediate and late erythroid progenitors
	TPO	Endothelial cells of liver sinusoids, myeloid stromal cells	Megakaryocyte progenitors, megakaryocytes
	G-CSF	Macrophages, fibroblasts, endothelial cells	Late neutrophil progenitors
	M-CSF	Macrophages, fibroblasts, endothelial cells	Intermediate and late monocyte progenitors
	IL-5	T cells	Late eosinophil progenitors

* Excluding inhibitory factors; *IL* denotes interleukin, *CSF* denotes colony stimulating factor, *EPO* denotes erythropoietin, and *TPO* denotes thrombopoietin.
** Fibroblast-like reticular cells are listed here as fibroblasts.
*** Precise cell type is uncertain.

manner. When erythrocytes age and are withdrawn from the circulation, the body's tissues suffer a slight deficit of oxygen. The kidneys compensate for this oxygen deficit by releasing erythropoietin, which stimulates the erythroid progenitor **CFU-E** to produce a colony of more differentiated erythroid cells that go on to synthesize hemoglobin and become erythrocytes. Other later-acting growth factors regulate platelet production and formation of the various leukocytes (see Table 7-2).

Progeny of the different hematopoietic progenitors are morphologically recognizable in marrow films. Forming blood cells that are not yet mature are often referred to as **blood cell precursors.** Without requiring further changes in gene expression, these precursors mature into fully functional **blood cells.**

B cell production from the B cell progenitor occurs in myeloid tissue. T cell production from T cell progenitor requires the special microenvironment of the thymic cortex.

Microscopically Recognizable Erythroid Precursors

The various stages of erythroid differentiation and maturation that are morphologically identifiable are listed in Table 7-3. The earliest recognizable precursor is the **proerythroblast**, a comparatively

TABLE 7-3

MATURATION OF ERYTHROCYTIC PRECURSORS

Proerythroblast
↓
Basophilic erythroblast
↓
Polychromatophilic erythroblast
↓
Normoblast
↓
Polychromatophilic erythrocyte
= Reticulocyte
↓
Mature erythrocyte

TABLE 7-4

MATURATION OF GRANULOCYTIC PRECURSORS

Myeloblast
↓
Promyelocyte
↓
Myelocyte
↓
Metamyelocyte
↓
Band form
↓
Mature (segmented) granulocyte

large cell with a large spherical nucleus, prominent nucleoli, and strikingly basophilic cytoplasm (Plate 7-1*A*). Present in greater frequency are the progeny of proerythroblasts, which are termed **basophilic erythroblasts.** These cells are slightly smaller than proerythroblasts. Their spherical nucleus is proportionately smaller and their chromatin is relatively more condensed (see Plate 7-1*B*). Their cytoplasm is diffusely basophilic because of an abundance of free ribosomes engaged in globin synthesis (see Fig. 3-6). At the next stage, known as the **polychromatophilic erythroblast,** the cell is smaller and the cytoplasmic staining is polychromatophilic because it represents both diffuse blue (basophilic) staining of RNA and diffuse pink (acidophilic) staining of hemoglobin. The net result is an intermediate bluish pink to muddy-gray (see Plate 7-1*C*). The spherical nucleus is proportionately smaller and its chromatin stains more intensely. The polychromatophilic erythroblast is the last stage of the erythroid series to undergo mitosis. At the following stage, termed the **normoblast,** the spherical nucleus is small, pyknotic, and dark-staining (see Plate 7-1*D*). The maturing red blood cell extrudes its pyknotic nucleus at a stage when the cytoplasm is still slightly polychromatophilic, producing a **polychromatophilic erythrocyte** (see Plate 7-1*E*). Erythrocytes that are still at this enucleated, immature stage can be discerned more readily as **reticulocytes** (see Plate 6-2 and Chap. 6 under Reticulocytes). Maturing erythrocytes enter the circulation by penetrating the endothelium of stromal sinusoids. After circulating for about 2 days, polychromatophilic erythrocytes lose their residual RNA and become fully mature erythrocytes (see Plate 7-1*F*).

Microscopically Recognizable Granulocytic Precursors

The morphologically identifiable stages of granulocytic differentiation and maturation are listed in Table 7-4 and shown in Figure 7-3. The largest cell in this series is the **promyelocyte**, which is the progeny cell of a less easily recognized precursor called the **myeloblast** (see Plate 7-1*G*). Promyelocytes possess an expansive, slightly indented nucleus with rather light-staining chromatin and a prominent nucleolus or nucleoli. Their copious cytoplasm, also light-staining, contains **azurophilic (primary) granules** (see Plate 7-1*H*). A promyelocyte's specific lineage (neutrophil, eosinophil, or basophil) is not yet perceptible, so only a single indeterminate type is recognized. At the subsequent **myelocyte** stage, however, the cell acquires an additional complement of distinctive **specific (secondary) granules** that stain the lineage-specific color. Myelocytes are smaller than promyelocytes,

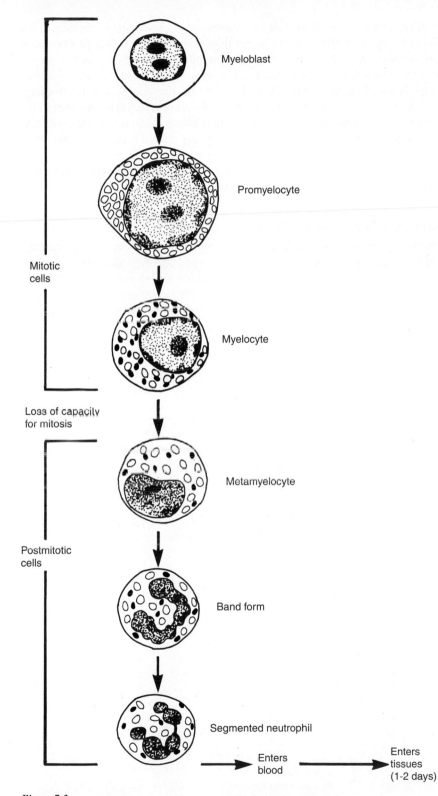

Myeloblast

Promyelocyte

Mitotic
cells

Myelocyte

Loss of capacity
for mitosis

Metamyelocyte

Postmitotic
cells

Band form

Segmented neutrophil

Enters
blood

Enters
tissues
(1-2 days)

Figure 7-3
Maturation of neutrophils (specific granules indicated in color).

and their granules are more abundant (see Plate 7-1*I*). Furthermore, most myelocytes belong to the neutrophilic series. The capacity for mitosis is lost at the myelocyte stage. The nucleus first becomes ovoid in shape and then develops an indentation. At the **metamyelocyte** stage (Gk. *meta*, beyond), the nucleus appears more or less kidney-shaped. Again, the distinction between the three different types of metamyelocytes is based on the color imparted to the specific granules. A neutrophilic metamyelocyte is shown in Plate 7-1*J*. Subsequent maturation of granulocytes involves overall reduction in size and change of nuclear shape, first to the **band** (horseshoe) form (see Plate 7-1*K*) and then to the progressively **segmented** (lobed) shape characterizing the mature granulocyte (see Plate 6-1*D* and *E*).

The precursors of monocytes and lymphocytes are harder to recognize than granulocytic precursors. Mature **lymphocytes** and **plasma cells** are also present among the hematopoietic cells.

Megakaryocyte Maturation and Platelet Formation

Platelets are derived from megakaryocytes, which are massive cells with a very large, dark-staining nucleus that consists of many interconnected lobes (see Fig. 7-2 and Plate 7-2). Careful focusing is sometimes necessary to distinguish megakaryocytes from osteoclasts, which are large multinucleated cells that resorb bone. But unlike osteoclasts, which lie along bone surfaces, megakaryocytes are distributed throughout myeloid tissue, and many of them are closely associated with stromal venous sinusoids (see Fig. 7-2). A hematopoietic growth factor called **thrombopoietin** (TPO) stimulates megakaryocyte production and maturation. In the process of maturing, the majority of megakaryocytes acquire eight times the typical somatic (diploid) number of chromosomes. Such extreme polyploidy is attained in the following way. Every time the megakaryocyte replicates its DNA

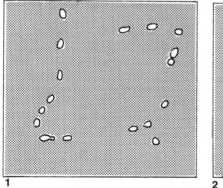
1

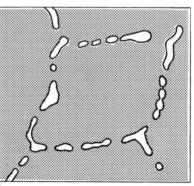
2

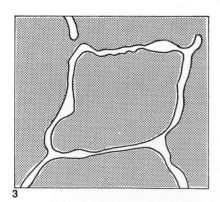
3

Figure 7-4
Platelet demarcation channels develop from rows of vesicles in the megakaryocyte cytoplasm.

and enters mitosis, its cytoplasm fails to divide. This **endoreduplication** leads to endogenous generation of multiple diploid sets of chromosomes. The resulting daughter chromosomes, however, fail to segregate and do not form separate nuclei. Instead, they recombine into a single massive nucleus that as a result becomes increasingly multilobed, a unique form of chromosomal rearrangement termed **endomitosis**. Megakaryocytes produce platelets only after they have attained a significant degree of polyploidy. Electron micrographs indicate that megakaryocytic cytoplasm can fragment through the formation of tiny channels arising from rows of vesicles (Fig. 7-4). The vesicles fuse with their neighbors and establish continuity with the cell membrane, producing an extensive system of tubular **platelet demarcation channels** that subdivide the cytoplasm into platelet-sized portions (Fig. 7-5). Separation along these channels can produce hundreds of platelets each with its covering membrane. Cytoplasmic processes of megakaryocytes are also able to protrude into sinusoids as **proplatelet processes** that can constrict to form strings of detaching platelets. Large numbers of platelets are liberated by progressive fragmentation of megakaryocytic cytoplasm. This is the likely fate of any whole megakaryocytes (or substantial cytoplasmic masses detaching from them) that on entering the circulation from myeloid stromal sinusoids subsequently become trapped in pulmonary capillary beds.

LYMPHOID TISSUE AND IMMUNE SYSTEM

Lymphoid tissue, the second hematopoietic tissue, is represented by the group of body organs and related structures listed in Table 7-5. Lymph nodes, which filter lymph passing through lymphatics before its return to the blood, are not only a form of lymphoid tissue and therefore a part of the **immune system,** but also a part of the **lymphatic system,** which is the lymph-draining part of the circulatory system.

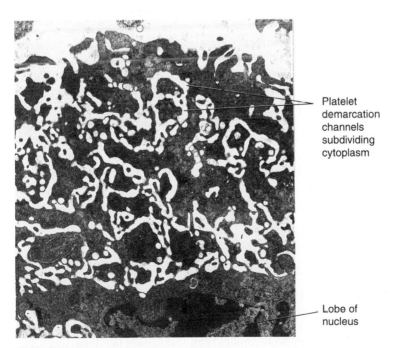

Platelet
demarcation
channels
subdividing
cytoplasm

Lobe of
nucleus

Figure 7-5
Electron micrograph of a megakaryocyte (mouse), showing platelet demarcation channels along which it subdivides, producing platelets.

TABLE 7-5

LYMPHOID ORGANS AND TISSUES

Thymus

Lymphoid follicles (nodules)
    Solitary type
    Aggregate type
        Tonsils
        Peyer's patches
        Appendix

Lymph nodes

Spleen

A distinctive feature of the various lymphoid organs is that they are all heavily populated with lymphocytes. This is reflection of the roles that these organs play in producing lymphocytes or mediating immune responses. The **thymus** is considered a **primary lymphoid organ** because its chief role is T cell production, and it is not specifically designed to facilitate immune responses. Such responses are, however, facilitated to various extents by the other lymphoid organs, which are termed **secondary lymphoid organs** because when their constituent lymphocyte populations expand, it is a consequence of antigenic stimulation of pre-existing responsive cells.

Strategically situated lymphoid tissue represent an essential part of the **immune system** (a *system* is a group of components that collectively carry out some special function for the body as a whole). An important function of the immune system is the mounting of resistance to disease-causing microorganisms. Tell-tale traces of foreign antigens, released from infecting microorganisms or from atypical cells that express unusual antigens, can build up locally in tissue fluid and elicit immune responses. Diffusely distributed **lymphoid follicles** or **lymphoid (lymphatic) nodules** are unencapsulated groups of B cells that are involved in responses to such local accumulations of antigens. Lymphoid follicles are often present in the loose connective tissue layer (**lamina propria**) bordering on a wet epithelium that is either subject to infection or openly exposed to exogenous antigens. Since excess tissue fluid and any antigens that it may contain collects as lymph, these antigens reach **lymph nodes,** the small bean-shaped structures that filter the lymph flowing along lymphatics. Lymphocytes that become suitably exposed to foreign antigens present in lymph can mediate immune responses to them. Hence, immune responses to lymph-borne antigens occur in lymph nodes. Lymph flowing through lymph nodes also comes into contact with numerous macrophages that engulf infecting microorganisms and other suspended particulate matter. The role of the **spleen** is complementary to that of lymph nodes. The lymphocytes in the spleen become exposed to any foreign antigens that may be present in the blood. Hence, immune responses to blood-borne antigens occur in the spleen. In addition, the spleen efficiently eliminates worn-out blood cells and suspended particulate matter from the blood.

Functional Roles of B and T Cells

Lymphocytes cross over from the peripheral blood to lymph and then return to the bloodstream on a continual basis. Also, vast numbers of them temporarily reside in secondary lymphoid organs. Lymphocytes are able to escape from the blood circulation by way of unusual blood vessels in lymph nodes. Many of these liberated cells join the resident lymphoid cell populations in lymph nodes, but others are swept away in the lymph flow and return to the blood along with lymph. The dual pathway taken by these continuously **recirculating** lymphocytes (blood to lymph, then back to blood again) increases the likelihood that they will encounter any foreign antigens entering the body. Such encounters can lead to immune responses, indicating that lymphocytes are **immunocompetent.**

Immune responses are of two main types. One type (already mentioned in Chapter 5 in connection with plasma cells) leads to the production of antigen-specific **circulating immunoglobulins (antibodies)** and is termed the **humoral antibody response.** Primarily a response to infectious bacteria, it is mediated by B cells and their progeny (plasmablasts and plasma cells), but T cells have to help by producing certain cytokines as well. The second type of immune response is chiefly a response to infectious viruses, antigenically different or foreign cells, or fungi. Termed the **cell-mediated immune response,** it produces antigen-specific **killer cells,** which are **cytotoxic** (cell-killing) **T cells** capable of destroying antigenically altered cells. Mediated by a particular subset of T cells, the cell-mediated immune response does not depend on the participation of B cells. Each type of immune response is the outcome of various interactions between lymphocytes and the specific antigens that they recognize.

B lymphocytes are so named because in chickens they are derived from a cloacal lymphoid organ called the **bursa of Fabricius** (*B* for *bursa*). Human and other mammalian B cells, however, arise from progenitor cells (**pre-B cells**) that in postnatal life are present in **red bone marrow.** Many B cells subsequently congregate in secondary lymphoid organs. **T cells,** on the other hand, are derived from progenitor cells (**prothymocytes** or **prethymocytes**) that enter the **thymus** (*T* for *thymus*). A critical step in the differentiation of both B cells and T cells is individual **programming** for antigen recognition. This process confers a particular **antigenic specificity** on the developing lymphocyte. Programming for antigen recognition occurs independently in each lymphocyte, and all progeny of each programmed lymphocyte retain the identical antigenic specificity. The initial programming process takes place without requiring the participation of the antigen concerned. In this manner, the body builds up and maintains an extensive repertoire of both types of lymphocytes, each type having the potential to recognize every conceivable foreign antigen. Hence, for any given foreign antigen that might enter the body, there are likely to be pre-existing lymphocytes capable of recognizing it.

Morphologically, small lymphocytes individually respond to specific antigens by acquiring intense cytoplasmic basophilia and then enlarging rapidly. This induced change in their histological appearance reflects accelerated synthesis of RNA and proteins. Each responding lymphocyte then enters the S phase of the cell cycle and undergoes a series of divisions that produces a clone of cells with the same antigenic specificity (a *clone* is the progeny of a single cell). The antigen-induced process that leads to such clonal expansion is known as **lymphocyte activation.** Lymphocytes that are responding to antigen (**activated lymphocytes**) can enlarge to a diameter of 30 μm, thereby becoming even larger than the large lymphocytes of peripheral blood. Next, we shall discuss how each type of small lymphocyte responds to a specific antigen.

Role of B Cells in Humoral Immune Responses

B cells programmed to recognize a particular antigen express small patches of **surface membrane immunoglobulin** specific for that antigen. Known also as the **B cell antigen receptor,** the surface membrane immunoglobulin is an integral cell membrane protein of the B cell. It provides the molecular basis for specific antigen recognition and serves as a distinctive B cell recognition marker.

B CELL ACTIVATION

Few foreign antigens activate B cells unless these cells receive synergistic signals. For most antigens, the B cells in G_0 need to come into contact not only with their specific antigen but also with certain cytokines secreted by helper T cells activated by the same antigen. Furthermore, a number of other interleukins from helper T cells are necessary 1) to induce activated B cells to proliferate and 2) to enable resulting B cell progeny to mature. The chief cytokines involved are listed in Table 7-6. In general, then, B cells produce substantial clones of antibody-producing cells only after becoming exposed to the necessary T cell lymphokines as well as the specific antigen. These stringent multiple requirements minimize the risk of accidental humoral immune responses.

TABLE 7-6

INTERLEUKIN INVOLVEMENT IN IMMUNE RESPONSES

Factor	Chief Sources	Principal Responding Lymphoid Cells
IL-1	Macrophages, keratinocytes, fibroblasts, hepatocytes, glial cells, B cells	T cells, B cells, macrophages
IL-2	Activated helper T cells	T cells, B cells
IL-4	Activated helper T cells	B cells, T cells
IL-5	Activated helper T cells	B cells
IL-6	Activated helper T cells, B cells, macrophages, fibroblasts, endothelial cells, hepatocytes	Immature B cells, T cells
IL-7	Myeloid stromal cells, thymic cortical epithelial reticular cells	Immature B cells, immature T cells
IL-9	Activated T cells	T cells
IL-10	Activated helper T cells	T cells, B cells
IL-12	Monocytes	T cells
IL-13	Activated T cells	B cells, monocytes
IL-14	Activated T cells	B cells
IL-15	Monocytes	B cells, T cells

Many progeny cells of activated B cells mature into **plasma cells,** the presence of which is considered histological evidence of humoral antibody responses. Plasma cells and their immediate precursors **(plasmablasts)** are able to synthesize and secrete relatively large amounts of specific immunoglobulin. Other progeny cells resemble small lymphocytes and persist chiefly in the secondary lymphoid organs as long-lived **memory B cells.** Because they represent clonally expanded descendants of B cells already activated by antigen, memory B cells produce quicker, more extensive **secondary responses** during subsequent challenges with the same antigen.

Roles of T Cells in Cell-Mediated and Humoral Immune Responses

The long-lived, recirculating T cells that represent 65% to 80% of the peripheral blood lymphocytes do not synthesize immunoglobulins. The molecular structure of the antigen-specific **T cell antigen receptor** (TCR) on their cell surface is different from that of the surface membrane immunoglobulin on B cells. Another difference between T cells and B cells lies in the **CD antigens** (*CD* denoting a *c*luster of *d*ifferentiation) that T cells express during and following their differentiation in the thymic cortex. The surface markers **CD4** and **CD8**, for example, facilitate identification of various functional subsets of T cells.

The process of intrathymic T cell differentiation produces a number of different T cell subsets, including effector cells of the cell-mediated immune response and cells that can regulate both types of immune responses. Further details now follow.

Cytotoxic T cells are effector cells of the cell-mediated immune response. Known also as **killer cells,** they specifically recognize antigenically different or altered target cells and can destroy these cells, chiefly by ravaging the selective permeability of their cell membrane. One mechanism by which this is achieved is through release of **perforin,** a potentially cytolytic protein present in the killer cell's secretory granules. When this cell adheres to its target cell, rearrangement of its cytoplasmic microtubules shifts its Golgi apparatus and secretory granules to the lethal contact area. Perforin is then discharged by exocytosis into the intercellular space at the site of contact. Recognition of the target cell is highly specific, but the ensuing cell destruction is nonspecific.

The liberated perforin molecules become inserted into the lipid bilayer of the target cell membrane, and during their incorporation they polymerize into open cylindrical transmembrane channels. Another way in which cytotoxic T cells destroy their target cells is through induction of the apoptotic pathway.

Regulatory T cells are of two contrasting types. **Helper T cells** up-regulate immune responses by producing a broad range of lymphokines capable of inducing proliferation, secretion, differentiation, and maturation in lymphocytes (see Table 7-6). A separate population of helper T cells up-regulates each main type of immune response. **Suppressor T cells** downregulate each main type of immune response. In general, helper T cells express CD4 whereas cytotoxic T cells and suppressor T cells express CD8. **Memory T cells,** the counterpart of memory B cells, are long-lived progeny of T cells. **Delayed hypersensitivity T cells** produce lymphokines that bring about delayed hypersensitivity reactions.

T CELL ACTIVATION

T cells do not become activated unless several necessary rigorous conditions are met. Whereas B cells can be triggered into cell cycle by direct contact with foreign antigens, T cells respond to few antigens unless they are suitably presented in the form of enzymatically processed **peptide fragments.** Furthermore, it is necessary for the peptide fragments to be co-presented on the surface of an **antigen-presenting cell** in intimate molecular association with certain integral membrane glycoproteins encoded by genes of the **major histocompatibility complex (MHC).** In other words, co-recognition of a peptide fragment of the foreign antigen along with a self-MHC encoded glycoprotein (MHC Class II glycoprotein in the case of helper T cells) on the same cell surface is required. The essential molecular association between a self-MHC glycoprotein and a foreign antigen-derived peptide that is recognized during T cell activation is often described as a **T cell recognition complex.** Besides providing this recognition complex, antigen-presenting cells such as macrophages produce **interleukin-1** (IL-1 in Table 7-6) and alternative **co-stimulatory signals** (notably the **B7-1** and **B7-2** surface molecules on antigen-presenting cells) that by interacting with co-receptors on helper T cells act as a supplementary part of the T cell activation signal.

To a certain extent, localization of B and T cell activation in the development of immune responses accounts for the histological organization of the secondary lymphoid organs in the immune system, soon to be considered. Another factor that to some extent determines lymphocyte distribution outside and within lymphoid organs is **targeted lymphocyte migration.** In contrast to antigenically unstimulated lymphocytes, which recirculate continuously through the secondary lymphoid organs, it is common for **memory cells** and **effector lymphocytes** to show a *tissue-selective* pattern of accumulation. This is because they have a tendency to **home** to body sites where they are likely to re-encounter the same specific antigen. For example, plasma cell precursors ready to secrete IgA accumulate in the loose connective tissue layer (lamina propria) under wet epithelial surfaces. Generally, lymphocyte homing involves up-regulation or induced expression of microenvironmental **homing receptors** on the cell surface as part of the lymphocyte's activation response to specific antigen.

Lymphoid Organs

Lymphoid tissue is distributed widely throughout the body, chiefly in these lymphoid organs.

Thymus

The **thymus,** a primary lymphoid organ, is a bilobed endocrine gland that lies mostly within the superior mediastinum, behind the upper part of the sternum. During childhood the thymus is active, but from puberty to old age it undergoes progressive atrophy and produces declining numbers of T cells. In addition, this organ produces a number of **thymic hormones** that support proliferation and differentiation of **T cell progenitors (prothymocytes).** Besides its densely packed content of differentiating T cells, the thymus is characterized by **thymic epithelial reticular cells** that are mostly arranged in a loose network. This epithelial network is supported by a connective tissue **capsule** and **septa.** The outer, dark-staining region of the thymus is known as its **cortex** and the inner, pale-staining region is called its **medulla** (Plate 7-3*A*). The reticular cells of the thymus are heterogeneous and dendritic in shape, with long cytoplasmic processes. They lack associated reticular fibers but are held together by desmosomes. Derived mostly from the endodermal lining of the third pharyngeal pouches of the embryo, the epithelial cells of the thymic cortex are the source of at least three thymic hormones (**thymosin, thymulin,** and **thymopoietin**) and several other differentiation-inducing cytokines. In the thymic medulla, the epithelial cells are also partly arranged as spherical structures known as **thymic (Hassal's) corpuscles** (see Plate 7-3*B*). Consisting of concentric layers of flat nonsecreting epithelial cells that eventually keratinize, these distinctive whorls of acidophilic cells are unique to the thymic medulla.

The thymus is incompletely subdivided into lobules by septa that extend inward from the fibrous capsule (see Plate 7-3*A*). The only blood vessels supplying the thymic cortex are looped capillaries that extend out into the cortex from arterioles at the corticomedullary border. Each cortical capillary is invested by a perivascular epithelial sheath made up of processes of epithelial reticular cells. These processes constitute a part of the **blood–thymus barrier** that limits the concentration of blood-borne antigens reaching T cells differentiating in the cortex. Furthermore, no afferent lymphatics supply the thymus, as they do in the case of lymph nodes. The thymus is provided only with **efferent lymphatics** that transport lymph and lymphocytes away from the organ.

THYMIC T CELL PRODUCTION

T cells differentiate exclusively in the thymic cortex. In response to the thymic hormones, T cell progenitors proliferate in the outer cortex and the differentiating T cells accumulate between progenitor-associated epithelial reticular cells. The thymic medulla is relatively pale in appearance (see Plate 7-3*A*). T cells are able to pass from the thymic cortex into the venules and efferent lymphatics along the corticomedullary border. Many of them, however, pass into the thymic medulla where they undergo further selection and maturation before leaving the thymus by entering its medullary venules and efferent lymphatics. The circulating T cells then undergo several days of extra-thymic maturation.

Although the thymic cortex continues to generate T cells with diverse antigenic specificities, only 5 percent of the forming T cells survive. T cells that are double-positive for CD4 and CD8 generally perish. The only T cells that endure are those able to recognize self-MHC encoded surface glycoproteins, and therefore antigen-presenting cells belonging to the same person. Programming for antigen recognition does not require presence of the antigen. Indeed, the thymic microenvironment in which it occurs contains comparatively low levels of blood-borne or lymph-borne antigens. Lymphoid follicles resulting from B cell activation are lacking in the thymus. Plasma cells are uncommon even in the thymic medulla where both types of recirculating lymphocytes abound. The thymic medulla contains marrow-derived **thymic dendritic cells** believed to be involved in 1) T cell selection and maturation and 2) tolerance development (i.e., specific non-reactivity to a foreign antigen). The medulla differs from the cortex in that it is not a site where T cells with new antigenic specificities are generated. Macrophages present in both the cortex and the medulla produce differentiation-inducing cytokines. They also dispose of cellular debris and residual macromolecules not carried away by the comparatively permeable medullary blood vessels.

In contrast to the thymus, the **secondary lymphoid organs** of the immune system are to a variable extent designed to *facilitate immune responses.* The simplest arrangement is found in lymphoid follicles.

Lymphoid Follicles

The loose connective tissue associated with the epithelial linings of the digestive, respiratory, and urinary tracts commonly contains more or less spherical groups of small lymphocytes (Plate 7-4). Known as **lymphoid follicles (nodules)**, these accumulations of lymphocytes are not confined by surrounding connective tissue capsules. Most lymphoid follicles are solitary, small, and discrete, with a diameter approaching 1 mm or so. At certain sites, however, lymphoid follicles are multiple, large, and confluent. Such sites include 1) the **tonsils**, which are aggregates of more or less unencapsulated lymphoid tissue that lie in the walls of the pharynx and nasopharynx and at the base of the tongue, constituting an incomplete ring around the crossing paths of the gastrointestinal and respiratory tracts; 2) **Peyer's patches,** which are large masses of confluent lymphoid follicles situated mostly in the walls of the ileum, a region of the small intestine; and 3) the **appendix**, which can have conspicuously large unencapsulated lymphoid follicles in its walls. Under low power, lymphoid follicles are distinguishable as rounded accumulations of dark blue nuclei (see Plate 7-4). The boundaries of the follicles are diffuse because the lymphocytes lie free in loose connective tissue without a surrounding capsule.

Although wet epithelia have certain structural adaptations for excluding foreign materials from the body, temporary discontinuities may develop in them as a result of epithelial cell death, or accidental leakage may occur between the constituent cells, admitting foreign antigens or infectious microorganisms. Solitary lymphoid follicles represent sites where B cells exposed to such antigens have produced a number of clonal progeny. The presence of a lighter-staining **germinal center** in a lymphoid follicle indicates that some of its activated B cells are still enlarged and proliferating. Also, the presence of **plasma cells** under wet epithelial membranes is related to the fact that many progeny cells of activated B cells become plasma cells.

The solitary, discrete lymphoid follicles present in loose connective tissue form whenever B cells become activated through fortuitous exposure to the antigen for which they are programmed. Solitary lymphoid follicles are transitory structures. The permanent secondary lymphoid organs have a more complex organization that 1) increases the likelihood that their transient internal lymphocyte population will encounter and respond to foreign antigens and 2) expedites the necessary diverse interactions between antigen-presenting accessory cells, T cells, and B cells.

GUT-ASSOCIATED LYMPHOID TISSUE

A marginally higher level of complexity is present in permanent aggregates of lymphoid follicles that are multiple, confluent, and large. Foreign antigens that penetrate a mucosal epithelium diffuse through the lamina propria. Furthermore, the epithelial coverings of the palatine tonsils and Peyer's patches, and also the epithelial lining of the appendix, are provided with special flat epithelial cells known as **M** (*membrane-like*) **cells** or **FAE** (*follicle-associated epithelial*) **cells**. These thinly stretched dome-shaped cells ingest tiny amounts of antigens entering the gut lumen and deliver them to antigen-presenting cells and lymphocytes of the **gut-associated lymphoid tissue** (Fig. 7-6). Antigen sampling by these flat epithelial cells is an important preliminary stage in the formation of IgA-producing plasma cells. The **secretory IgA** secreted onto the free surface of mucosal epithelia represents a primary mucosal defense mechanism against infection because appropriate antigen-specific IgAs are able to decrease microbial adhesion to host cells and neutralize bacterial toxins and viruses.

Lymph Nodes

Strategically positioned along the length of large lymphatics are kidney-shaped structures up to 2 cm long known as **lymph nodes.** In common with the thymus, lymph nodes have a **capsule, cortex,** and **medulla**. In contrast to the thymus, however, the cortex of lymph nodes contains **lymphoid follicles** (Plate 7-5). Progeny cells of B cells proliferating in the follicles pass directly into the medulla. The organization of lymph nodes enables them to carry out two useful functions at the same time. First, their abundant macrophages are able to clear the lymph by removing any bacteria or other particulate matter that it may contain. In cancer patients, the trapping and filtering function of lymph nodes can lead to colonization of individual nodes or groups of nodes by lymph-borne cancer cells that have dissociated from a primary tumor. Hence, lymph nodes tend to be a site of secondary (metastatic) malignant growth. The second major function of lymph nodes is that they are a site of local cell-mediated and humoral immune responses. As a result of activation by one or more foreign antigens present in the lymph, their lymphocyte content undergoes clonal expansion. Killer cells,

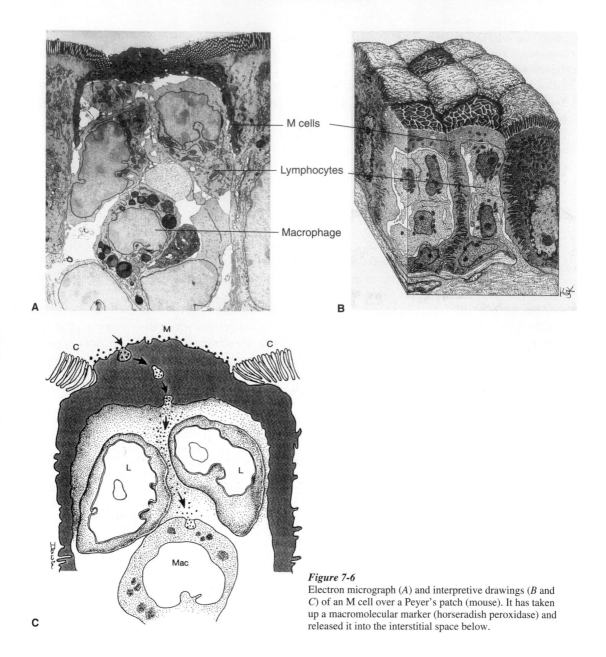

M cells

Lymphocytes

Macrophage

Figure 7-6
Electron micrograph (*A*) and interpretive drawings (*B* and *C*) of an M cell over a Peyer's patch (mouse). It has taken up a macromolecular marker (horseradish peroxidase) and released it into the interstitial space below.

plasma cell precursors, and other progeny of activated lymphocytes may leave the node and enter the recirculating pool by way of the efferent lymph. Germinal centers that form in response to foreign antigens do not persist when the antigens disappear, hence sections of lymph nodes provide only static, transitory impressions of the various functional activities taking place in these structures.

The substantial limiting **capsule** of a lymph node is composed of dense connective tissue. It is most evident under low power (Fig. 7-7). Lymph enters by way of **afferent lymphatics** that open onto the convex surface of the node. It leaves by way of **efferent lymphatics** that are situated in the recess (**hilum**) on the concave surface of the node. Connective tissue **trabeculae** extending from the capsule into the node provide substantial support and convey large blood vessels. Within the node,

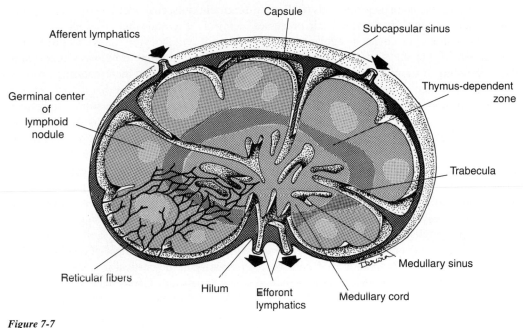

Figure 7-7
Basic histologic organization of a lymph node.

lymphocytes are held in place by a delicate stroma that consists chiefly of reticular fibers, with associated stromal cells that include macrophages, reticular cells, and fibroblasts. The macrophages are highly phagocytic and serve as antigen-presenting cells, the role of which is described earlier under T Cell Activation. Also present in the cortex is a second type of antigen presenting cell. Known as the **follicular dendritic cell** or **dendritic reticular cell,** it possesses long, pale-staining cytoplasmic processes (Gk. *dendron*, tree). Similar dendritic cells are also found in Peyer's patches and white pulp of the spleen (see later). Although only mildly phagocytic, the dendritic cells of lymph nodes are able to trap antigens and present them on their surface as antigen—antibody complexes.

Lymph reaching the node from the afferent lymphatics enters the **subcapsular sinus,** a narrow lymph space that lies just deep to the capsule (see Fig. 7-7). From this sinus, lymph passes by way of narrow channels termed **cortical sinuses** into **medullary sinuses** and leaves through efferent lymphatics. All these sinuses are lined by a discontinuous layer of simple squamous endothelium, and in addition to lymph they contain lymphocytes and macrophages. The capsule, trabeculae, and intimate supporting stroma of the node (including the endothelial lining of the sinuses) constitute its connective tissue component.

The interstices of the reticular fiber meshwork between cortical sinuses house abundant small lymphocytes (see Plate 7-5 and Fig. 7-7). The medullary reticular meshwork is packed with small lymphocytes and maturing plasma cells. In response to antigenic stimulation, the cortical lymphocyte population forms rounded aggregates, many of which have a pale spherical **germinal center.** Called **lymphoid follicles,** these rounded accumulations have a transitory existence. Lymphoid follicles without germinal centers are termed **primary follicles,** whereas those with germinal centers are termed **secondary follicles.**

The **germinal centers** of secondary follicles are sites of antigen-elicited B cell proliferation, and their presence is indicative of immune responses that are either prolonged or secondary. Within germinal centers it is possible to find mitotic figures and large, activated B cells with basophilic cytoplasm. Also present are dendritic cells (**follicular dendritic cells,** characterized by a large, pale-staining nucleus and indistinct cytoplasmic processes), a few T cells, and some macrophages.

From the lymphoid follicles, irregular tapering columns of lymphocytes, known as **paracortical cords,** extend into the medulla. Here, the columns subdivide into multiple wavy **medullary cords** representing tortuous stromal channels packed with lymphocytes and their maturing progeny (see Plate 7-5). A special feature of the deep cortical region of lymph nodes is that it contains distinctive **postcapillary venules** that elsewhere in the body would be lined with a simple squamous endothelium. In the deep cortex (**paracortex**) of lymph nodes, these vessels are lined with **simple cuboidal endothelium** instead (Fig. 7-8). The distinctive venules are accordingly known as **high endothelial venules (HEVs).** The functional significance of HEVs is that large numbers of circulating blood lymphocytes (e.g., unstimulated T cells) recognize and adhere to adhesion molecules on their high endothelial cells and then migrate between these cells into the deep cortical region of nodes. The term **thymus-dependent zone** (see Fig. 7-7) was originally used for the paracortical region to indicate that it is heavily populated with T cells entering from HEVs. Also present in this region are antigen-presenting cells called **interdigitating dendritic cells.**

HEVs represent the crossover point where small lymphocytes pass from peripheral blood into lymph nodes and lymph. Activation of T cells occurs primarily in the cortical regions that lie between lymphoid follicles. Following antigen-elicited clonal expansion, T cells leave by way of the efferent lymph. B cells passing into nodes from HEVs become preferentially incorporated into cortical follicles. In the primary follicles B cells predominate, and they are present along with T cells in the **follicular mantle** that surrounds the germinal center in secondary follicles. Medullary cords contain B cells, along with large numbers of **plasma cells** that arise from B cells activated in the cortex. For their entire lifespan of approximately 3 days, most of these plasma cells stay in the medullary cords, liberating their immunoglobulin in the efferent lymph. Fully differentiated plasma cells are not abundant in lymph and they are only rarely found in the peripheral blood. The main class of immunoglobulin produced by lymph nodes is IgG.

Spleen

The left upper quadrant of the abdominal cavity contains the spleen, the body's largest lymphoid organ. The major splenic blood vessels enter or leave the spleen at its **hilum,** a shallow recess that ex-

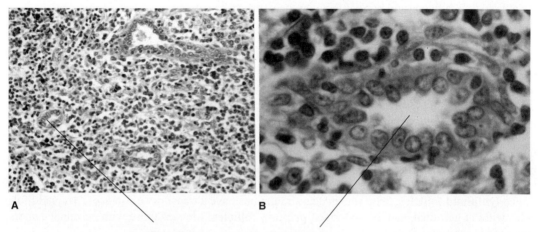

A   B

Postcapillary venules lined with simple
cuboidal endothelium

Figure 7-8
Postcapillary venules in a lymph node. (*A*) Low power view. (*B*) High power view.

tends along its medial border. In common with the thymus, the spleen possesses only **efferent** lymphatics, which also leave at its hilum. The general organization of the spleen is understandable if two of its major functions are appreciated. The first important function is **antibody formation.** Splenic B cells activated by blood-borne antigens give rise to vast numbers of plasma cells. So many plasma cells are produced in the spleen that it represents the body's chief source of circulating antibodies. The second key function of the spleen is to *dispose of defective blood cells.* Easy access of the spleen's vast population of avidly phagocytic macrophages to cells circulating in the peripheral blood facilitates efficient removal of blood cells or platelets that are deteriorating, along with debris and suspended particulate matter. The spleen also concentrates and stores certain blood cells and platelets. Yet if surgical removal of the spleen becomes necessary, its key functions are carried out by other hematopoietic tissues.

One major component of the spleen facilitates immune responses to blood-borne antigens; another eliminates worn-out blood cells and platelets. Both components lie within a fibrous **capsule** covered by simple squamous mesothelium (Fig. 7-9 and Plate 7-6). The capsule contains smooth muscle cells and elastic fibers as well as collagen fibers, but in the human spleen it is only minimally contractile. Extending in from the hilum and capsule are connective tissue **trabeculae** that provide internal support for the spleen and convey its blood vessels. Internal to the capsule lies soft **splenic pulp** of two distinct types, distinguishable with the unaided eye on a cut surface of the spleen. In the fresh state, **white pulp** appears as tiny pale islands scattered throughout the **red pulp,** which appears bright red. The splenic pulp is internally supported by reticular fibers. However, it is not organized into cortical and medullary regions or subdivided into lobules. Spleen sections disclose that the tiny islands of white pulp are primarily **lymphoid follicles** (Fig. 7-10). The contrasting red color of the red pulp is due to its abundant content of erythrocytes. This second major component of the spleen serves as a blood filter that removes worn-out blood cells, platelets, and suspended particulate matter from the circulation.

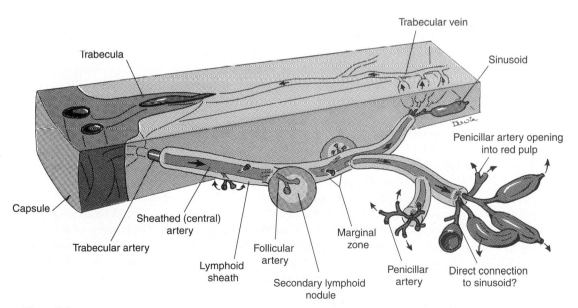

Figure 7-9
Basic histologic organization of the spleen, showing the close association of splenic white pulp with arterial vessels. Penicillar arteries open into an extensive extravascular reticular meshwork lying between venous sinusoids of the red pulp. Blood cells entering sinusoids return through trabecular veins.

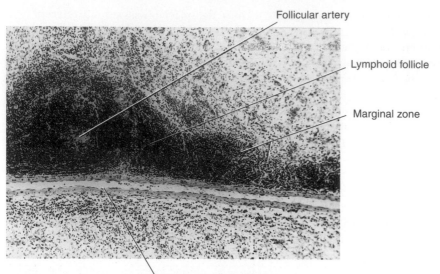

Figure 7-10
Sheathed (central) artery of the spleen, showing the associated lymphoid sheath, a lymphoid follicle and follicular artery, and the border between the white pulp and red pulp (marginal zone).

SPLENIC WHITE PULP

Splenic trabeculae constitute an irregularly branching, tree-like structure that conveys branches of the splenic artery to all internal regions of the spleen. Small arterial branches projecting from the trabeculae supply oxygen and nutrients to the splenic pulp. Each extending artery is invested by a **lymphoid sheath** consisting of a reticular fiber network with a dense population of **small lymphocytes** and some antigen-presenting **dendritic cells** in its interstices (see Fig. 7-9 and Plate 7-6). Scattered along the **sheathed (central) arteries** and **arterioles** supplying the pulp are multiple **lymphoid follicles** (see Figs. 7-9 and 7-10). A distinguishing feature of the splenic lymphoid follicle is its unique association with a fine branch of the splenic artery (see Fig. 7-10). The so-called **follicular artery** supplying follicular capillaries is in fact an arteriole. Hence, the splenic **white pulp** consists of **lymphoid sheaths** and **lymphoid follicles** intimately associated with arterial extensions emerging from trabeculae to supply the splenic pulp.

Periarterial and periarteriolar lymphoid sheaths are abundantly populated with **T cells.** These cells reach the sheaths by way of terminal arterioles that extend radially from sheathed arteries and open into the **marginal zone,** which is the extensive interface between white pulp and red pulp (see Figs. 7-9 and 7-10). In contrast, the lymphoid follicles of the white pulp are densely populated with **B cells.** Some B cells also remain in the marginal zone, near their site of discharge from radial terminal arterioles. Formation of secondary follicles with germinal centers (see Fig. 7-9) indicates persistent or secondary exposure of follicular B cells to blood-borne antigens. The progeny of activated B cells are progressively displaced toward the red pulp, the site where mature plasma cells are finally produced. Hence large numbers of plasma cells lie in the marginal zone and red pulp of the spleen. The immunoglobulin they produce is predominantly IgG, as is the case in lymph nodes.

SPLENIC RED PULP

Blood reaches the red pulp from continuations of the splenic sheathed arteries (see Fig. 7-9). The outer boundary of the red pulp is supplied by **penicillar arteries** (L. *penicillus*, painter's brush), which fan out like the bristles of an artist's brush. Arterioles from these vessels open into a vast meshwork of reticular fibers, the interstices of which constitute an extensive extravascular compartment in the red pulp.

Distal to its arterial supply, the **red pulp** consists of 1) thin-walled, wide venous vessels termed **sinusoids**, with numerous associated macrophages, that drain into trabecular veins, and 2) an extensive, ramifying **extravascular compartment** supported by reticular fibers with associated reticular cells and countless extravasated blood cells lying free in its interstices.

In contrast to the typical closed pathway of blood circulation through the body, the spleen's circulatory pathway is described as being *open* because most of the splenic arterial blood is not delivered directly to splenic sinusoids. Nevertheless, in vivo studies of splenic blood flow suggest that from time to time, a small proportion of the blood arriving from arterioles is channeled more directly to sinusoids, as depicted in a simplified manner at bottom right in Figure 7-9. This may mean that when necessary, some of the blood usually delivered to the extravascular compartment may be permitted to bypass it.

The endothelial cells that line the splenic sinusoids are relatively long and narrow, with wide slit-shaped gaps between their lateral margins (Figs. 7-11 and 7-12). Anastomosing rings of basement membrane support the endothelial cells, much as metal hoops support the wooden staves of a barrel. In this case, however, the barrel is very leaky because of the open slits in its lining. This sieve-like arrangement provides an effective *filter* through which enormous numbers of blood cells are required to pass before they can leave the spleen by way of the splenic sinusoids, trabecular veins, and splenic vein (see Fig. 7-9).

From the peripheral blood, erythrocytes, leukocytes, and platelets continuously pass into the interstices of the reticular meshwork that lies outside the splenic sinusoids. In subsequently gaining access to sinusoids, any worn-out or defective erythrocytes are severely damaged when they have to pass through the narrow intercellular slits. Together with dead leukocytes, senescent platelets, and extraneous particles, they are phagocytosed by the numerous macrophages in the red pulp, many of which are intimately associated with sinusoids (see Fig. 7-11).

The respective phagocytic and lining roles of 1) sinusoid-associated macrophages and 2) sinusoid-lining endothelial cells of the *spleen, bone marrow,* and *liver* were initially dually ascribed to the *endothelium.* This led to the misrepresentation that the elimination of debris accumulating in the bloodstream is carried out by a **reticuloendothelial system (RES)** made up entirely of phagocytic endothelial cells.

The sieve-like design of the sinusoids also accounts for the so-called **pitting** function of the spleen. Any superfluous particles that may be present in erythrocytes become extruded when these cells squeeze through the open intercellular slits. Such particles include denatured hemoglobin, iron-containing granules, nuclear remnants, and the malarial parasite. The extruded particles are promptly engulfed by the sinusoid-associated macrophages.

The two main functions of the red pulp are therefore 1) to produce immunoglobulins in response to blood-borne foreign antigens, and 2) to filter out and dispose of worn-out blood cells and

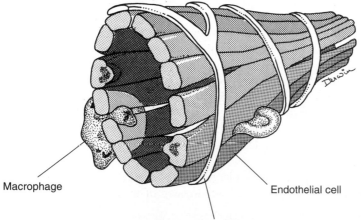

Macrophage   Endothelial cell

Basement membrane

Figure 7-11
Sinusoid in splenic red pulp, showing its endothelial lining cells and their supporting hoop-like segments of basement membrane. The slit-shaped gaps between these cells admit blood cells to the lumen.

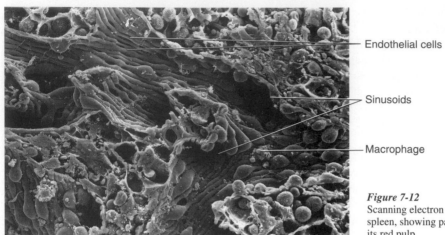

Endothelial cells

Sinusoids

Macrophage

Figure 7-12
Scanning electron micrograph of the
spleen, showing parts of sinusoids in
its red pulp.

suspended particles that otherwise might clutter up the bloodstream. The first function involves
plasma cells that although residing in the red pulp, arise in the white pulp. The second function involves sinusoid-associated macrophages that are avidly phagocytic. In addition, the red pulp behaves as a temporary reservoir for blood cells and platelets that are not circulating.

Summary

The hematopoietic tissues generate replacements for senescent or lost blood cells, most of which are
specialized, short lived, and unable to divide. The stroma of myeloid tissue consists chiefly of en-
dothelially lined sinusoids, with macrophages, fibroblasts, and reticular cells. Its cells produce several important myeloid growth factors (see Table 7-2). The hierarchy of hematopoietic cells (shown
in Table 7-1) begins with pluripotential hematopoietic stem cells originating from yolk sac mesenchyme that in due course seed red bone marrow, where they remain in adult life. Undifferentiated
and capable of self-renewal, these stem cells have great proliferative potential. They give rise to all
the blood cells and also platelets (and, by extension, to plasma cells and macrophages). Their
progeny become increasingly restricted to specific lines of myeloid or lymphoid differentiation, producing unipotential (committed) progenitors and functional end-cells. Proliferation and differentiation within the various blood cell lineages is regulated by a series of hematopoietic growth factors
(see Table 7-2).

The morphologically recognizable stages of erythroid and granulocytic maturation are listed in
Tables 7-3 and 7-4 and illustrated in Plate 7-1. Granulocytic precursors outnumber erythroid precursors because granulocytes have a shorter life span than erythrocytes. In general, the diameter of
blood cell precursors diminishes as their maturation proceeds. Relative to overall cell size, nuclear
diameter diminishes more markedly in erythroid precursors, and at the normoblast stage the nucleus
is extruded. Chromatin condensation is another sign of maturation in both the erythroid and the granulocytic series. Granulocytic precursors acquire their specific granules at the myelocyte stage. Progressive indentation and constriction of the nucleus leads to the distinctive segmented nuclear shape
that characterizes mature neutrophils.

Megakaryocytes are massive polyploid cells with a large multilobed nucleus. Commonly, they
lie adjacent to sinusoids. When they become polyploid, subdivision of their cytoplasm produces
platelets.

TABLE 7-7

B AND T CELLS: PRINCIPAL DIFFERENCES

Feature	B Cells	T Cells
Directly involved in humoral antibody responses	Yes	Yes; upregulate or down-regulate the response
Directly involved in cell-mediated immune responses	No	Yes
Effector cells produced in immune responses	Plasma cells	Cytotoxic T cells = killer cells
Distinctive markers	Surface immunoglobulin	T-cell receptor; CD4 and CD8

Whereas B cells arise in myeloid tissue, T cells are produced in the thymic cortex. The major differences between B cells and T cells are summarized in Table 7-7. The T cell receptor differs in important respects from the surface membrane immunoglobulin on B cells. The different T cell subsets also express the surface markers CD4 or CD8. To produce an effective humoral antibody response, B cells generally require exposure to certain T cell lymphokines as well as antigen. For T cells to become activated, the antigen must be appropriately presented as peptide fragments and other stringent conditions must be met as well. B cell activation results in production of plasma cells and B memory cells. T cell subset activation results in production of cytotoxic T cells (killer cells), regulatory T cells (i.e., helper or suppressor T cells), memory T cells, and delayed hypersensitivity T cells.

Solitary lymphoid follicles may be found under wet epithelia when B cells become activated by foreign antigens in tissue fluid. Confluent aggregates of lymphoid follicles characterize certain sites in the gastrointestinal tract, notably the tonsils, ileum (Peyer's patches), and appendix. The main features of the other lymphoid organs are summarized in Table 7-8.

TABLE 7-8

DISTINGUISHING FEATURES OF LYMPHOID ORGANS

Feature	Thymus	Lymph Node	Spleen
Functional role	Primary	Secondary	Secondary
Connective tissue capsule, septa, and trabeculae	Present	Present	Present
Cortex and medulla	Present	Present	Absent
Lymphatics	Efferent only	Afferent and efferent	Efferent only
Major epithelial component*	Epithelial reticular cells and thymic corpuscles	Absent	Absent
Main derivatives	T cells; thymic hormones	Immunoglobulins; killer cells	Immunoglobulins
Exposure to foreign antigens	Partly shielded cortex	Antigens in lymph	Antigens in blood
Lymphoid follicles	Absent from cortex	Present in cortex	Present in white pulp (associated with arteries)
Plasma cells	Absent from cortex; uncommon in medulla	Present in medulla	Present in red pulp
Recirculating lymphocytes	Present in medulla only	Present	Present

* Excluding vascular endothelium or covering mesothelium.

Bibliography

Myeloid Stroma

Tavassoli M. Marrow adipose cells and hemopoiesis: an interpretive review. Exp Hematol 12:139, 1984.

Weiss L. The haemopoietic microenvironment of bone marrow: an ultrastructural study of the interactions of blood cells, stroma, and blood vessels. Ciba Found Symp 71:13, 1980.

Weiss L, Chen LT. The organization of hematopoietic cords and vascular sinuses in bone marrow. Blood Cells 1:617, 1975.

Hematopoietic Cells and Growth Factors

Bekkum van DW, Van den Engh GJ, Wagemaker G et al. Structural identity of the pluripotential hemopoietic stem cell. Blood Cells 5:143, 1979.

Burke F, Naylor MS, Davies B, Balkwill F. The cytokine wall chart. Immunol Today 14:165, 1993.

Dexter TM, Spooncer E. Growth and differentiation in the hemopoietic system. Annu Rev Cell Biol 3:423, 1987.

Erickson N, Quesenberry PJ. Regulation of erythropoiesis. The role of growth factors. Med Clin North Am 76(3):745, 1992.

Heyworth CM, Vallance SJ, Whetton AD, Dexter TM. The biochemistry and biology of the myeloid hemopoietic cell growth factors. J Cell Sci Suppl 13:57, 1990.

Johnson GR. Erythropoietin. Br Med Bull 45:506, 1989.

Koury ST, Bondurant MC, Koury MJ. Localization of erythropoietin synthesizing cells in murine kidneys by in situ hybridization. Blood 71:524, 1988.

Metcalf D. Haemopoietic regulators. Trends Biochem Sci 17:286, 1992.

Metcalf D. Thrombopoietin—At last. Nature 369:519, 1994.

Sims RB, Gewirtz AM. Human megakaryocytopoiesis. Annu Rev Med 40:213, 1989.

Morrison SJ, Uchida N, Weissman IL. The biology of hematopoietic stem cells. Annu Rev Cell Biol 11:35, 1995.

Spangrude GJ. Biological and clinical aspects of hematopoietic stem cells. Annu Rev Med 45:93, 1994.

Witte ON. Steel locus defines new multipotent growth factor. Cell 63:5, 1990.

Leukocyte Maturation

Bainton DF, Farquhar MC. Segregation and packaging of granules in eosinophilic leukocytes. J Cell Biol 45:54, 1970.

Bainton DF, Ullyot JL, Farquhar MC. The development of neutrophilic polymorphonuclear leukocytes in human bone marrow: origin and content of azurophil and specific granules. J Exp Med 134:907, 1971.

Nichols BA, Bainton DF, Farquhar MG. Differentiation of monocytes. Origin, nature and fate of their azurophilic granules. J Cell Biol 50:498, 1971.

Megakaryocytes and Platelet Formation

Becker RP, De Bruyn PPH. The transmural passage of blood cells into myeloid sinusoids and the entry of platelets into the sinusoidal circulation: a scanning electron microscopic investigation. Am J Anat 145:183, 1976.

Penington DG. The cellular biology of megakaryocytes. Blood Cells 5:5, 1979.

Yamada E. The fine structure of the megakaryocyte in the mouse spleen. Acta Anat 29:267, 1957.

Lymphoid Tissue (General)

Abbas AK, Lichtman AH, Pober JS. Cellular and Molecular Immunology, ed 2. Philadelphia, W.B. Saunders, 1994.

Roitt I, Brostoff J, Male D. Immunology, ed 5. London, Mosby, 1998.

B Cells, T Cells, and Antigen-Presenting Cells

Askonas BA, Openshaw PJM. MHC and antigen presentation. Immunol Today 10:396, 1989.

Boehmer von H. The developmental biology of T lymphocytes. Annu Rev Immunol 6:309, 1988.

Brodsky FM, Guagliardi LE. The cell biology of antigen processing and presentation. Annu Rev Immunol 9:707, 1991.

Butcher EC, Picker LJ. Lymphocyte homing and homeostasis. Science 272(5258):60, 1996.

Clevers HC, Owen MJ. Towards a molecular understanding of T cell differentiation. Immunol Today 12:86, 1991.

Davis MM. Molecular genetics of T-cell antigen receptors. Hosp Pract 23:157, 1988.

Dinarello CA, Mier JW. Lymphokines. N Engl J Med 317:940, 1987.

Dinome MA, Young JD. How lymphocytes kill tumor and other cellular targets. Hosp Pract 22:59, 1987.

Engelhard VH. How cells present antigens. Sci Am 271:54, 1994.

Gallagher R. Sandoz prize: T-B collaboration. Immunol Today 11:228, 1990.

Grey HM, Sette A, Buus S. How T cells see antigen. Sci Am 261:56, 1989.

Helinek DF, Lipsky PE. Regulation of human B-lymphocyte activation, proliferation and differentiation. Adv Immunol 40:1, 1987.

King PD, Katz DR. Mechanisms of dendritic cell function. Immunol Today 11:206, 1990.

Littman DR. Role of cell-to-cell interactions in T lymphocyte development and activation. Curr Opin Cell Biol 1:920, 1989.

Lotze MT, Thomson AW, eds. Dendritic Cells: Biology and Clinical Applications. San Diego, Academic Press, 1999.

Noelle RJ, Snow EC. Cognate interactions between helper T cells and B cells. Immunol Today 11:361, 1990.

Pellas TC, Weiss L. Migration pathways of recirculating murine B cells and CD4+ and CD8+ T lymphocytes. Am J Anat 187:355, 1990.

Parker DC. T cell-dependent B cell activation. Annu Rev Immunol 11:331, 1993

Reinherz EL, Schlossman SF. Regulation of the immune response—inducer and suppressor T-lymphocyte subsets in human beings. N Engl J Med 303:370, 1980.

Reinherz EL, Schlossman SF. The characterization and function of human immunoregulatory T lymphocyte subsets. Immunol Today 2:69, 1981.

Smith KA. Interleukin-2. Sci Am 262(3):50, 1990.

Tonegawa S. The molecules of the immune system. Sci Am 253(4):122, 1985.

Young JD, Cohn ZA. How killer cells kill. Sci Am 258(1):38, 1988.

Young LHY, Liu C-C, Joag S, Rafii S, Young JD. How lymphocytes kill. Annu Rev Med 41:45, 1990

Young M, Geha RS. Human regulatory T-cell subsets. Annu Rev Med 37:165, 1986.

Thymus

Boyd RL, Hugo P. Towards an integrated view of thymopoiesis. Immunol Today 12:71, 1991.

Gorgollón P, Ottone-Anaya M. Fine structure of canine thymus. Acta Anat 100:136, 1978.

Hwang WS, Ho TY, Luk SC, Simon GT. Ultrastructure of the rat thymus: a transmission, scanning electron microscope, and morphometric study. Lab Invest 31:473, 1974.

Kendall MD. Functional anatomy of the thymic microenvironment. J Anat 177:1, 1991.

Raviola E, Karnovsky MJ. Evidence for a blood—thymus barrier using electron-opaque tracers. J Exp Med 136:466, 1972.

Lymph Nodes and Lymphoid Follicles

Anderson AO, Anderson ND. Lymphocyte emigration from high endothelial venules in rat lymph nodes. Immunology 31:731, 1976.

Befus AD, Bienenstock J. The mucosa-associated immune system of the rabbit. In Hay JB, ed. Animal Models of Immunological Processes. London, Academic Press, 1982, p 167.

Belisle C, Sainte-Marie G. Blood vascular network of the rat lymph node: Tridimensional studies by light and scanning electron microscopy. Am J Anat 189:111, 1990.

Crouse DA, Perry GA, Murphy BO, Sharp JG. Characteristics of submucosal lymphoid tissue located in the proximal colon of the rat. J Anat 162:53, 1989.

Ferguson A. Mucosal immunology. Immunol Today 11:1, 1990.

Girard JP, Springer TA. High endothelial venules (HEVs): specialized endothelium for lymphocyte migration. Immunol Today 16:449, 1995.

Jarry A, Robaszkiewicz M, Brousse N, Potet F. Immune cells associated with M cells in the follicle-associated epithelium of Peyer's patches in the rat. An electron- and immuno-electron-microscopic study. Cell Tissue Res 255:293, 1989.

Liu YJ, Grouard G, De Bouteiller O, Banchereau J. Follicular dendritic cells and germinal centers. Int Rev Cytol 166:139, 1996.

Luk SC, Nopajaroonsri C, Simon GT. The architecture of the normal lymph node and hemolymph node. A scanning and transmission electron microscopic study. Lab Invest 29:258, 1973.

Nopajaroonsri C, Luk SC, Simon GT. Ultrastructure of the normal lymph node. Am J Pathol 65:1, 1971.

Owen RL. Sequential uptake of horseradish peroxidase by lymphoid follicle epithelium of Peyer's patches in the normal unobstructed mouse intestine. An ultrastructural study. Gastroenterology 72:440, 1977.

Owen RL, Bhalla DK. Lympho-epithelial organs and lymph nodes. In Hodges GM, Carr KE (eds): Biomedical Research Applications of Scanning Electron Microscopy, vol 3. New York, Academic Press, 1983.

Szakal AK, Kosco MH, Tew JG. Microanatomy of lymphoid tissue during humoral immune responses: structure function relationships. Annu Rev Immunol 7:91, 1989.

Volk P, Meyer LM. The histology of reactive lymph nodes. Am J Surg Pathol 11:866, 1987.

Spleen

Barnhart MI, Lusher JM. The human spleen as revealed by scanning electron microscopy. Am J Hematol 1:243, 1976.

Blue J, Weiss L. Vascular pathways in non-sinusal red pulp: an electron microscope study of cat spleen. Am J Anat 161:135, 1981.

Chen L-T, Weiss L. The role of the sinus wall in the passage of erythrocytes through the spleen. Blood 41:529, 1973.

Fujita T, Kashimura M, Adachi K. Scanning electron microscopy (SEM) studies of the spleen: normal and pathological. Scanning Electron Microscopy 1982(1):435, 1982.

Song SH, Groom AC. Scanning electron microscope study of the splenic pulp in relation to the sequestration of immature and abnormal red cells. J Morphol 144:439, 1974.

Weiss L. A scanning electron microscopic study of the spleen. Blood 43:665, 1974.

CHAPTER 8

Dense Connective Tissue, Cartilage, Bone, and Joints

OBJECTIVES

When you have studied the contents of this chapter, you should be able to do the following:

- Name body sites where each form of dense ordinary connective tissue is found
- Outline the chief similarities and differences between bone and cartilage, and specify the subtypes of each tissue
- Outline the two different ways by which bones develop
- Discuss the structural and functional differences between osteoblasts and osteoclasts
- Distinguish between cancellous bone and compact bone in histological sections
- Recognize the four constituent zones and diaphyseal trabeculae of an epiphyseal plate and state their respective functional significance
- Distinguish between sites of bone growth and sites of bone resorption
- Explain how microscopic structure and tissue function are interdependent in two kinds of joints

This chapter is concerned mostly with cartilage and bone, which are skeletal tissues that can support the body's full weight. Before considering these two special connective tissues, however, we shall describe the dense ordinary connective tissue that constitutes tendons and ligaments and the fibrous investments of organs and various other parts of body.

DENSE ORDINARY CONNECTIVE TISSUE

Dense ordinary connective tissue contains fewer cells than loose connective tissue and is less vascular. Because dense connective tissue is characterized by a relative abundance of inextensible collagen fibers, it is also known as **fibrous connective tissue.** Two distinct forms of dense ordinary connective tissue are recognized, based on the arrangement of their collagen fibers. In the **regular** form, bundles of parallel fibers extend in the direction of tension and constitute effective arrangements for transmitting unidirectional pull. The regular arrangement is characteristic of the various tendons and aponeuroses (wide, flat tendons expanded into fibrous sheets) that transmit the force of muscular contractions to bones or cartilages. It is also characteristic of ligaments, which are the tough fibrous bands present in synovial joints that hold articulating bones together, provide necessary support, and limit joint motion to appropriate ranges and directions. As we shall see, bone growth entails further deposition of bone matrix on the bone surface, with the result that any associated tendon and ligament insertions become increasingly embedded in bone matrix. Such embedded collagen bundles are called **Sharpey's fibers.** Where collagen bundles insert into cartilage, they become a matrix component of a distinctive cartilage subtype called **fibrocartilage** (described later).

In the **irregular** form of dense ordinary connective tissue, fiber bundles lie oriented in a number of planes, that is, they are not all parallel (Plate 8-1). Accordingly, they resist stretch from various directions. This sort of tissue is suited for many purposes. It constitutes 1) the fibrous protective covering of bones and cartilages; 2) the innermost part of the skin (reticular layer of dermis); 3) the deep fascia of the body; 4) the tough fibrous wrappings of the heart, brain, spinal cord, nerves, and skeletal muscles; 5) the supporting elements (fibrous capsule and septa or trabeculae) of glands and organs; and 6) the fibrous valves that ensure one-way flow in the circulatory system.

Tendons

Tendons consist of tightly packed bundles of parallel extracellular collagen fibers, with interposed rows of compressed nuclei representing fibrocytes that produced this collagen (Fig. 8-1). Capillaries are present but rarely evident. In addition, tendons are provided with sensory receptors called **Golgi tendon organs** that register tension in the tendon. Some tendons are surrounded by a **tendon sheath** consisting of two concentric sheaths, which are made of comparatively cellular connective tissue that is separated by a narrow space. Whereas the inner sheath is attached to the tendon, the outer sheath merges with the surrounding connective tissue. Composed chiefly of collagen, the apposed smooth gliding surfaces are often described as **synovium.** Friction between them is minimized by a thin film of slippery **synovial fluid** (described under Synovial Joints).

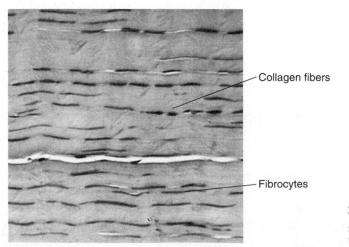

Collagen fibers

Fibrocytes

Figure 8-1
Tendon (longitudinal section). This tissue represents dense ordinary connective tissue, regularly arranged.

CLINICAL IMPLICATIONS

Tendon Repair

Tendon damage is a relatively common complication in penetrating trauma of the extremities, especially in severe laceration of the hands. Yet tendons heal successfully when suitably managed. If severed, they need to be rejoined surgically and sometimes require a tendon graft. The key cells responsible for tendon repair are fibroblasts derived from the inner sheath or, where no tendon sheath exists, from the loose connective tissue layer around the tendon. When these fibroblasts penetrate the defect, they produce abundant new collagen that effectively restores tendon continuity and strength. Tendon grafts become incorporated into rejoined tendons in a similar manner.

Ligaments

Ligaments have a similar composition to tendons, with parallel bundles of extracellular fibers and intervening rows of flattened fibrocyte nuclei. Most ligaments have substantial, longitudinal collagen fibers interwoven with fine collagen fibers and some elastic fibers. This renders ligaments sufficiently inextensible to provide strong support and limit excessive or misaligned joint motion without impeding the normal range of motion. The ligaments at a few joints are more extensible (e.g., **ligamenta flava** of the vertebral column, interconnecting the laminae of adjacent vertebral arches). The substantial, parallel fibers that resist the strain in these more extensible ligaments are elastic fibers, and the subsidiary fibers that weave these longitudinal fibers together are collagen fibers. Such ligaments are called **elastic ligaments.**

CLINICAL IMPLICATIONS

Ligament Repair

During the course of certain sports activities, immense strain is occasionally placed on the weight-bearing ligaments of a knee or ankle. Ligaments torn by excessive joint strain repair fairly readily provided the injury is properly managed. Effective healing requires tight apposition of the torn ligament ends. This is usually achieved by taping the joint in a position that approximates the torn ends of the ligament. Following more severe trauma, the torn ligament should be reunited directly using surgical sutures to ensure adequate repair. Satisfactory return of strength to the torn ligament depends on adequate deposition of strong new collagen across the joint, as in tendon repair, but in this case the source of the cells that produce the necessary collagen is not firmly established.

CARTILAGE

Cartilage, a strong but slightly flexible semirigid supporting tissue, is resilient enough to withstand compression forces resulting from locomotion and weight bearing and yet can bend. Much of the cartilage that develops prenatally is subsequently replaced by bone tissue. Thus, cartilage plays a key role in the development and growth of long bones, but the cartilaginous growth plates in these bones disappear when postnatal growth is over. The articulating ends of bones nevertheless remain capped by articular cartilages that provide polished gliding surfaces for unimpeded joint motion. Cartilage also persists 1) in some joints that are not freely movable, 2) as costal cartilages interconnecting the top ten pairs of ribs with the sternum, and 3) in the walls of the major airways and respiratory passages (nose, trachea, larynx, and bronchi), where it provides flexible support and guards against airway collapse as a result of respiratory movements or external compression.

Like epithelial tissue, cartilage *has no capillary blood supply* of its own, so its cells must obtain their oxygen and nutrients by *long-range diffusion*. This arrangement strongly contrasts with the way bone cells are nourished, because bone tissue is provided with abundant capillaries.

Three different forms of cartilage exist. In the fresh state, **hyaline cartilage** (the most common form) has a pearly white translucent appearance resembling that of frosted glass (Gk. *hyalos*, glass). Tendon insertions and intervertebral discs of the vertebral column are characterized by a particularly strong form of cartilage reinforced with parallel bundles of collagen fibers and hence known as **fibrocartilage**. The cartilage of the external ear and epiglottis, structures that are subjected to a great deal of bending, is highly flexible and resilient because it contains elastic fibers as well as collagen. It is called **elastic cartilage.**

Hyaline Cartilage

Incorporated within the hard, bluish-white extracellular matrix of hyaline cartilage are cells called **chondrocytes** (Plate 8-2) that become embedded in the matrix in the following manner. Embryonic **chondroblasts** differentiating at sites of developing cartilages begin to secrete macromolecular constituents of cartilage matrix. Cells at the periphery of such sites give rise to a fibrous covering known as the **perichondrium** (Gk. *peri*, around). The inner part of this covering is described as **chondrogenic** because it repeatedly gives rise to new chondroblasts that build up more matrix, adding to that already formed. The cells in the outer part of the perichondrium differentiate into collagen-producing **fibroblasts**, and as a result the developing cartilage becomes covered with a layer of **fibrous perichondrium.** This outer part of the perichondrium typically remains in adult life, but there are a few instances where both layers of the perichondrium disappear. Articular cartilages, for example, are devoid of a perichondrium.

Chondroblasts buried in cartilage matrix are described as **chondrocytes**. Their tiny matrix-enclosed compartments are termed **lacunae** (L. for small pits). In growing cartilages, chondrocytes divide and a partition of matrix begins to form between the daughter cells, resulting in a so-called **cell nest** of two or four cells (see Plate 8-2). Each living chondrocyte virtually fills its lacuna, but fixation usually results in a shrinkage artifact between the cell border and the lacunar wall. Mature chondrocytes are large secretory cells with a spherical nucleus and prominent nucleolus. Initially their cytoplasm is basophilic, indicating an extensive rER, but later it contains numerous fat droplets and appears vacuolated.

Cartilages can grow in two different ways at the same time. **Interstitial growth,** the net result of population increase of proliferative chondrocytes and accompanying supplementary matrix production, causes cartilages to expand within like rising dough. Interstitial growth is a feature of cartilage, but does not occur in bones. **Appositional growth,** the second growth mechanism, occurs in cartilages and bones. It is due to addition of new surface layers of matrix to the preexisting matrix. Thus, the appositional growth of cartilages is a result of 1) continuing production of new chondroblasts from the perichondrium and 2) incorporation of the supplementary matrix constituents that they produce at the periphery of the cartilage.

Hyaline Cartilage Matrix

With optimal staining, the matrix of hyaline cartilage has a slightly basophilic appearance in H&E-stained sections (see Plate 8-2). Its resilient gel structure has a distinctive macromolecular organization. **Cartilage proteoglycan,** the chief macromolecular constituent, is supplemented by several proteins and glycoproteins. Most of the proteoglycan exists as large supramolecular **proteoglycan aggregates** that confer on cartilage matrix much of its characteristic resilience. Another distinctive feature of cartilage matrix is that it is intimately reinforced with abundant fibrils of **type II collagen** strong enough to resist stretch. Because these fine fibrils are widely dispersed they are not seen with the LM. Collagen accounts for 40% to 70% of the dry weight of the matrix. **Tissue fluid**, partly trapped and partly bound by matrix constituents, accounts for 65% to 80% of the wet weight of the matrix. Cartilage, as noted, is *avascular* (i.e., it lacks capillaries), even though a few larger vessels may course through it (within connective tissue tunnels) without providing nourishment. Also, there are no lymphatics in this tissue. The substantial volume of tissue fluid held in its matrix, however, facilitates long-range diffusion of oxygen and nutrients to all the constituent chondrocytes from capillaries that lie *outside* the cartilage. Metabolic byproducts follow a reverse diffusion path to these vessels. Dependence on such long diffusion paths is hazardous, especially if matrix proteoglycans become displaced by insoluble calcium salts. Cartilage that undergoes heavy calcification and endochondral ossification (described later) is replaced by bone.

Fibrocartilage

A distinctive feature of fibrocartilage is its conspicuous parallel bundles of type I collagen fibers, which are strong enough to resist stretching under extreme tension. Because these bundles are noticeable, they can mislead beginners into mistaking regular dense ordinary connective tissue for fibrocartilage unless care is taken to distinguish between flat fibrocytes and larger, more rounded chondrocytes within lacunae (compare Fig. 8-1 and Plate 8-3). Many tendon attachments to cartilages are made of fibrocartilage. The chondrocyte lacunae present in the somewhat basophilic matrix typically lie in rows between the collagen bundles (see Plate 8-3). Fibrocartilage is avascular. In adult life, it lacks a perichondrium. Besides constituting tendon insertions, this extremely strong form of cartilage is found in the pubic symphysis, intervertebral disks of the vertebral column, and intra-articular menisci (described under Synovial Joints).

Elastic Cartilage

An even more resilient kind of cartilage, known as **elastic cartilage,** is adapted primarily to withstand repetitive bending. It supports the epiglottis and external ear, which are required to be flexible but capable of springing back when bent. Elastic cartilage resembles hyaline cartilage except that in addition to its content of fine type II collagen fibrils, the matrix contains acidophilic **elastic fibers** (Plate 8-4). The chondroblasts that produce the various matrix constituents (including the elastin) become embedded in matrix as chondrocytes. Situated in lacunae, the chondrocytes are in some cases arranged as cell nests, as in hyaline cartilage. Also, the fibrous layer of perichondrium persists in elastic cartilages.

BONE

A basic similarity between bone and cartilage is that they both contain living cells embedded in an extracellular matrix reinforced by collagen fibrils. Bone matrix, however, is heavily calcified, making bone harder and less supple than cartilage. Like chondrocytes, the embedded cells of bone, termed **osteocytes** (Gk. *osteon*, bone), occupy spaces called **lacunae.** Another similarity is that bones have a fibrous connective tissue covering called a **periosteum** that is the counterpart of the perichondrium. Lastly, both osteocytes and chondrocytes are indirectly derived from mesenchyme. However, osteocytes differentiate close to capillaries and chondrocytes differentiate in regions that are essentially devoid of such vessels.

The stone-like composition of bone matrix does not permit sectioning until bones have been *decalcified* (prior to this, the tissue is called **undecalcified bone**). Unfortunately, this procedure spoils the histological appearance of osteocytes, leaving only their nucleus and occasional shrunken remnants of cytoplasm (Fig. 8-2A). Living osteocytes fill their lacunae.

Several key differences between bone and cartilage relate to the way osteocytes are nourished, since the high mineral content of bone matrix severely limits long-range diffusion through it. A special arrangement that enables osteocytes to survive in such an environment is evident in thin slices

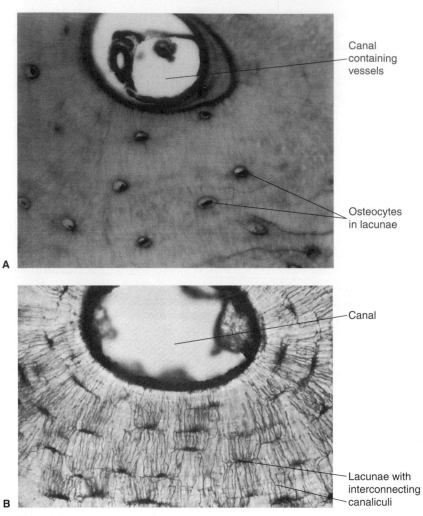

Figure 8-2
(*A*) Bone tissue (decalcified bone). (*B*) Undecalcified bone. Canaliculi appear distinct but the cells are not retained (ground section).

of undecalcified bone that have been ground down until transparent (**ground bone sections**). Tiny canals termed **canaliculi** (see Fig. 8-2*B*) interconnect the lacunae with one another and link them to bone surfaces bathed by tissue fluid. Within each canaliculus, a slender osteocyte process is also bathed in tissue fluid (see Fig. 8-3*C*). The canaliculi are miniature lifelines that bring tissue fluid, oxygen, and nutrients to all the osteocytes, enabling them to thrive in a heavily mineralized environment.

Bone is a *highly vascular* tissue. In marked contrast to cartilage, it is extensively permeated with blood capillaries that become incorporated during its development. As a consequence, all the osteocytes are situated within a 0.2-mm radius of a capillary, and the tissue fluid that this capillary produces reaches the surrounding osteocyte population by way of the canaliculi.

Bone development is known as **ossification** or **osteogenesis** (Gk. *gennan*, to produce). All bones are derived from mesenchyme, but by two different processes, depending on which bones they are. The flat bones that constitute the cranium develop directly in areas of vascularized mesenchyme by the process of **intramembranous ossification**, which is so named because the site where they develop is considered an embryonic *connective tissue membrane*. Other bones that develop intramembranously are the facial bones, and also the clavicles and mandible, though these subsequently acquire cartilaginous ends. In contrast, long bones develop indirectly from mesenchyme through an elaborate process termed **endochondral ossification**. Each long bone is preceded by a temporary **cartilage model.** Bone tissue then replaces most of the cartilage in the model during fetal life. The details of this process need not be addressed until we deal with bone growth. It is nevertheless important to understand that that although intramembranous ossification and endochondral ossification occur in different local environments, they both give rise to the *same kinds of bone tissue.*

Intramembranous Ossification

An example of a bone that develops intramembranously is a parietal bone of the skull. The mesenchymal cells on each lateral site on the head are initially loosely packed and pale-staining, with slender cytoplasmic extensions (shown at the periphery of Fig. 8-3A). At a site already supplied by capillaries a center of osteogenesis (ossification) begins to form. Mesenchymal cells in this center give rise first to osteoprogenitor or osteogenic cells (stem cells of skeletal tissue) and then to rounded, basophilic **osteoblasts**. These basophilic cells are called osteoblasts because they produce the organic matrix constituents of bone (Gk. *blastos*, germ). Once embedded in matrix, they are called **osteocytes** (see Fig. 8-3B). When the organic matrix calcifies, osteocytes receive oxygen and nutrients through canaliculi formed in the following manner.

Osteoblasts have numerous interconnecting processes (see Fig. 8-3A), so the organic matrix that they secrete becomes molded around their cell bodies and cytoplasmic processes, forming lacunae

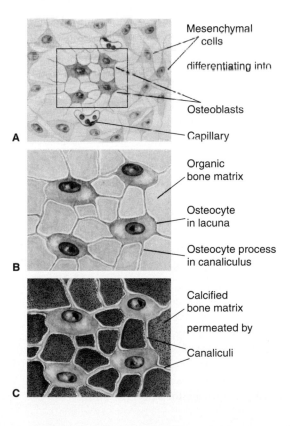

Mesenchymal
cells

differentiating into

Osteoblasts

Capillary

Organic
bone matrix

Osteocyte
in lacuna

Osteocyte process
in canaliculus

Calcified
bone matrix

permeated by

Canaliculi

A

B

C

Figure 8-3
Key stages in the process of intramembranous ossification.

and canaliculi (see Fig. 8-3*B*). Following calcification, the matrix remains riddled with interconnecting canaliculi that bring fresh tissue fluid and nutrients to each lacuna from bone capillaries by way of tiny extracellular spaces between osteocyte processes and canalicular walls (see Fig. 8-3*C*).

Organic bone matrix first appears at the site as small irregularly shaped **spicules** that subsequently lengthen into anastomosing long structures called **trabeculae** (L., small beams). Bone spicules and trabeculae are bright pink in H&E-stained sections and are covered with basophilic **osteoblasts** (see Plate 3-2). The trabeculae grow out radially from the center of osteogenesis, in the curved plane of the developing skull (see Fig. 8-6*A*). Such plate-like masses of anastomosing trabeculae are described as consisting of **spongy** or **cancellous bone** (L. *cancellus*, lattice). The lattice-like arrangement that characterizes this type of bone may be seen in Plate 8-5 and Figure 8-5*B*.

Some of the cells on the bone surfaces are small flat **osteoprogenitor (osteogenic) cells.** These **bipotential stem cells** give rise to osteoblasts and bone tissue only if an extensive local capillary blood supply is established. In the absence of such a supply, they give rise to chondroblasts and cartilage instead. Since osteoprogenitor cells are self-renewing, they persist in adult life and constitute a potential source of new skeletal tissue for the repair of broken bones.

Bone Matrix

Bone matrix can withstand bending, twisting, compression, and stretch. Besides being rock-hard owing to insoluble calcium salts, it is highly resistant to tensile stresses due to an abundance of collagen fibrils. The collagen is mostly type I, with small amounts of type V. It accounts for more than 90% of the organic content of bone matrix (a higher proportion than in cartilage matrix), and it imparts a pink to red color to bone matrix in H&E-stained sections (see Plate 8-9). The proteoglycan content of bone matrix, however, is much lower than that of cartilage matrix. Only about 25% of bone matrix is water. Other organic constituents of the matrix are glycosaminoglycans, glycoproteins, **osteonectin** (a protein that anchors bone mineral to collagen), and **osteocalcin** (a calcium-binding protein). In addition, bone resorption releases certain other matrix proteins that have the capacity to *induce bone formation*. Finally, almost 70% of the wet weight of bone matrix is **bone mineral,** primarily crystalline **hydroxyapatite**.

Until the organic matrix of bone becomes calcified, the tissue is known as **osteoid** (meaning *bone-like*) **tissue** or **prebone**. For this tissue to calcify, the local combined concentration of calcium and phosphate ions has to reach the level required for calcium phosphate deposition. Thus, in the bone disorder **rickets** (considered later), impaired mineralization leads to marked accumulation of osteoid tissue.

Bone Cells

The four cell types characterizing bone tissue are bone matrix producers, bone matrix maintaining cells, the osteogenic stem cells (osteoprogenitors) producing these cells, and bone matrix-resorbing cells.

Osteoprogenitor (Osteogenic) Cells

Originally referred to as **osteogenic cells, osteoprogenitor cells** are small spindle-shaped cells residing on all nonresorptive bone surfaces. They constitute the deep layer of the **periosteum** that invests each bone and also the **endosteum** that lines the medullary cavity, haversian canals, and other soft tissue spaces. The **periosteum** is a tough yet highly vascular connective tissue membrane that covers the bone but not its articulating surfaces. The thick outer layer of this membrane, termed its **fibrous layer**, is composed of irregular dense ordinary connective tissue. The thin, poorly defined inner region, termed its **osteogenic layer**, is made up of osteoprogenitor cells. The **endosteum** is a single layer of flat osteoprogenitor cells without a fibrous layer. Its osteoprogenitor cells are nevertheless able to participate with those of the periosteum in repairing broken bones.

Osteoprogenitor cells of the periosteum or endosteum that are stimulated to proliferate give rise to **osteoblasts** in regions that are well vascularized and to **chondroblasts** in regions that are unvascularized. Self-renewal of these bipotential stem cells maintains the supply of osteoprogenitor cells for further bone growth and fracture repair.

Osteoblasts

Fully differentiated **osteoblasts** are specialized nondividing cells that synthesize and secrete the organic constituents of bone matrix. Their cell bodies and cytoplasmic processes create the lacunae and canaliculi in this matrix (see Fig. 8-3). They characterize *growing* surfaces and are distinguishable from osteoprogenitor cells by their large size, rounded to polygonal outline, and eccentric nucleus. Their cytoplasm is markedly basophilic, usually with a distinct negative Golgi image (see Plate 3-4).

The fine structure of osteoblasts is typical of actively secreting cells. Numerous ribosomes bound to an extensive rER account for their cytoplasmic basophilia. Procollagen and other matrix constituents synthesized by the rER are packaged into secretory vesicles in the large Golgi complex and released by exocytosis from all parts of the cell surface, as in fibroblasts. Also, osteoblasts (together with chondrocytes and odontoblasts, the cells that produce dentin in teeth) are implicated in the process of **matrix calcification.** Furthermore, osteoblasts have the additional role of mediating bone resorption, as discussed later in the chapter (see Hormone Regulation of Bone Growth and Bone Resorption).

Osteocytes

Osteocytes are less basophilic and somewhat smaller than osteoblasts. Their numerous interconnecting cytoplasmic processes (see Fig. 8-3B) are usually indistinguishable in H&E-stained sections, but the canaliculi they create are evident in ground bone sections (see Fig. 8-2). Osteocyte lacunae generally retain a thin, unmineralized lining layer of osteoid tissue. The osteocytes within them are nondividing, so cell nests such as those seen in cartilage are not found in bone. Most osteocytes have a minimal amount of rER and a relatively small Golgi apparatus and are believed to maintain the bone matrix in good repair. They represent the final stage of maturation of the bone cell lineage.

Osteoclasts

Osteoclasts (Gk. *klan*, to break) are large nondividing motile cells that resorb surplus or inferior bone matrix. They are required for the remodeling that occurs during bone growth and repair, and also for the removal of substandard or weakened matrix that needs to be replaced. Osteoclasts are characteristic of **resorptive surfaces.** Instead of appearing smooth and evenly covered by a layer of cells, resorptive surfaces are etched or scalloped, and bare except for scattered osteoclasts on their surface (Plate 8-6). Such surfaces can be found at the site labeled 2 on the left of Figure 8-10. Some osteoclasts fit into recesses, known as **Howship's lacunae** or **resorption bays,** that they have eroded in the matrix. In general, osteoclasts are recognizable by their large size, multiple nuclei (several may be seen per cell in an LM section), and proximity to a bone surface (see Plate 8-6). However, osteoclasts sometimes detach from a bone surface because of shrinkage artifact. A frayed border on bone matrix may indicate a resorption site (see Plate 8-6).

The area of osteoclast surface responsible for bone matrix resorption is termed a **ruffled border** (Fig. 8-4), but its "ruffles" are really branching finger-like processes that poke into the surface of the matrix. Peripheral to the ruffled border is a ring-shaped region called the **clear zone** that if

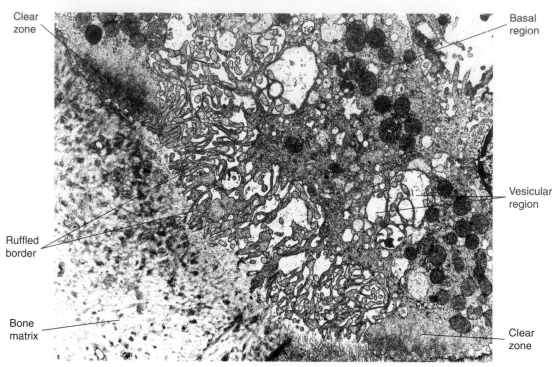

Clear zone
Basal region
Ruffled border
Vesicular region
Bone matrix
Clear zone

Figure 8-4
Electron micrograph showing an osteoclast's ruffled border (× 8500). An edge of one of the many nuclei is included at middle right.

seen in transverse section is represented on both sides of the border. It is described as clear because it lacks organelles other than microfilaments, which are abundant enough to give it a mottled appearance. Deep to the ruffled border is the **vesicular region** containing vesicles of various shapes and sizes. However, most of the so-called vesicles are really oblique sections of clefts extending into the cytoplasm between finger-like processes of the ruffled border. Farthest away from the bone surface is the **basal region** of the cell, which contains its nuclei, numerous mitochondria, and multiple Golgi stacks.

RUFFLED BORDER

The fine structure of the osteoclast indicates that it is a secretory type of cell. At the ruffled border, an extensive area of cell membrane is presented to the matrix surface. The ring-like clear zone effectively localizes and seals off the cell's working area. Its numerous microfilaments suggest possible limpet-like attachment of the cell to the matrix or agitation of the ruffled border to facilitate the resorptive process. The cell's numerous Golgi stacks package hydrolytic enzymes into vesicles that subsequently discharge their contents through clefts of the ruffled border into the tiny extracellular working compartment sealed off between the ruffled border and the apposed matrix surface. For efficient degradation of organic matrix constituents by the liberated hydrolases, prior acidification and matrix demineralization is necessary. Carbonic anhydrase, an enzyme that catalyzes the production of carbonic acid from CO_2 and H_2O, is present in the vicinity of the ruffled border. The H^+ ions produced by this enzyme are transported by a proton-ATPase in the ruffled border membrane to the extracellular digestion compartment sealed off by the clear zone. Here, the locally acidified conditions cause the matrix to decalcify and increase the enzymatic activities of the acid hydrolases. Hence, bone resorption involves 1) **focal decalcification** by acid secreted by the ruffled border and 2) **extracellular digestion** by acid hydrolases liberated at this border. Since osteoclasts are not intensely phagocytic, other kinds of cells assist them in disposing of the residual debris.

OSTEOCLAST PRECURSORS

Osteoclasts arise from **blood monocytes.** Cells of the monocyte–macrophage lineage become attracted toward bare bone surfaces, where they form osteoclasts by fusing with one another or by fusing with preexisting macrophage-like or osteoclast-like cells. Thus, instead of belonging to the osteoprogenitor cell family, osteoclasts represent an extension of the **monocyte—macrophage-multinucleated giant cell** line of differentiation. An essential maturation regulator for osteoclasts has recently been identified.

Bone Growth

In contrast to cartilages, which grow both interstitially and by apposition, bones grow only by apposition. This is because osteocytes, unlike chondrocytes, do not divide. Moreover, organic bone matrix calcifies soon after it is laid down and this prevents further internal expansion of the tissue. Hence, bone growth takes place exclusively on some preexisting surface.

Some of the cells on a bone's growing surfaces are osteoprogenitor cells. In their vascular environment, the progeny of these stem cells may persist as osteoprogenitor cells or they may differentiate into osteoblasts that deposit a new layer of matrix on the preexisting surface. Throughout the process, however, the osteoprogenitor cells stay in the necessary superficial position to repeat the process when the need arises. Referred to as the **appositional growth mechanism,** this simple process builds up bone tissue one layer at a time and is the only way in which bone tissue can grow. Each new generation of osteoblasts adds new canaliculi, so that when these cells become osteocytes they are linked to the bone surface above and the osteocytes below (Fig. 8-5A, *stage 3*). Furthermore, in the process of trabecular widening as a result of appositional growth, trabeculae incorporate adjacent capillaries that then nourish their more deeply situated osteocytes.

Bone growth involves more than bone deposition. It depends on close coordination between two opposing processes. Osteoclasts compensate for the addition of new bone by removing a similar amount of old bone from unnecessary places, thus preventing excessive buildup of bone tissue. The process that leads to the change in shape of a growing bone as a result of deposition at certain sites and resorption at others is described as **bone remodeling.**

Dense (Compact) Bone Formation

Continuing appositional growth of bony trabeculae can eventually change cancellous bone into a more solid form of bone known as **dense** or **compact bone.** A general working rule that is helpful for distinguishing between these two forms of bone is that 1) cancellous bone has a higher content of soft tissue spaces than of bone matrix, and 2) compact bone has a higher content of bone matrix than of soft tissue spaces (compare *B* and *C* in Fig. 8-5). The soft tissue is initially loose connective tissue but later this becomes replaced by bone marrow.

Every new layer of matrix produced makes the bony trabeculae one layer wider and the spaces they surround one layer narrower, as shown in Figure 8-5A. Much as lime building up inside water pipes diminishes their bore, cancellous bone can become converted into **dense (compact) bone** with narrow soft tissue spaces (see Fig. 8-5C). However, there is still some cancellous bone in the medullary regions of most bones. The progressive filling-in process that changes cancellous bone into compact bone creates numerous narrow canals lined by osteoprogenitor cells. Within these canals lie the vessels that formerly supplied the soft tissue spaces in the cancellous network.

The bone tissue that builds up layer upon layer on the bony walls of a soft tissue space constitutes a cylindrical structural unit of compact bone called a **haversian system** or **osteon.** Each concentric ring in the system is a **lamella** (layer) of bone tissue (see Fig. 8-5A, *stage 3*). The axial **haversian canal** in the system houses one or two small blood vessels, responsible for nourishing the

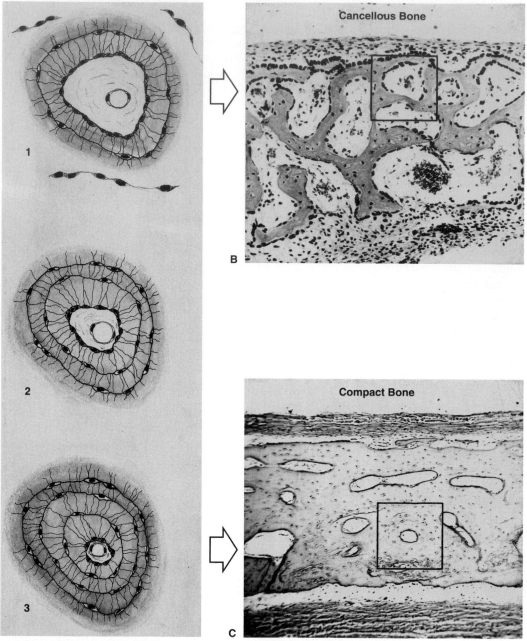

Figure 8-5
Key stages in the process of conversion of cancellous bone to compact bone (developing skull). (*A*) Soft tissue spaces fill in with concentric lamellae that accumulate and become a haversian system. (*B*) Developing cranial bone *(stage 1 in A)*. (*C*) Growing cranial bone *(stage 3 in A)*.

osteocytes by diffusion through interconnecting canaliculi, a few nerve fibers, and a single lining layer of osteoprogenitor cells.

Haversian system formation in developing flat bones converts their cancellous network (see Fig. 8-5*B*) into plates of compact bone (see Fig. 8-5*C*). Such bony plates may then undergo further remodeling at a later date. Meanwhile, to accommodate the expanding brain, the bones constituting the cranial vault increase in diameter and alter their curvature.

Flat Bone Growth

Figure 8-6 illustrates how flat bones of the cranial vault grow and it should be referred to throughout this section. To facilitate enlargement of the head, the margins of the flat bones constituting the cranial vault are interconnected by a type of joint that is composed entirely of dense ordinary connective tissue. Each joint is a seam of dense fibrous tissue (indicated in light gray in Fig. 8-6*A*). Such a skull **suture** (L. *sutura*, seam) enables the contiguous flat bones to grow and remodel independently. Continuing expansion of the cranial cavity is the combined result of 1) growth at the perimeter of these bones so that they spread into the sutures that join them and 2) bone deposition along the broad convex surface of these bones. Accompanying compensatory resorption along their concave surface prevents their becoming too thick. It also matches their curvature to that of the growing brain. The skull of the newborn has soft spots called **fontanelles** representing sites where the sutures are still rather wide. An example is the **anterior fontanelle** present at the junction of the frontal and parietal bones (see Fig. 8-6*A*). During childhood, the bones of the cranial vault that initially were composed of compact bone undergo internal remodeling. By the age of 8 years or so, the single plates are converted into double plates of compact bone with a central layer of cancellous bone. This distinctive arrangement is described as the **diploë** of the skull (Gk. meaning double). By the time the head is fully grown, bone tissue replaces the skull sutures and the formerly separate bones fuse and become the cranial vault.

Earlier in the chapter it was noted that there are two different ways in which bones develop. Flat bones arise directly from mesenchyme, but long bones are formed indirectly by a process called **endochondral ossification.** An understanding of this more elaborate process is necessary for appreciation of the growth processes occurring in long bones and the healing mechanisms occurring in such bones after their fracture.

Endochondral Ossification

Embryonic mesenchymal cells condense locally and differentiate into chondroblasts, delineating the site of a future bone (Plate 8-7*A*). The chondroblasts produce matrix, converting the model into hyaline cartilage, and a peripheral perichondrium develops (see Plate 8-7*B*). Interstitial and appositional

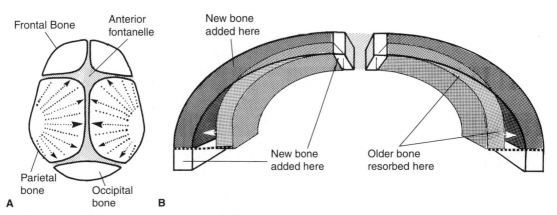

Figure 8-6
Flat bones in the growing cranial vault. (*A*) Superior view of the fetal skull (sutures and fontanelles indicated in *gray*). (*B*) Curvature changes in the growing cranial vault (coronal section).

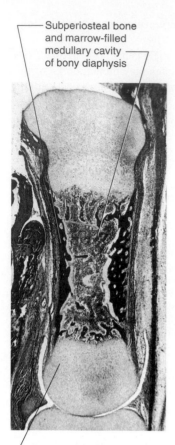

Subperiosteal bone
and marrow-filled
medullary cavity
of bony diaphysis

Figure 8-7
A developing long bone in which the subperiosteal bone and enlarging medullary cavity may be recognized.

Cartilaginous epiphysis
at each end of diaphysis

growth of the cartilage ensue. Lengthening of the model is largely the result of continuing chondrocyte division with further matrix production by the daughter cells. Widening is primarily due to the peripheral addition of matrix by new chondroblasts differentiating from the perichondrium.

In the midregion of the model, chondrocytes enlarge (hypertrophy) and mature, and hydroxyapatite becomes deposited in the matrix partitions between their lacunae (see Plate 8-7*B*). Following this stage, the chondrocytes die, probably as a consequence of activation of their apoptotic pathway. Many of the large lacunae become vacant, and the thin partitions between them begin to break down. At this stage, numerous capillaries vascularize the perichondrium. Differentiation of the osteoprogenitor cell progeny then occurs in a vascular environment. The surrounding membrane becomes a **periosteum**, producing osteoblasts that lay down a thin shell of bone matrix around the midregion. A strong collar of **subperiosteal bone** gradually builds up under the periosteum around the weakened midsection of the model.

Primary Ossification Center

Periosteal capillaries grow into the calcified cartilage of the midsection, supplying its interior (see Plate 8-7*C*). Together with associated osteoprogenitor cells, these capillaries constitute the **periosteal bud** (which is typically, but not always, a single structure). The internal capillaries set up a primary center of ossification, so named because the resulting bone tissue will replace most of the cartilage in the model. The osteoprogenitor cells brought into this newly vascularized environment give rise to osteoblasts that begin to deposit bone matrix on persisting remnants of calcified cartilage (see Plate 8-7, stages 3 and 4). The bone tissue initially formed is **cancellous bone** that has remnants of calcified cartilage in its trabeculae. In H&E-stained sections, the calcified cartilage remnants in the cores of the trabeculae usually stain pale blue to mauve in contrast to the bright pink to red color of the bone matrix covering their surfaces (see Plate 8-7*C* and *D*). Almost all the cancellous bone in the innermost midregion is subsequently resorbed, leaving a **medullary cavity** (see Plate 8-7*C*) surrounded by **bone cortex.** The forming medullary cavity becomes populated with **myeloid tissue** (Fig. 8-7).

A long collar of subperiosteal bone now extends along the midsection of the bone, but the ends are still cartilaginous. The midsection is known as the shaft or **diaphysis**; the cartilaginous ends are called **epiphyses.** The primary center of ossification is accordingly also known as the **diaphyseal center of ossification.**

The bone continues to elongate as a result of interstitial cartilaginous growth in its epiphyses. However, this does not cause lengthening of the epiphyses because the cartilage present at each end of the diaphyseal center of ossification progressively matures, calcifies, and becomes replaced by bone. Hence, elongation of the diaphyseal center of ossification keeps pace with the growth of the cartilaginous epiphyses, which remain more or less constant in size whereas the bony diaphysis between them lengthens.

Secondary Ossification Centers

Most **secondary** (i.e., **epiphyseal**) **centers of ossification** develop postnatally. The chondrocytes in the midregion of an epiphysis hypertrophy, and the matrix between them calcifies and begins to break down. Capillaries with associated osteoprogenitor cells then grow into cavities developing in the calcified cartilage (see Plate 8-7*D*). Osteoblasts are produced that deposit bone matrix on the cartilage remnants. Thus, as previously occurred in the diaphysis, the cartilage in the midregion of the epiphysis becomes replaced by bone tissue. Cartilage nevertheless persists as 1) an **articular cartilage** on the articular surface (Fig. 8-8*A*) and 2) an **epiphyseal plate**, which is a transverse disk of hyaline cartilage that remains between the epiphysis and the diaphysis. The epiphyseal plates enable

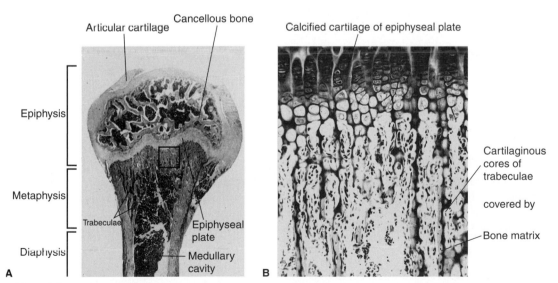

Figure 8-8
(*A*) Proximal end of a growing long bone (low power). (*B*) Area indicated in *A*, showing bony trabeculae on the diaphyseal side of the epiphyseal plate. The dark cores of calcified cartilage are covered with a layer of lightly stained bone matrix.

the bone to keep lengthening until full stature is attained, at which time they become replaced by bone tissue. Whereas the foramen of the nutrient artery of a bone marks the site of entry of the periosteal bud, the foramina of the epiphyseal arteries indicate where capillaries grew in to initiate secondary centers of ossification (compare Plate 8-7D with Fig. 8-16). Most long bones develop two secondary centers of ossification as well as a primary center (see Plate 8-7E), but a few bone develop a secondary center at one end only (see Plate 8-7F). Typical short bones ossify solely from their primary center (see Plate 8-7G).

Postnatal Long Bone Growth

Long bones continue to lengthen as a result of interstitial growth of their cartilaginous growth plates. Yet the formation of new cartilage matrix in epiphyseal plates does not increase their thickness. This is because cartilage production is compensated for by cartilage loss through calcification, vascularization, and bony replacement on the diaphyseal side of the plate. By growing on one side and becoming replaced by bone on the other, the epiphyseal plates are progressively separated, lengthening the diaphysis. Cartilage replacement eventually supersedes cartilage production, so when bones are approaching full size their epiphyseal plates disappear.

Epiphyseal Plates

The **epiphyseal plates** have a distinctive histological organization. From epiphysis to diaphysis, they consist of merging **zones** of 1) **resting** or **reserve cartilage,** 2) **proliferating cartilage,** 3) **maturing cartilage,** and 4) **calcifying cartilage** (Plate 8-8 and Fig. 8-9). Extending down into the diaphysis from the fourth zone are remnants of calcified cartilage with a thin layer of bone matrix deposited on their surface.

ZONE OF RESTING (RESERVE) CARTILAGE

The zone of cartilage that borders on bone tissue of the epiphysis (see Plate 8-8) is *resting* in the sense that its chondrocytes are not actively contributing to bone growth. Its chief role is to anchor the rest of the epiphyseal plate to the bony epiphysis. Capillaries interposed between it and the adjacent bony epiphysis supply oxygen and nutrients not only to the bone tissue in the epiphysis but also to all the chondrocytes in the plate as far down as the zone of calcifying cartilage.

ZONE OF PROLIFERATING CARTILAGE

Chondrocytes in the zone of proliferating cartilage (more appropriately called the zone of proliferative chondrocytes) divide and supply new chondrocytes to replace those lost from the diaphyseal side of the plate. The proliferating cells build up into characteristic longitudinal columns resembling stacks of coins (see Plate 8-8 and Fig. 8-9) and these columns contain occasional mitotic figures.

ZONE OF MATURING CARTILAGE

In this zone, known also as the **zone of hypertrophic cartilage,** the maturing chondrocytes remain arranged in longitudinal columns, but they have hypertrophied and are filled with accumulated glycogen and lipid. They are therefore large and pale-staining (see Plate 8-8). The enzyme **alkaline phosphatase** that they produce is widely believed to facilitate calcification of the extracellular matrix.

ZONE OF CALCIFYING CARTILAGE

Alternatively known as the **zone of provisional calcification,** this zone is so called because insoluble calcium salts become deposited in the cartilage matrix. In LM sections, some lacunae appear

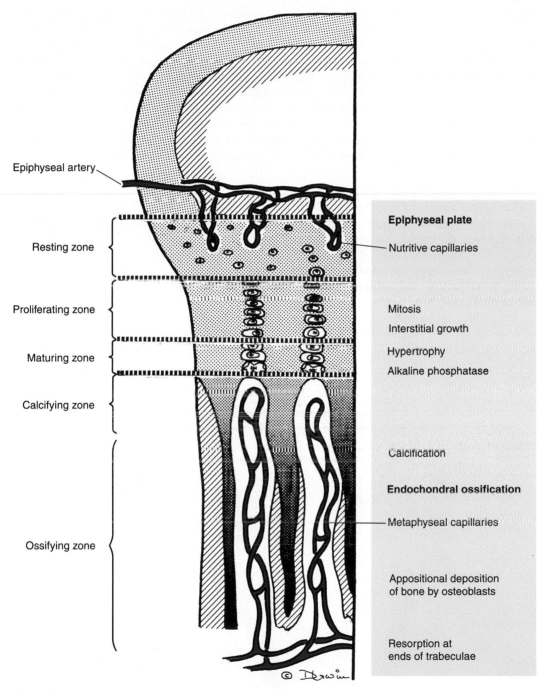

Epiphyseal artery

Epiphyseal plate

Resting zone — Nutritive capillaries

Proliferating zone — Mitosis
Interstitial growth

Maturing zone — Hypertrophy
Alkaline phosphatase

Calcifying zone

Calcification

Endochondral ossification

Metaphyseal capillaries

Ossifying zone

Appositional deposition
of bone by osteoblasts

Resorption at
ends of trabeculae

Figure 8-9
Constituent zones of the epiphyseal plate, showing the key processes occurring in them.

empty and fragile, and many of the thin transverse partitions show signs of breaking down (see Fig. 8-9). EM studies indicate that the majority of chondrocytes in this zone are structurally intact and viable. Apoptotic chondrocytes, however, are found in the terminal row adjacent to the vascular invasion front. Whereas typical cartilage matrix contains angiogenic inhibitors (Gk. *angeion*, vessel; *genesis*, production), the zones of hypertrophic and calcifying cartilage have angiogenic activator activity. Capillaries with associated osteoprogenitor cells accordingly grow into this zone from the diaphysis, providing a vascular environment in which osteoblasts differentiate and lay down bone matrix on the remaining calcified cartilage scaffold, as described in the next section. Although the apoptotic response in terminal chondrocytes is functionally coupled to vascularization and ossification, it is not clear whether such apoptosis leads to vascular invasion or vice versa.

Bone Formation At Epiphyseal Plates

Unlike the thin transverse matrix partitions between chondrocytes of the epiphyseal plate, the more substantial longitudinal partitions remain fairly intact when the matrix calcifies (see Figs. 8-8*B* and 8-9). The residual longitudinal remnants of calcified cartilage on the diaphyseal side of the plate serve as a scaffolding on which diaphyseal osteoblasts begin to lay down bone matrix. Long tapering spikes of bone known as **trabeculae** are seen projecting from the diaphyseal side of the epiphyseal plate. In H&E-stained sections, their cores of calcified cartilage appear pale blue to mauve in contrast to the pink bone matrix covering them (see Plate 8-8).

Continuing replacement of the cartilage matrix produced by both epiphyseal plates lengthens the bony diaphysis. However, while new bone is formed at the upper, wider end of the growing trabeculae, a similar amount of bone is resorbed from their trailing end (Fig. 8-10). Accordingly, the

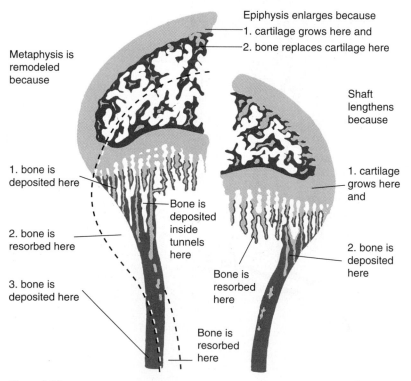

Figure 8-10
Sites of bone deposition and resorption in the process of lengthening and remodeling of long bones. Bone is shown in gray, cartilage in color.

trabeculae remain fairly uniform in length while the bony diaphysis and its medullary cavity elongate. Under the periphery of each epiphyseal plate, however, the trabeculae *become incorporated* into the diaphysis instead of becoming shortened as a result of resorption.

Bone Remodeling at Metaphyses

Lying at the ends of long bones are flared regions, the **metaphyses**, where the diaphyseal diameter increases to that of the epiphyses (see Fig. 8-8A). The flared region corresponds to the level where bony trabeculae are present on the diaphyseal side of the epiphyseal plate during bone growth. The cartilaginous growth plate is considered a part of the epiphysis. Throughout bone growth, the metaphyses retain the same general shape because osteoclasts resorb bone from the periphery of the metaphysis until its diameter is reduced to that of the shaft. Such resorption occurs at the sites shown in Figure 8-10 (the former outline of the epiphysis is indicated by the dotted line). The external surface of a metaphysis remains an active resorption site throughout bone growth, and osteoclasts can usually be found there. New bone concurrently built up on the medullary surface of the metaphysis compensates for bone removal from the periphery (see Figs. 8-8A and 8-10). Such ongoing readjustment of the shape of a growing bone is termed **bone remodeling**. Paradoxically, the distinctive shape of the growing bone would not be retained without remodeling.

Bony trabeculae cut in longitudinal sections appear to project from the diaphyseal side of the epiphyseal plate much as stalactites hang from the roof of a cave (see Plate 8-6D). However, it is really only the free ends of the trabeculae that do this. Nearer to the epiphyseal plate, the trabeculae are still interconnected in a honeycomb-like arrangement (Fig. 8-11B) that is riddled with long spaces. These spaces develop in the following way.

In the lower part of the epiphyseal plate, the chondrocytes are arranged in parallel longitudinal columns (see Fig. 8-11A). Breakdown of the thin transverse matrix partitions between them creates long tubular spaces (see Plate 8-6, 3 and 4, and Fig. 8-11A and B). The bony trabeculae seen adjacent to this region are therefore essentially the walls of longitudinal tunnels. Each intervening wall appears as a trabecula with a core of calcified cartilage covered by a layer of bone. However, the bone tissue that seems to *cover* the cores of trabeculae is really the *lining* of cartilaginous tunnels (see Fig. 8-11B and C).

Under the periphery of an epiphyseal plate, the cartilaginous tunnels fill in with successive layers of bone (see Fig. 8-10). The tunnels become reduced to narrow **haversian canals** that contain osteoprogenitor cells, osteoblasts, one or two small blood vessels, and in some cases, peripheral

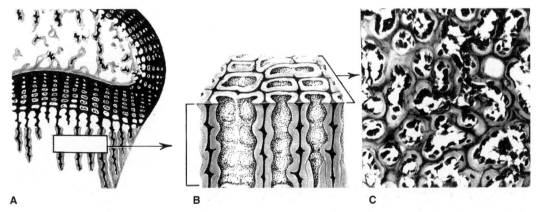

A   **B**   **C**

Figure 8-11
(*A*) Metaphyseal trabeculae on the diaphyseal side of the epiphyseal plate (longitudinal section). (*B*) Region indicated in *A* (longitudinal section) with these trabeculae depicted as tunnel walls (cartilage shown in black, bone in gray). (*C*) Region indicated in *A* seen in transverse section.

nerve fibers. Concentric lamellae of bone now surround the central canals as **haversian systems** (see Fig. 8-14 and Plate 8-9) that typically contain up to six lamellae. Most haversian systems that form under the periphery of the plate become incorporated into cortical bone of the diaphysis, but the bony trabeculae that form under the central part of the plate undergo resorption, with resulting elongation of the medullary cavity.

Bone Widening

Each new generation of osteoblasts that arises from osteoprogenitor cells of the periosteum can add another layer of bone matrix to the outer surface of the diaphysis (see Fig. 8-10, *site 3*). Such appositional growth widens the shaft and is compensated for by similar widening of the medullary cavity (see Fig. 8-10). New haversian systems form under the periosteum as depicted in Figure 8-12. First, longitudinal ridges and grooves form along the diaphysis (see Fig. 8-12*A*). Additional bone matrix then extends adjacent ridges toward each other (see Fig. 8-12*B*) until they meet and fuse (see Fig. 8-12*C*). In this manner, each former groove becomes a bony tunnel. Subsequent buildup of additional bone layers on the walls of the tunnel results in formation of a new haversian system (see Fig. 8-12*D–F*).

The new haversian systems that form under the periosteum are built up around periosteal vessels that then become haversian vessels in haversian canals. The haversian vessels continue to receive blood from the periosteum by way of small vessels that enter the cortex through other canals called **Volkmann's canals** (see Fig. 8-14). Two distinctive features of Volkmann's canals, some of which lead from the medullary cavity, are 1) they extend either obliquely or transversely in a *radial* direction through the diaphysis, not in the longitudinal direction characterizing the haversian canals that they interconnect; and 2) in contrast to haversian canals, they are not surrounded by concentric lamellae.

When a bone approaches its full size, the rough outer and inner circumferential surfaces of the shaft (still rough at the stage shown in Fig. 8-13) become smoothed off by a few **outer** and **inner circumferential lamellae** (Fig. 8-14 and Plate 8-9). The remainder of the compact bone consists mostly of haversian systems, but between these systems lie small remnants of preexisting haversian

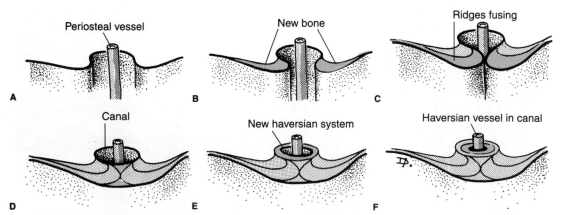

Figure 8-12
Bone widening occurs when new haversian systems are added to the periphery of the growing diaphysis. Periosteal vessels become incorporated in the new haversian canals.

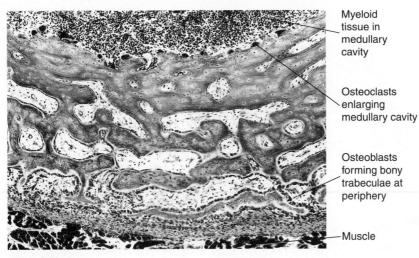

Myeloid tissue in medullary cavity

Osteoclasts enlarging medullary cavity

Osteoblasts forming bony trabeculae at periphery

Muscle

Figure 8-13
Diaphysis of growing long bone (kitten femur, transverse section). Cancellous bone constitutes the diaphyseal periphery. Osteoclasts are widening the medullary cavity.

systems that were largely replaced by new haversian systems during remodeling. Such incomplete remnants are known as **interstitial lamellae** (see Fig. 8-14).

Bone Remodeling

Bones are not the static structures they appear to be, even when fully grown. Long bones, for example, can adapt continuously to prevailing stresses by remodeling their internal structure. Any substantial rearrangement of stresses is compensated for by appropriate deposition or resorption of compact bone or appropriate realignment of the bony trabeculae. Thus, at the upper end of a femur, thin plates and columns of trabecular bone become aligned so as to counteract the strains imposed by weight-bearing and locomotion, and this creates a distinctive trabecular pattern for each person. Moreover, if a limb is not used for a long time, its bones cease to be subjected to the usual stresses. The remodeling process that ensues may result in excessive bone resorption with consequent weakening, a degenerative change in underused bones known as **atrophy of disuse.**

Another reason why bones undergo lifelong internal remodeling is that their matrix gradually weakens and therefore requires a certain amount of daily replacement. Permanent as it may seem, even compact bone is resorbed a little at a time by osteoclasts and then immediately replaced by new compact bone. This is laid down in the form of new haversian systems within **resorption tunnels (resorption cavities)** left by the osteoclasts. Resorption tunnels can usually be distinguished from haversian canals or Volkmann's canals by 1) their *irregular, etched outlines* and 2) the presence of *osteoclasts* along their borders. However, resorption tunnels are rapidly invaded by osteoprogenitor cells and osteoblasts, and promptly become filled in with new haversian systems.

CLINICAL IMPLICATIONS

Osteoporosis

Day-to-day maintenance of an almost constant total bone mass is virtually guaranteed by a distinctive regulatory mechanism that matches the amount of new bone formed during remodeling to the amount of older bone lost through resorption. There is evidence that certain differentiation and growth factors, present in

(continued)

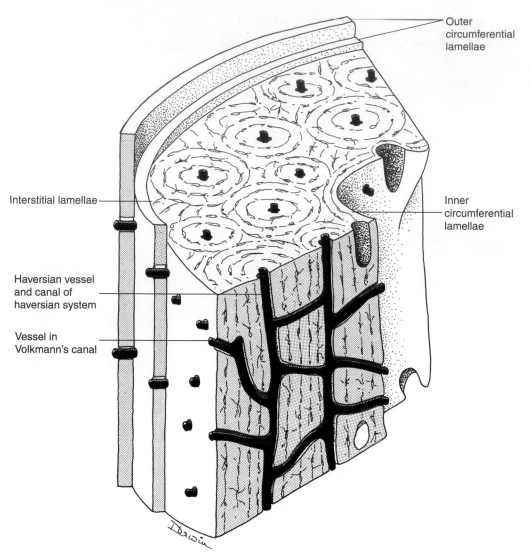

Figure 8-14
Histological organization of compact bone (diaphyseal cortex of a long bone). For clarity, haversian systems are reduced in number.

bone matrix and liberated during bone resorption, directly **couple** new bone formation to bone loss. The net result is bone **turnover** rather than bone **loss**. Imbalance between bone loss and bone replacement leads to **osteoporosis**, a common disorder in the elderly that is characterized by an absolute **reduction of total bone mass.**

Immature Bone

The bone tissue initially formed, known as **immature bone,** has only a transitory existence. In post-natal life, almost all of it is replaced by bone of a more permanent kind known as **mature bone.** In H&E-stained sections, occasional persisting regions of immature bone are recognizable by the fact that the matrix appears unevenly streaked or mottled with purple, in contrast to the matrix of mature bone, which stains a uniform pink to red (Fig. 8-15). Also, the osteocytes in immature bone lie closer

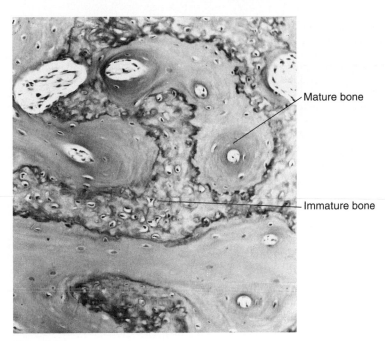

Mature bone

Immature bone

Figure 8-15
Comparison between sites of mature bone and immature bone.

together and are distributed more randomly than those in mature bone. The **mature bone** that characterizes adult bones is more obviously deposited as consecutive layers or **lamellae**. Its matrix stains evenly, and compared with immature bone it contains somewhat fewer osteocytes (see Fig. 8-15). The parallel collagen fibrils that spiral through each lamella crisscross with those of the adjacent lamellae in an arrangement that resembles the laminated woodgrains of plywood.

It should be understood that no clear-cut correlation exists between *immature* or *mature* bone on the one hand and *cancellous* or *compact* bone on the other. Conversion of cancellous bone to compact bone is a consequence of repeated deposition of consecutive bone layers on the bony walls of soft tissue spaces. Deposition of mature bone, on the other hand, follows resorption of immature bone, which may be either compact or cancellous in form. Hence replacement of immature bone can occur independently of consolidation. The latter process is an outcome of extensive appositional growth of cancellous bone, whereas the former process is a consequence of remodeling that introduces a superior type of bone.

Next, we briefly consider some critical dietary requirements for bone formation and the hormones that regulate calcium homeostasis.

CLINICAL IMPLICATIONS

Nutritional Requirements for Bone Growth
The process of endochondral ossification is profoundly influenced by factors that interfere with either 1) the *secretion* of organic constituents of bone matrix or 2) the *calcification* of organic extracellular matrix. Thus, a dietary deficiency of **vitamin C** can result in a disease called **scurvy**. Vitamin C promotes proline hydroxylation and is required for adequate collagen formation. If vitamin C is in short supply, the epiphyseal

(continued)

plates and bony shaft of growing long bones stay thin and fragile, predisposing to fractures. Insufficient bone maintenance (an adult manifestation of scurvy) plagued many a seafarer until the daily requirement of leafy green vegetables and fresh citrus fruits was fully appreciated.

Vitamin D is also necessary because its active metabolite, 1-α,25-dihydroxyD$_3$ (**calcitriol**), promotes absorption of calcium and phosphate from the gut. Infants deprived of this vitamin and also sunshine (because long-wave ultraviolet light reaching the skin promotes production of vitamin D$_3$ from 7-dehydrocholesterol) may develop the bone disorder **rickets**, which can lead to permanent skeletal deformities. Most noticeably affected are the weight-bearing bones, which being poorly calcified are semirigid and bend under the strain of supporting the body. Common indications of rickets are bowing of the legs or the development of knock-knees. A scarcity of calcium or phosphate delays calcification of the epiphyseal plates, which become unduly thick as a result of excessive growth. Also, the bone matrix produced on the diaphyseal side of the plates remains insufficiently calcified, with the result that comparatively weak osteoid tissue, in contrast to properly mineralized bone, accumulates in the metaphyses.

Hormonal Regulation of Bone Growth and Bone Resorption

The blood calcium level is dually regulated through the actions of **parathyroid hormone** (PTH) and **calcitonin**. A key effector cell in bone tissue responses to these two hormones is the **osteoclast**. The chief consequence of stimulation by **PTH** is that it **promotes bone resorption** through enlargement of active ruffled borders on osteoclasts. This action is largely an *indirect* response mediated by osteoblast-derived factors, because PTH induces osteoblasts to secrete a peptide mediator and various cytokines that all enhance resorptive activity in osteoclasts. The action of **calcitonin** on osteoclasts, on the other hand, is *direct*. Calcitonin **inhibits bone resorption** by diminishing the size and activity of the ruffled borders on osteoclasts. Hence, PTH induces osteoblasts to promote resorption by osteoclasts, liberating more calcium from bone matrix and consequently raising the blood calcium level. Conversely, calcitonin depresses resorption by osteoclasts, reducing the amount of calcium they liberate from bone matrix and causing the blood calcium level to drop. These and other opposing actions of the two hormones maintain the blood calcium level within closely regulated limits.

It should be noted also that an important effect of **somatotropin (growth hormone**, GH) is to **augment bone growth** by stimulating proliferation, secretion, and maturation of the chondrocytes in epiphyseal plates. This action of GH is primarily an indirect one mediated by insulin-like growth factors (chiefly **IGF-1**, known also as **somatomedin C**). Overproduction of GH causes children to grow exceptionally tall, whereas underproduction stunts growth. **1,25-Dihydroxycholecalciferol** is now recognized as the circulating (i.e., hormonal) form of vitamin D$_3$ responsible for 1) conserving calcium and phosphate and 2) promoting bone mineralization.

Blood Supply and Fracture Repair in Long Bones

The diaphysis, metaphyses, and marrow of a long bone are supplied primarily by the **nutrient artery** or arteries (Fig. 8-16). A supplementary blood supply reaches the metaphyses from the **metaphyseal arteries.** Furthermore, oxygen and nutrients from adjacent periosteal capillaries diffuse to osteocytes in the outermost lamellae by way of superficial canaliculi. Hence, viability of superficial osteocytes depends primarily on blood supplied by way of **periosteal arteries.** The epiphyses receive their blood mainly from the **epiphyseal arteries.** These various arteries became incorporated as follows. The nutrient artery is derived from the principal vessel of the periosteal bud that grew in and initiated the primary center of ossification. The epiphyseal arteries are the equivalent vessels initiating the secondary centers. The metaphyseal arteries are former periosteal arteries that became incorporated into bone tissue when the metaphyses widened. At the end of bone growth, the

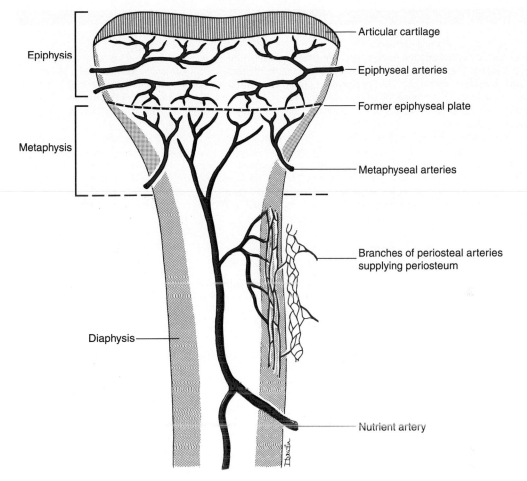

Figure 8-16
Blood supply of an adult long bone (tibia).

epiphyseal plates disappear. Anastomoses are consequently formed between terminal branches of the nutrient, metaphyseal, and epiphyseal arteries. Because each long bone receives blood from several arteries, most parts of it remain viable if the nutrient arterial main blood supply becomes interrupted.

Maintenance of Epiphyseal Plates
The growth plates of a growing bone are have no internal capillaries since they are made of hyaline cartilage. The bony trabeculae on the diaphyseal side of these plates are associated with an extensive capillary supply, but diffusion to the growth plate chondrocytes from these vessels is minimal because the cartilage matrix is heavily calcified on the diaphyseal side of the plate. The primary source of nourishment for these chondrocytes is the closest network of capillaries lying at the **epiphyseal border** of the growth plate, adjacent to the zone of resting cartilage. These essential capillaries, indicated in Figure 8-9, receive blood supplied by the **epiphyseal arteries.**

No description of bone tissue is complete without mention of bone fractures. The following section summarizes the repair process that occurs in a simple fracture healing in a plaster cast.

Healing of Long Bone Fractures

On either side of a realigned fracture site, trabeculae of cancellous bone grow out from adjacent undamaged regions of the bone and begin bridging the gap between the apposed broken ends. Meanwhile, a sleeve of hyaline cartilage forms. This cartilage provides temporary additional support for the fracture site. The cartilage then undergoes endochondral ossification and in due course becomes totally replaced by bone tissue. Finally, the new bone tissue that unites the broken ends becomes consolidated. The stages of this repair process are as follows.

First, the tearing of blood vessels results in substantial bleeding into the fracture site. Interruption of the blood supply leads to ischemic necrosis of osteocytes on either side of the fracture line (nonviable bone and remnants of the blood clot are depicted in Fig. 8-17). Next, osteoprogenitor cells in the endosteum and periosteum begin to proliferate. The environment near the damaged bone tissue is still vascular, so here their progeny cells differentiate into osteoblasts that begin to lay down bony trabeculae (Fig. 8-18). More superficial to the damaged bone tissue, however, the progeny cells differentiate in an environment that is avas-

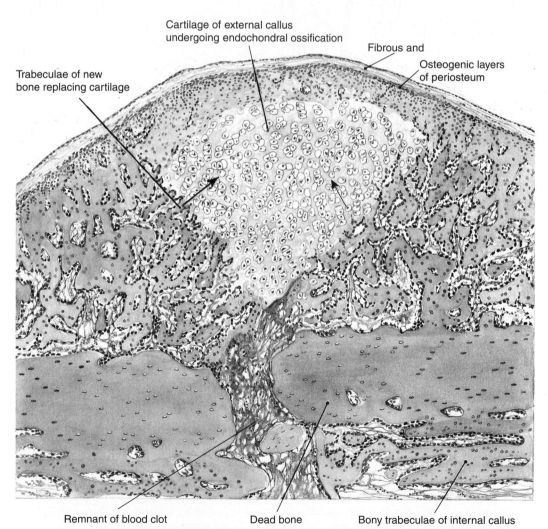

Cartilage of external callus
undergoing endochondral ossification

Fibrous and

Osteogenic layers
of periosteum

Trabeculae of new
bone replacing cartilage

Remnant of blood clot   Dead bone   Bony trabeculae of internal callus

Figure 8-17
Healing fracture of a rib, showing ossification of the cartilaginous external callus. This quantity of cartilaginous external callus indicates undue fracture mobility during healing.

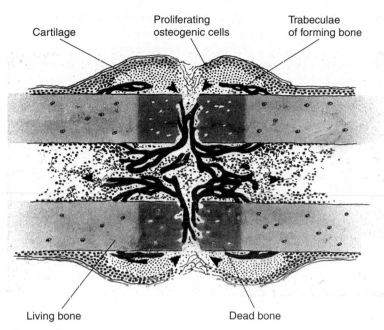

Cartilage | Proliferating osteogenic cells | Trabeculae of forming bone

Living bone | Dead bone

Figure 8-18
Healing fracture of a rib (later stage). Cancellous bone is indicated in black; cartilage is shown lightly stippled. *Arrowheads* indicate direction of trabecular growth in internal and external callus.

cular, so here they become chondroblasts, with resulting formation of some cartilage. As a result, an external sleeve of hyaline cartilage forms around the apposed fractured ends, providing supplementary support while new bony trabeculae form, both in the medullary cavity and subsequently in this so-called **external callus,** eventually reuniting the broken ends of the bone.

The last stage of repair involves progressive replacement of the cartilage collar by cancellous bone through endochondral ossification. This begins with chondrocyte maturation followed by calcification of the cartilage matrix, and proceeds as depicted in Figure 8-17. The newly formed bone tissue is initially all cancellous, but that destined for the cortex becomes converted into compact bone, and subsequent remodeling accurately restores the former shape and composition of the fractured bone.

JOINTS

Where bones lie in contact they are held together by connective tissue arrangements called **joints,** most of which are composite structures designed to facilitate free articulation between the bones. The common type of joint permits a considerable range of movement that in many cases occurs in more than one plane. At such joints, the articulating surfaces are covered by shiny **articular cartilages** that glide smoothly over each other with minimal friction because they are lubricated by **synovial fluid,** a viscous fluid resembling the white of an egg (L. *ovum,* egg). Joints of this type are accordingly termed **synovial joints.**

A different type of joint, called a modified **symphysis**, is present in the vertebral column. In the anterior intervertebral joints, contiguous vertebrae are held together by **intervertebral disks.** Consisting mainly of fibrocartilage, these tough cushion-like pads have the capacity to withstand substantial compression forces while allowing a limited range of joint movement.

A third type of joint, already mentioned, facilitates skull growth. In the newborn, the individual flat bones constituting the vault of the skull are still joined by cranial **sutures** (see Fig. 8-6*A*). These bands of dense fibrous tissue represent a type of joint known as the **syndesmosis** (Gk. *syn*, together; *desmos*, band or bond). When the head is fully grown, the flexible fibrous joints are replaced by rigid bony ones called **synostoses** that by cementing the individual cranial bones together produce the completed bony case.

Degenerative disorders of synovial and anterior intervertebral joints are fairly common.

Synovial Joints

A representative example of the synovial joint is the knee, the general structure of which is indicated in Figure 8-19. The articulating surfaces are capped by **articular cartilages** (*cross-striped* in Fig. 8-19). Enclosing the articulating joint is the **fibrous capsule,** a strong sleeve of dense ordinary connective tissue that is continuous with the fibrous periosteum of the articulating bones. Lining the joint capsule is an inner connective tissue layer called the **synovial membrane,** a major function of which is to produce synovial fluid. A small amount of this fluid is present in the narrow intra-articular space, which is termed the **joint cavity** (appearing dark in Fig. 8-19). A thin film of synovial fluid between the articular cartilages minimizes resulting friction when they glide over each other.

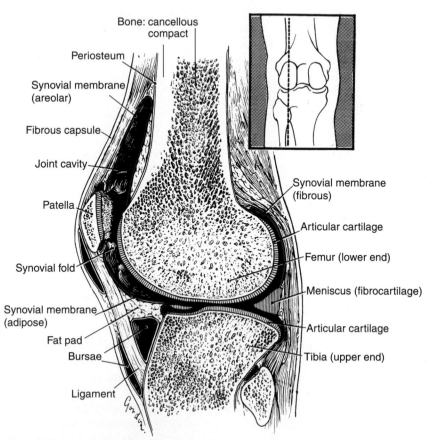

Figure 8-19
Knee joint (sagittal section indicated by inset). This is an example of a synovial joint.

Cord-like thickenings of the fibrous capsule constitute the **ligaments** of the joint. Some ligaments are integral to the capsule itself. Others are separated from the capsule by **bursae**, which represent minor extensions of the joint cavity. At sites where ligaments and tendons attach to cartilages, there is generally a transitional region of **fibrocartilage** (Fig. 8-20A). At sites where they attach to bones, their strong bundles of collagen fibers are anchored in the collagen of bone matrix as typical **Sharpey's fibers** (see Fig. 8-20B). Many synovial joints are also provided with supplementary disk, ring-, or crescent-shaped cushions of fibrocartilage. The fibrocartilage cushions of the knee joint are termed **menisci** (see Fig. 8-19). The capsule ligaments and menisci are provided with mechano-receptive afferent nerve endings that include free nerve endings, Pacinian corpuscles, Ruffini corpuscles (see Chapter 12 under Cutaneous Sensory Receptors) and the ligamentous equivalent of Golgi tendon organs.

Articular Cartilage

Articular cartilage basically resembles hyaline cartilage present elsewhere in the body, but its free surface is not covered by a perichondrium, and the chondrocytes in its deeper layers lie in vertical columns that are arranged perpendicularly to this surface (Plate 8-10). In identifying sections of articular cartilage, it is advisable to confirm that one of its borders is free and that the other is attached to subchondral bone.

The characteristic arrangement of the chondrocytes in articular cartilage reflects a preferential distribution of the collagen fibrils in its matrix. Fibril bundles extend perpendicularly toward the surface from the deeper layers, hence the deeper chondrocytes are arranged in vertical columns between bundles. Near the articular surface, the fibril bundles arch over and run parallel to the surface, with chondrocytes scattered more randomly between them.

When the epiphyses are growing, the chondrocytes near the tops of the columns proliferate. In normal adult articular cartilages, however, the chondrocytes seldom divide. Farther down the columns, the chondrocytes hypertrophy. At the bottoms of the columns, they undergo apoptosis and their matrix becomes calcified. Relatively strong subchondral bone supports articular cartilage from below.

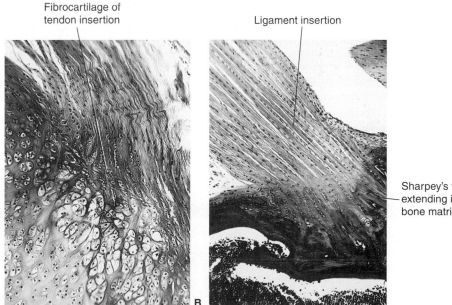

Fibrocartilage of
tendon insertion

Ligament insertion

Sharpey's fibers
extending into
bone matrix

A   B

Figure 8-20
(*A*) Tendon insertion (patellar tendon of rat). (*B*) Ligament insertion (anterior cruciate ligament of rat).

The **chondron**, defined as a chondrocyte and its surrounding region of pericellular matrix, is considered to be the microanatomical unit of articular cartilage. In contrast to the territorial and interterritorial regions of the cartilage matrix, where the collagen arrangement is multidirectional, the pericellular matrix in the chondron has an extensive network of collagen fibrils that virtually encloses and encapsulates the central chondrocyte. This stretch-resisting limiting network of collagen has a strong affinity for proteoglycans. The internal mass of hydrated matrix proteoglycan enveloped by the fibrillar network represents the central compartment of an efficient compression-resisting cushion. Damage to the chondron's peripheral encapsulating network of pericellular collagen fibrils severely compromises the unique hydroelastic properties of cartilage matrix.

Because articular cartilage is avascular, its nourishment depends on diffusion from outside the cartilage. The deepest part of the cartilage is heavily calcified, so diffusion from vessels of the underlying bone is limited. Most nourishment comes from the film of **synovial fluid** covering its free surface. Oxygen and nutrients reach this fluid by diffusing from capillaries of the synovial membrane.

Chondrocytes of fully grown articular cartilage hardly ever divide except under abnormal circumstances. However, they remain capable of secreting supplementary amounts of matrix constituents. This secretory response seems to be the chief normal compensatory mechanism for wear and tear in articular cartilages. Unfortunately, it leads to inadequate repair of damaged articular cartilages (another hazard in sports activities), making appropriate orthopedic management essential for the restoration of damaged cartilages.

Synovium

The **synovial membrane (synovium)** is a richly vascularized connective tissue membrane. It lines the joint cavity but does not cover the articular cartilages. This membrane is not considered an epithelial lining since its cells are not contiguous (i.e., they do not constitute a continuous layer). Thus, even the cells that border on the joint cavity lie among, and not on, the extracellular fibers of the membrane. In contrast to articular cartilage, the synovial membrane regenerates readily if damaged.

This membrane closely resembles fibrous, loose connective, or adipose tissue, depending on where it lies in the joint cavity. Its **fibrous** regions, which consist of irregular dense ordinary connective tissue with abundant collagen, cover ligaments, tendons, and other sites subject to pressure. **Areolar** regions are composed of highly vascular loose connective tissue, almost covered by a few layers of ovoid to cuboidal cells that lie among the superficial collagen and elastic fibers. Areolar regions also extend into the joint cavity as **synovial folds** and **villi** (see Fig. 8-19). Some of the superficial **synovial cells (synovocytes)** in these regions are secretory and contribute hyaluronic acid and glycoprotein to synovial fluid. The other synovial cells are more like macrophages. The loose texture of the areolar regions permits independent movement of the synovial lining relative to the fibrous capsule. Lastly, the **adipose** type of synovial membrane covers the intra-articular fat pads. Here, the superficial synovial cells are enmeshed in collagen fibers that are attached to the underlying fat cells.

Basically a viscous plasma dialysate containing additional **hyaluronic acid** and **glycoprotein, synovial fluid** has excellent lubricating properties. As well as minimizing friction 1) between articular cartilages and 2) between inner and outer tendon sheaths, this fluid plays a key role in nourishing articular cartilages. Suspended in it are a few cells, mostly monocytes, macrophages, and lymphocytes.

CLINICAL IMPLICATIONS

Osteoarthritis
Although the design of synovial joints minimizes wear and tear, their lifelong use commonly results in degenerative changes in the articular cartilages. These changes cause a certain amount of inflammation that, depending on its severity, is accompanied by stiffness, discomfort, or pain. Known as **osteoarthritis**, this disorder of the joints is a common cause of disability in the elderly. In particular, it affects joints such as the knees and hips that are required to support the full weight of the body. Progressive loss of the proteoglycan in cartilage matrix gradually compromises its substantial intrinsic resistance to compression. Also, inappropriate bony spurs (**osteophytes**) arise at the cartilage margins and progressively restrict joint mobility.

Intervertebral Joints

Each anterior intervertebral joint is a modified **symphysis,** which is a slightly movable joint where bones are held together by a combination of hyaline cartilage and fibrocartilage. Structures called **intervertebral disks** interconnect the bodies of the contiguous vertebrae (Fig. 8-21). Each vertebral body has a covering of **hyaline cartilage** (one vertebra is seen at the top and the other at the bottom of Fig. 8-21*A*), and interconnecting these coverings is the disk. Where the cartilage borders on the adjacent bone tissue it is calcified (see Fig. 8-21*B*). The soft gelatinous interior of the disk is termed the **nucleus pulposus** (see Fig. 8-21*C*). The strong ring-shaped fibrocartilaginous collar that supports the periphery of the disk is termed the **anulus fibrosus** (see Fig. 8-21*D*).

CLINICAL IMPLICATIONS

Intervertebral Disk Herniation
The semifluid nucleus pulposus and its surrounding inextensible anulus fibrosus constitute a tough compression-resisting cushion that permits limited movement between contiguous vertebrae. However, if those who are no longer young suddenly submit their spine to an inappropriate or excessive strain, the soft nucleus pulposus has a marked tendency to herniate (rupture) through the anulus fibrosus, a condition known as a **prolapsed** or **herniated intervertebral disk.** The resulting inflammation, generally severe and painful, may lead to spinal nerve root compression at the level involved and consequent peripheral nerve involvement.

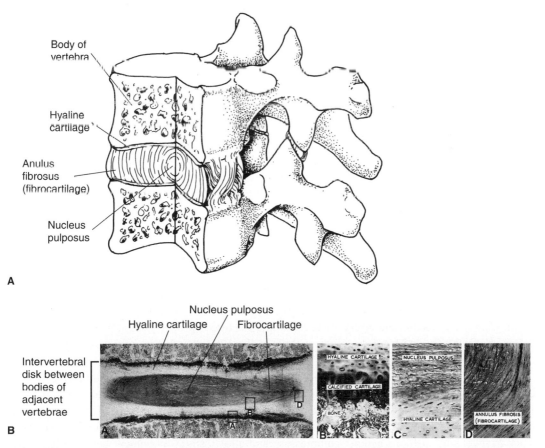

Figure 8-21
(*A*) Component tissues of the intervertebral disk, a modified symphysis. (*B*) Intervertebral disk (from a child, medium power) showing its internal histological organization.

Summary

The extracellular fibers of fibrous wrappings and supporting elements are irregularly arranged, whereas those of ligaments, tendons, and aponeuroses form parallel bundles. Ligaments (which join bones to other bones) and tendons (which join muscles to bones) insert as Sharpey's fibers into bone tissue or as fibrocartilage into articular cartilages.

Cartilage grows both interstitially and by apposition. Its matrix contains fine type II collagen fibrils and abundant tissue fluid. Because cartilage is avascular, its nourishment depends on long-range diffusion. Calcification of cartilage predisposes it to replacement by bone. Fibrocartilage is reinforced with substantial type I collagen bundles whereas elastic cartilage contains supplementary elastic fibers. In contrast, bone matrix is heavily calcified, contains more collagen, and is deposited only by apposition. Canaliculi facilitate diffusion from and to bone capillaries.

Osteoprogenitor cells are bipotential osteogenic stem cells present in the periosteum and endosteum. Their progeny cells differentiate into osteoblasts at vascular sites or chondroblasts at avascular sites. Osteoblasts on growing bone surfaces secrete the organic constituents of bone matrix. Osteocytes maintain the matrix. Neither mature osteoblasts nor osteocytes divide. Osteoclasts are multinucleated, nondividing cells with ruffled borders that demineralize foci of bone matrix and degrade some organic constituents. They belong to the monocyte—macrophage-multinucleated giant cell lineage.

Flat bones typically develop through intramembranous ossification in vascular connective tissue environments. The osteoblasts that differentiate produce trabeculae of cancellous bone that widen, incorporate vessels, and form a plate of compact bone. When this plate is remodeled, immature bone is replaced by mature bone, characterized by a uniformly staining matrix, comparatively widely spaced osteocytes, and concentric lamellae.

Long and short bones typically develop through endochondral ossification, meaning progressive replacement of a cartilage model by bone tissue. A bony supporting collar forms by apposition and the central region of the model calcifies. A periosteal bud grows in and supplies the cells and vessels necessary for ensuing osteogenesis. Cancellous bone is resorbed centrally from the midshaft, producing a medullary cavity. Most secondary centers of ossification develop postnatally. Each epiphysis retains an articular cartilage and epiphyseal plate. Cartilage production in this plate, which is made up of four recognizable zones, keeps pace with replacement by bone tissue. Epiphyseal plates are not present once bone growth is over.

Haversian systems (osteons) consist of concentric lamellae of bone arranged around central haversian canals. They are formed under the periphery of the epiphyseal plates and are also added to the periphery of the diaphysis as it widens. New haversian systems also form in resorption tunnels during remodeling.

Bone production is impaired if vitamins C or D or growth hormone are deficient. Resorption is augmented by parathyroid hormone and opposed by calcitonin. A long bone is supplied by several arteries, primarily its nutrient artery. When a simple fracture is properly set, it heals first with cancellous bone and then with compact bone. Cartilage also formed in this process is replaced by bone through endochondral ossification.

Synovial fluid lubricates and nourishes the articular cartilages, which are recognizable by their characteristic chondrocyte arrangement and the absence of a perichondrium on their articular surface. Synovial membrane provides the hyaluronic acid present in synovial fluid. The intervertebral disks of the anterior intervertebral joints have a soft center surrounded by a ring of fibrocartilage. This arrangement cushions against compression and allows slight movement between the vertebrae.

Bibliography

Dense Ordinary Connective Tissue, Cartilage, and Joints

Benjamin M, Evans EJ. Fibrocartilage. J Anat 171:1, 1990.

Carney SL, Muir H. The structure and function of cartilage proteoglycans. Physiol Rev 68:858, 1988.

Clark JM. The organization of collagen fibrils in the superficial zones of articular cartilage. J Anat 171:117, 1990.

Gardner E. Blood and nerve supply of joints. Stanford Med Bull 11:203, 1953.

Hall BK, ed. Cartilage, vols 1—3. New York, Academic Press, 1983.

Hall BK, Newman SA. Molecular Biology of Cartilage. Boca Raton, FL, CRC Press, 1991.

Heinegård D, Oldberg Å. Structure and biology of cartilage and bone matrix noncollagenous macromolecules. FASEB J 3:2042, 1989.

Honner R, Thompson RC. The nutritional pathways of articular cartilage. J Bone Joint Surg [Am] 53:4, 1971.

Hunziker EB. Growth plate structure and function. In: Woessner JF, Howell DS, eds. Joint Cartilage Degeneration: Basic and Clinical Aspects. New York, Marcel Dekker, Inc., 1993.

Hunziker EB. Mechanism of longitudinal bone growth and its regulation by growth plate chondrocytes. Microsc Res Tech 28:505, 1994.

Kuettner KE, Aydelotte MB, Thonar EJ-MA. Articular cartilage matrix and structure: a minireview. J Rheumatol 18(Suppl 27):46, 1991.

Poole CA. The structure and function of articular cartilage matrices. In: Woessner F, Howell D, eds. Joint Cartilage Degradation: Basic and Clinical Aspects. New York, Marcel Dekker, Inc., 1993, p 1.

Poole CA. Articular chondrons: form, function and failure. J Anat 191:1, 1997.

Potenza AD. The healing process in wounds of the digital flexor tendons and tendon grafts: an experimental study. In: Verdan C, ed. Tendon Surgery of the Hand, GEM Monograph 4. Edinburgh, Churchill-Livingstone, 1979, p 40.

Salter RB. Continuous Passive Motion (CPM). A Biological Concept for the Healing and Regeneration of Articular Cartilage, Ligaments, and Tendons. Baltimore, Md., Williams & Wilkins, 1993.

Salter RB, Hamilton HW, Wedge JH et al. The clinical application of basic research on continuous passive motion (CPM) for disorders and injuries of synovial joints: a preliminary report. J Ortho Res 1:325, 1983.

Sokolott L, ed. The Joints and Synovial Fluid. New York, Academic Press, 1978.

Vu TH, Shipley JM, Bergers G at al. MMP-9/gelatinase B is a key regulator of growth plate angiogenesis and apoptosis of hypertrophic chondrocytes. Cell 93:411, 1998.

Yahia L'H ed. Ligaments and Ligamentoplasties. Berlin, Springer, 1997.

Bone

Aarden EM, Burger EH, Nijweide PJ. Function of osteocytes in bone. J Cell Biochem 55:287, 1994.

Baron R. Molecular mechanisms of bone resorption by the osteoclast. Anat Rec 224:317, 1989.

Bellows CG, Ishida H, Aubin JE, Heersche JNM. Parathyroid hormone reversibly suppresses the differentiation of osteoprogenitor cells into functional osteoblasts. Endocrinology 127:3111, 1990.

Bonucci E. The structural basis of calcification. In: Ruggeri A, Motta PM, eds. Ultrastructure of the Connective Tissue Matrix. Boston, Martinus Nijhoff, 1984, p 165.

Brookes M. The Blood Supply of Bone: An Approach to Bone Biology. London, Butterworths, 1971.

Cruess RL. Healing of bone, tendon, and ligament. In Rockwood CA, Green DP, eds. Fractures in Adults, ed 2, vol 1. Philadelphia, JB Lippincott, 1984, p 147.

Emmanual J. A rapid method for producing stained sections of plastic embedded undecalcified bone specimens. Stain Technol 63:329, 1988.

Grills BL, Ham KN. Transmission electron microscopy of undecalcified bone. J Electron Microsc Tech 11:178, 1989.

Hall BK, ed. Bone: A Treatise, vol 5. Fracture Repair and Regeneration. Boca Raton, FL, CRC Press, 1991.

Holtrop ME. Light and electron microscopic structure of bone-forming cells. In: Hall BK, ed. Bone: A Treatise, vol 1. The Osteoblast and Osteocyte, Boca Raton, FL, CRC Press, 1989, p 1.

Holtrop ME. Light and electron microscopic structure of osteoclasts. In: Hall BK, ed. Bone: A Treatise, vol 2. The Osteoclast, Boca Raton, FL, CRC Press, 1990, p 1.

Holtrop ME, King GJ. The ultrastructure of the osteoclast and its functional implications. Clin Orthop 123:177, 1977.

Holtrop ME, King GJ, Cox KA, Reit B. Time related changes in the ultrastructure of osteoclasts after injection of parathyroid hormone in young rats. Calcif Tissue Int 27:129, 1979.

Kong Y, Yoshida H, Sarosi I et al. OPGL is a key regulator of osteoclastogenesis, lymphocyte development, and lymph node organogenesis. Nature 397:315, 1999.

Marks SC. The origin of osteoclasts: evidence, clinical implications and investigative challenges of an extraskeletal source. J Pathol 12:226, 1983.

Marks SC, Popoff SN. Bone cell biology: the regulation of development, structure, and function in the skeleton. Am J Anat 183:1, 1988.

Matthews JL. Bone structure and ultrastructure. In: Urist MR, ed. Fundamental and Clinical Bone Physiology. Philadelphia, JB Lippincott, 1980, p 4.

Sevitt S. Bone Repair and Fracture Healing in Man. Edinburgh, Churchill-Livingstone, 1981.

COLOR
PLATES

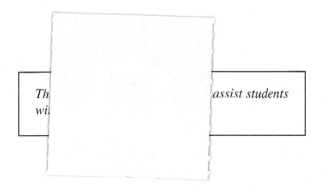

The *assist students* wit

Chapter 1

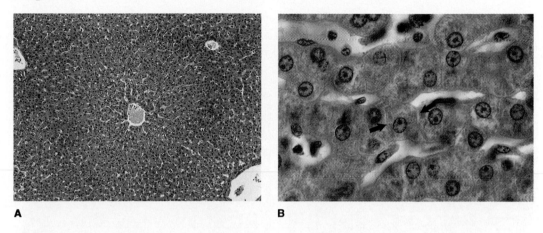

A
B

Plate 1-1
Microscopic appearance of hepatocytes (liver, H&E stain). (A) Low power (× 100); (B) oil-immersion (× 1,000). Arrows in B indicate lateral boundaries of a hepatocyte.

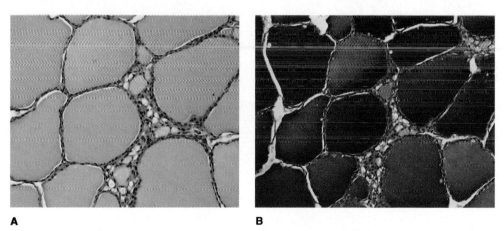

A
B

Plate 1-2
Microscopic appearance of thyroid follicles. (A) In H&E-stained sections, stored thyroglobulin is pink. (B) After PAS staining, it is magenta because it is a glycoprotein.

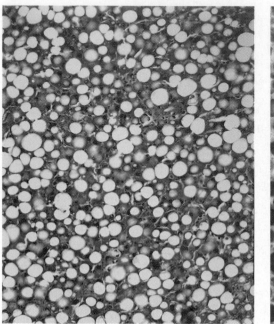
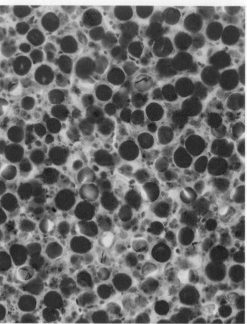

A   B

Plate 1-3
Hepatocytes with excess fat stored in their cytoplasm (fatty liver). (*A*) In H&E-stained sections, these round, empty spaces are left where the fat was present. (*B*) The large fat droplets are preserved in frozen sections. Here, they have been stained with a red, lipid-soluble Sudan dye.

Chapter 2

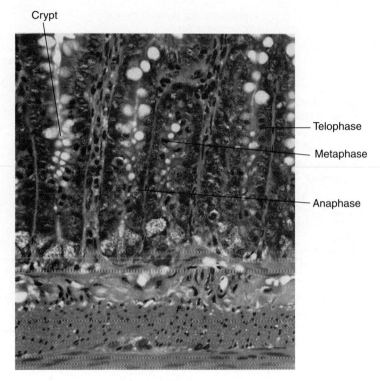

Crypt

Telophase

Metaphase

Anaphase

Plate 2-1
Mitotic figures in intestinal crypt epithelial cells.

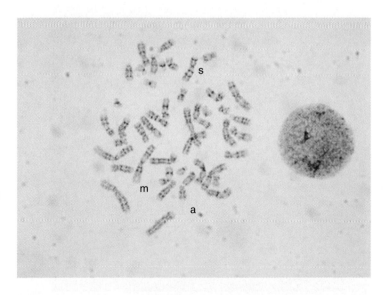

Plate 2-2
Chromosome spread (metaphase chromosomes of normal human male, Giemsa stain). Metacentrics (m), submetacentrics (s), and acrocentrics (a) are readily distinguished.

Chapter 3

Transmembrane protein (integral):
Uncharged region

Inner charged region

Outer charged
region

Peripheral membrane protein
(electrostatically associated)

Oligosaccharide
on glycoprotein

Oligosaccharide
on glycolipid

Multipass
transmembrane
protein (integral)

Cytoskeletal
linkage proteins

Glycolipid

Glycoprotein

Integral membrane
protein (attached
to phospholipid)

Phospholipids of
lipid bilayer

Cholesterol

Spectrin
(Cytoskeletal proteins)

Actin

Integral membrane protein
(with attached hydrocarbon chain)

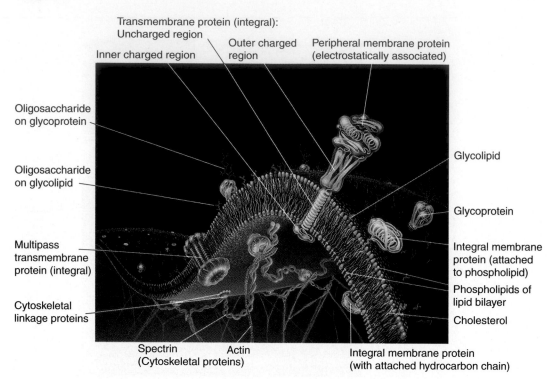

Plate 3-1
Molecular composition of the cell membrane, showing its associated membrane cytoskeleton
(model based in part on studies of the cell membrane of mammalian erythrocytes).

Basophilic
cytoplasm

Nucleus

Lumen

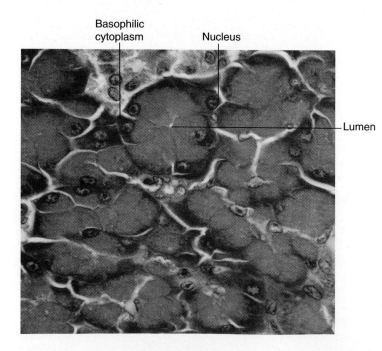

Plate 3-2
Pancreatic acinar cells showing
basal cytoplasmic basophilia.

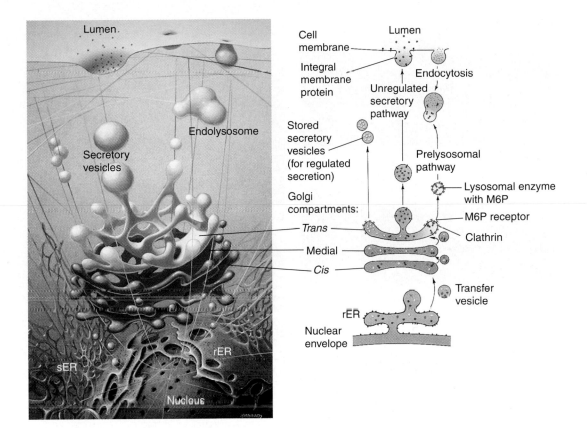

Plate 3-3
Secretory, lysosomal, and integral membrane proteins are synthesized by the rER and modified and sorted in the Golgi region.

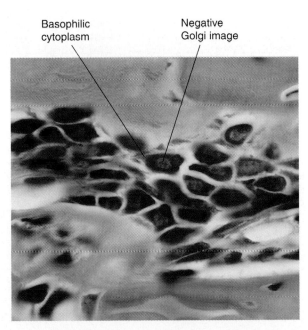

Plate 3-4
Osteoblasts showing a negative Golgi image in basophilic cytoplasm.

Chapter 4

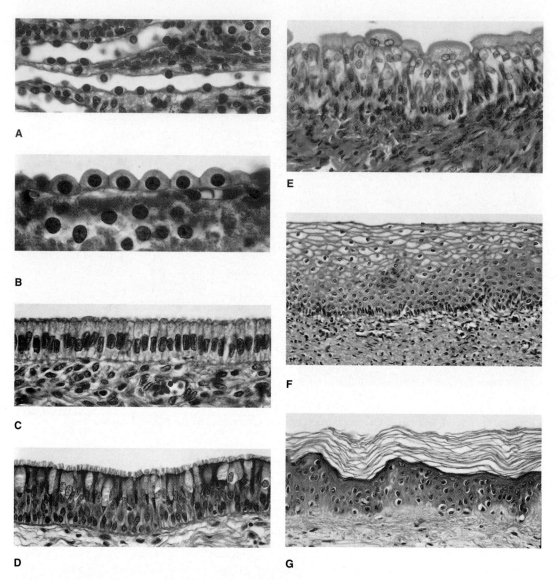

Plate 4-1
Types of epithelia. (*A*) Simple squamous; (*B*) simple cuboidal; (*C*) simple columnar;
(*D*) pseudostratified ciliated columnar, with goblet cells; (*E*) transitional; (*F*) stratified squamous
nonkeratinizing; (*G*) stratified squamous keratinizing.

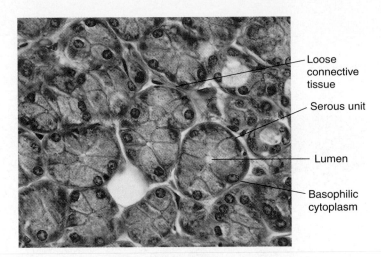

Loose
connective
tissue

Serous unit

Lumen

Basophilic
cytoplasm

Plate 4-2
Parotid gland showing serous
secretory units.

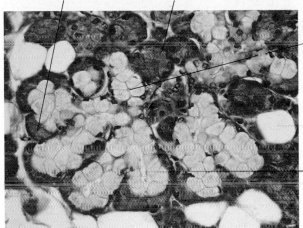

Serous
demilune

Serous
unit

Mucous
unit

Lipid in
fat cell

Lumen of
mixed
secretory
unit

Plate 4-3
Mixed salivary gland
showing mixed, mucous, and
serous secretory units. The
mixed secretory units are
capped by serous demilunes.

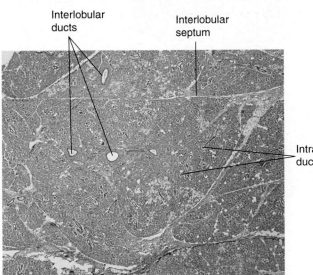

Interlobular
ducts

Interlobular
septum

Intralobular
ducts

Plate 4-4
General features of a compound
exocrine gland (submandibular,
low power).

Chapter 5

Mast cells   Capillary

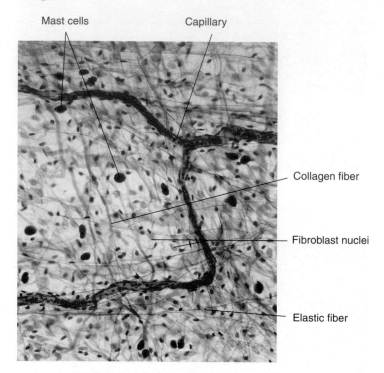

Collagen fiber

Fibroblast nuclei

Elastic fiber

Plate 5-1
Loose connective tissue (spread
stained with Weigert's
hematoxylin, eosin, and
resorcin-fuchsin).

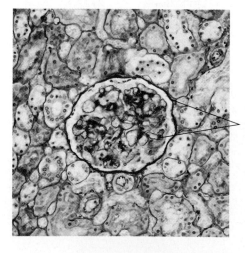

Basement membranes
of renal corpuscle

Plate 5-2
Basement membranes (renal
corpuscle of kidney; PAS stain).

Negative Golgi image

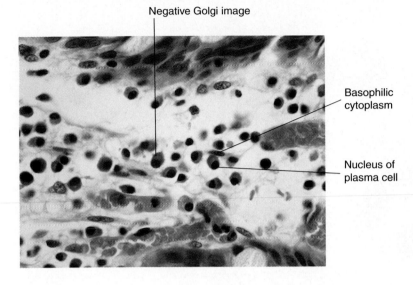

Basophilic
cytoplasm

Nucleus of
plasma cell

Plate 5-3
Plasma cells in loose connective tissue.

Blood vessels

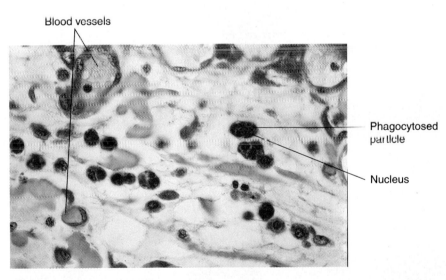

Phagocytosed
particle

Nucleus

Plate 5-4
Macrophages at a site of acute inflammation, showing their characteristic bean-shaped nucleus and
large ingested particles.

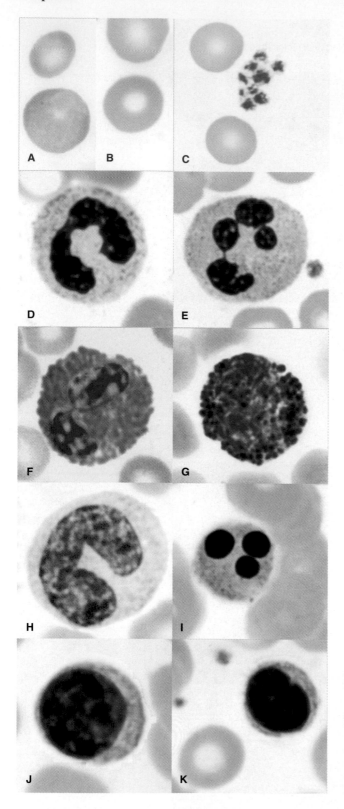

Chapter 6

Plate 6-1
Erythrocytes, leukocytes, and platelets
(peripheral blood film, Wright's blood
stain). (*A*) Polychromatophilic
erythrocyte; (*B*) erythrocyte (mature);
(*C*) platelets; (*D*) band neutrophil;
(*E*) neutrophil (mature); (*F*) eosinophil;
(*G*) basophil; (*H*) monocyte;
(*I*) degenerating neutrophil; (*J*) large
lymphocyte; (*K*) small lymphocyte.

Mature erythrocyte

Reticulocytes

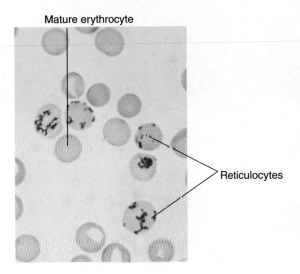

Plate 6-2
Peripheral blood reticulocytes (rabbit, reticulocyte count increased through prior bleeding; stained with brilliant cresyl blue). Residual RNA in reticulocytes appears as a wreath-like network or scattered particles.

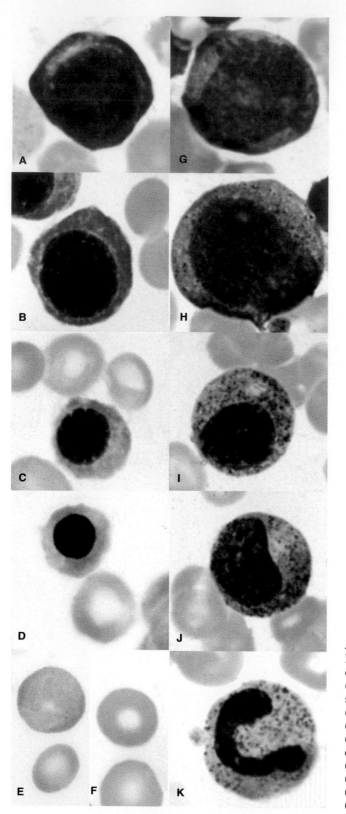

Chapter 7

Plate 7-1
Microscopically recognizable stages of erythroid and granulocytic maturation (bone marrow film, Wright's blood stain). (*A*) Proerythroblast; (*B*) basophilic erythroblast; (*C*) polychromatophilic erythroblast; (*D*) normoblast; (*E*) polychromatophilic erythrocyte; (*F*) erythrocyte (mature); (*G*) myeloblast; (*H*) promyelocyte; (*I*) neutrophilic myelocyte; (*J*) neutrophilic metamyelocyte; (*K*) band neutrophil.

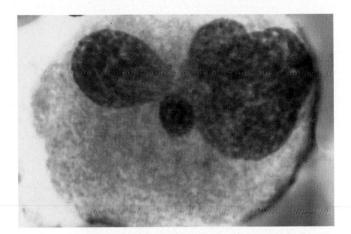

Plate 7-2
Megakaryocyte, showing its large
multilobed nucleus (bone marrow film,
Wright's blood stain).

Cortex   Medulla   Septum
between
lobules

Small lymphocytes in medulla

Blood
vessel

Thymic
corpuscle

Epithelial
reticular
cell

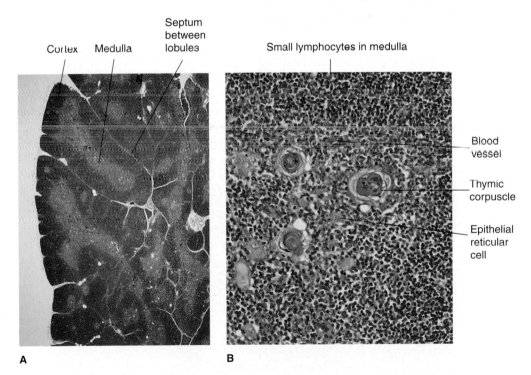

A   B

Plate 7-3
Thymus from a child. (*A*) Very low power; (*B*) medulla showing thymic corpuscles.

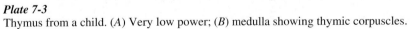

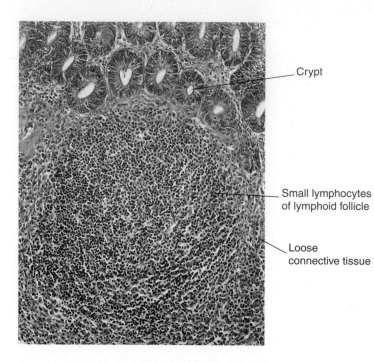

Crypt

Small lymphocytes
of lymphoid follicle

Loose
connective tissue

Plate 7-4
Lymphoid follicle associated
with epithelial lining of small
intestine.

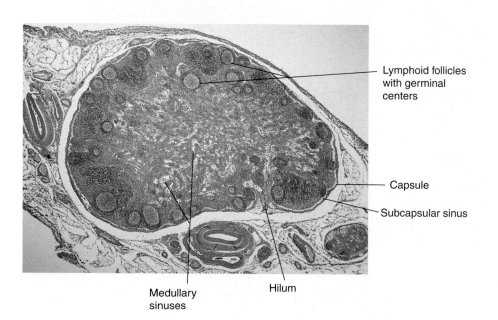

Lymphoid follicles
with germinal
centers

Capsule

Subcapsular sinus

Medullary
sinuses

Hilum

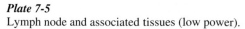

Plate 7-5
Lymph node and associated tissues (low power).

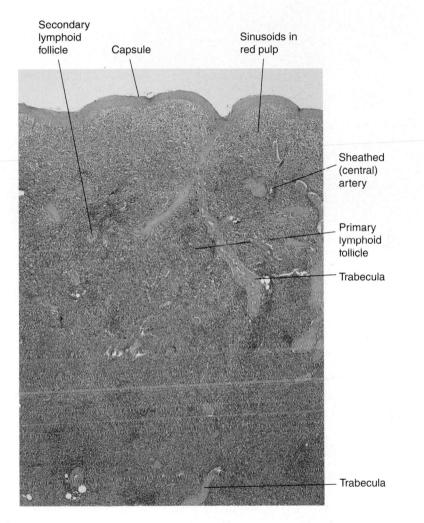

Secondary lymphoid follicle

Capsule

Sinusoids in red pulp

Sheathed (central) artery

Primary lymphoid follicle

Trabecula

Trabecula

Plate 7-6
Periphery of the spleen (low power). The splenic white pulp stains dark blue because it contains an abundance of small lymphocytes.

Chapter 8

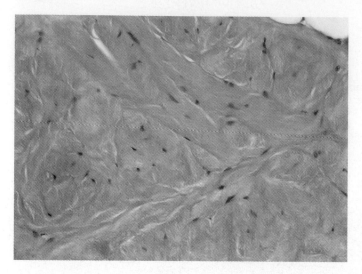

Plate 8-1
Reticular layer of dermis of thick skin, showing dense ordinary (fibrous) connective tissue, irregularly arranged. Substantial collagen bundles lie in various planes with compressed nuclei of fibrocytes scattered between them.

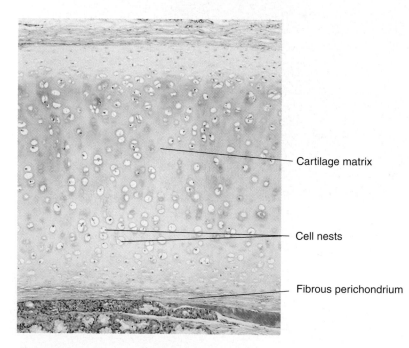

Cartilage matrix

Cell nests

Fibrous perichondrium

Plate 8-2
Tracheal cartilage, showing hyaline cartilage with perichondrium.

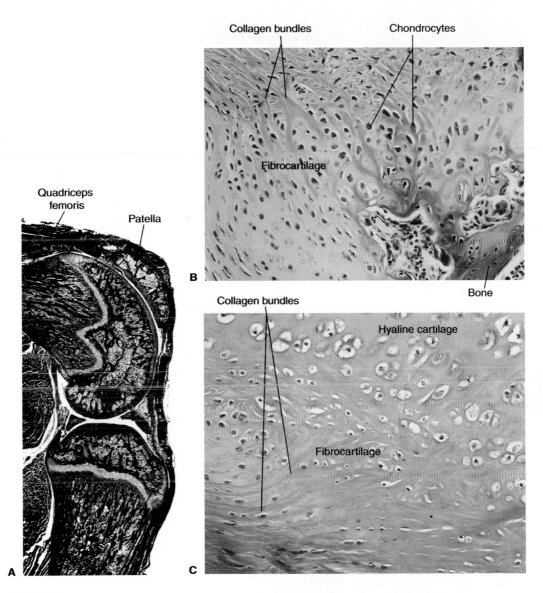

Plate 8-3
Fibrocartilage of the knee joint (rat). (*A*) Longitudinal section of the joint (scanning power for
orientation). *Upper box* indicates an attachment of the tendon of the quadriceps femoris muscle to
the patella. *Lower box* indicates another attachment site where fibrocartilage is commonly present.
(*B*) Fibrocartilage of the tendon attachment (high power). (*C*) Fibrocartilage attachment to hyaline
cartilage (high power).

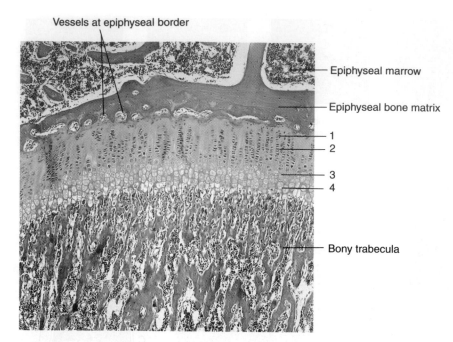

Vessels at epiphyseal border

Epiphyseal marrow

Epiphyseal bone matrix

1
2

3
4

Bony trabecula

Plate 8-8
Component zones and blood supply of an epiphyseal plate (rat). (*1*) Resting zone; (*2*) proliferating zone; (*3*) maturing zone; (*4*) calcifying zone.

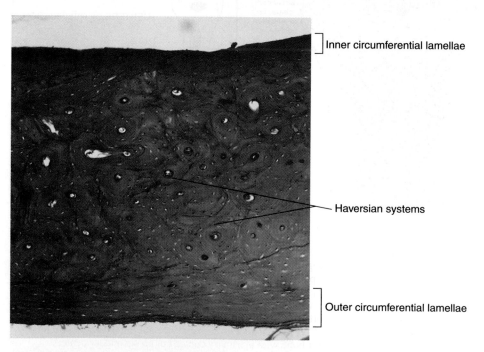

Inner circumferential lamellae

Haversian systems

Outer circumferential lamellae

Plate 8-9
Compact bone of the diaphyseal cortex (mature long bone, transverse section). Inner and outer diaphyseal surfaces are smoothed off with circumferential lamellae.

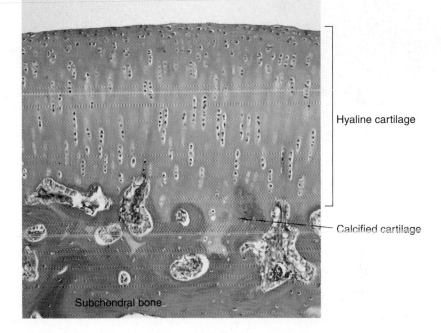

Hyaline cartilage

Calcified cartilage

Subchondral bone

Plate 8-10
Articular cartilage (knee joint of rabbit).

Chapter 9

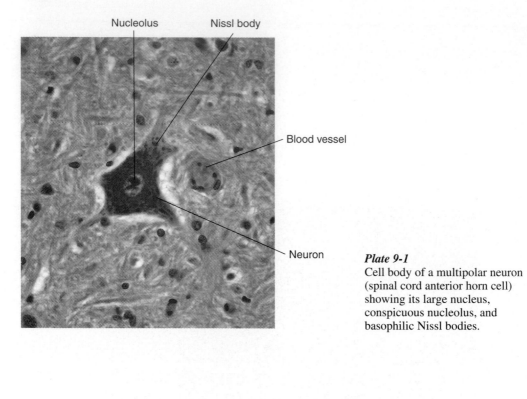

Nucleolus

Nissl body

Blood vessel

Neuron

Plate 9-1
Cell body of a multipolar neuron
(spinal cord anterior horn cell)
showing its large nucleus,
conspicuous nucleolus, and
basophilic Nissl bodies.

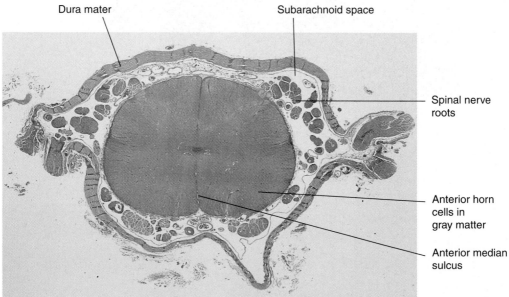

Dura mater

Subarachnoid space

Spinal nerve
roots

Anterior horn
cells in
gray matter

Anterior median
sulcus

Plate 9-2
Histologic features of the spinal cord and associated structures (low power).

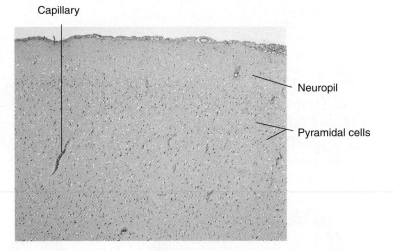

Capillary

Neuropil

Pyramidal cells

Plate 9-3
Cerebral cortex containing
pyramidal cells, other neurons,
neuroglia, and capillaries (motor
area, low power).

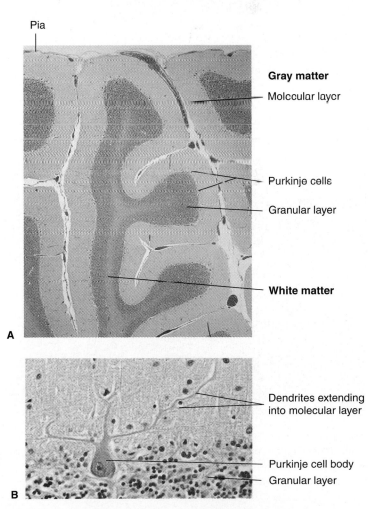

Pia

Gray matter
Molecular layer

Purkinje cells

Granular layer

White matter

A

Dendrites extending
into molecular layer

Purkinje cell body
Granular layer

Plate 9-4
(*A*) Three layers of gray matter
characterize the cerebellar cortex
seen under low power. (*B*) Cell
body and dendritic tree of a
Purkinje cell.

B

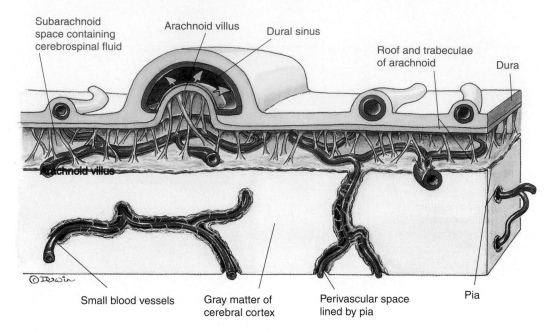

Subarachnoid space containing cerebrospinal fluid

Arachnoid villus

Dural sinus

Roof and trabeculae of arachnoid

Dura

Arachnoid villus

Small blood vessels

Gray matter of cerebral cortex

Perivascular space lined by pia

Pia

Plate 9-5
Schematic diagram of meninges, showing the pathway by which cerebrospinal fluid drains into dural sinuses from arachnoid villi.

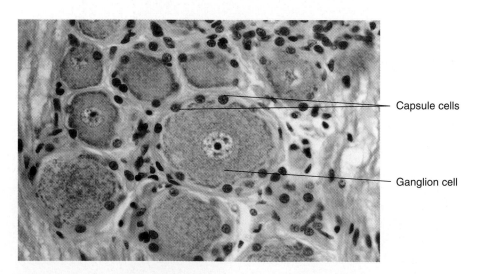

Capsule cells

Ganglion cell

Plate 9-6
Spinal (dorsal root or posterior root) ganglion, showing spinal ganglion cells enclosed by capsule cells.

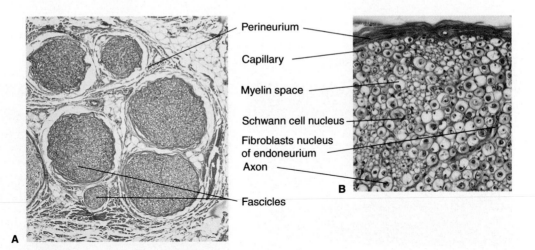

Perineurium

Capillary

Myelin space

Schwann cell nucleus

Fibroblasts nucleus
of endoneurium

Axon

Fascicles

A

B

Plate 9-7
Histologic appearance of a large peripheral nerve (transverse section). (*A*) Nerve fascicles and
perineurium (low power). (*B*) Part of a nerve fascicle, showing myelinated axons of various
diameters and the investing perineurium.

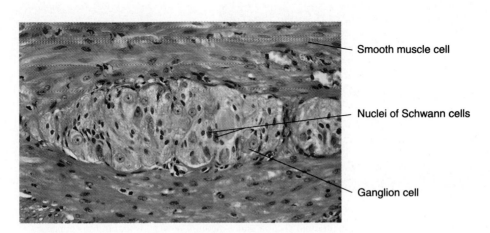

Smooth muscle cell

Nuclei of Schwann cells

Ganglion cell

Plate 9-8
Representative region of myenteric (Auerbach's) plexus in the duodenum, showing autonomic
ganglion cells and nuclei of plexus-associated Schwann cells. (To locate this plexus, refer to
Fig. 13-9.)

Chapter 10

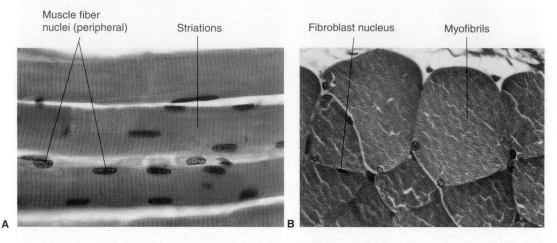

A Muscle fiber nuclei (peripheral)   Striations

B Fibroblast nucleus   Myofibrils

Plate 10-1
Skeletal muscle fibers seen in longitudinal section (*A*) and transverse section (*B*), showing striations, myofibrils, and peripheral nuclei (oil immersion).

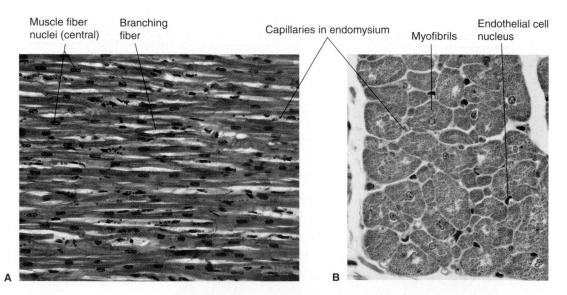

A Muscle fiber nuclei (central)   Branching fiber   Capillaries in endomysium

B Myofibrils   Endothelial cell nucleus

Plate 10-2
Cardiac muscle fibers seen in longitudinal section under medium power (*A*) and in transverse section under oil immersion (*B*), showing branching muscle fibers, myofibrils, central nuclei, and endomysium (sheep's heart).

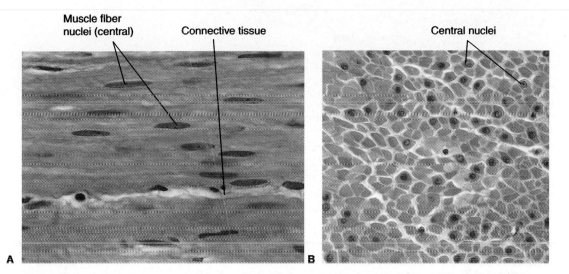

Plate 10-3
Intestinal smooth muscle fibers seen in longitudinal section (*A*) and transverse section (*B*), showing central nuclei and adjacent loose connective tissue (oil immersion).

Chapter 11

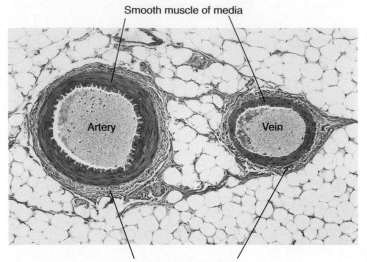

Smooth muscle of media

Artery

Vein

Connective tissue of adventitia

Plate 11-1
Muscular (distributing) artery
with accompanying vein
(abdominal mesenteric adipose
tissue, low power).

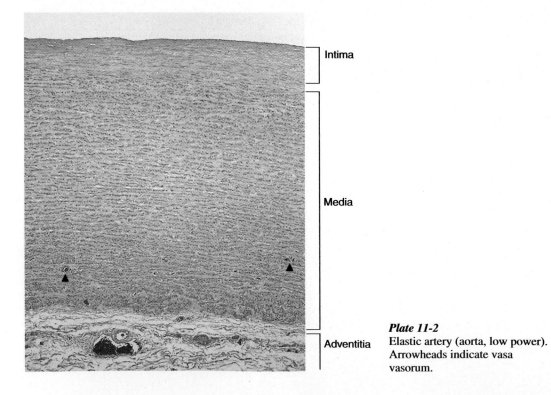

Intima

Media

Adventitia

Plate 11-2
Elastic artery (aorta, low power).
Arrowheads indicate vasa
vasorum.

Lymphatic   Capillary

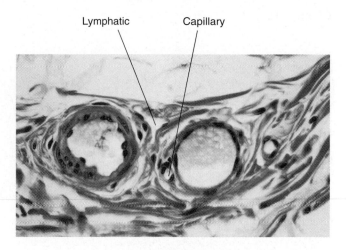

Plate 11-3
Arteriole and venule, along with
capillary and lymphatic (abdominal
mesenteric adipose tissue, high power).

Endothelium

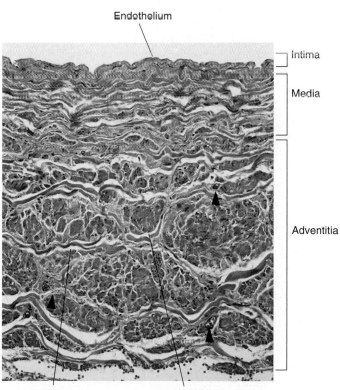

Intima

Media

Adventitia

Plate 11-4
Inferior vena cava, showing
smooth muscle and collagen
bundles of the adventitia (low
power). Arrowheads indicate vasa
vasorum.

Collagen
bundle

Longitudinal bundle
of smooth muscle

Chapter 12

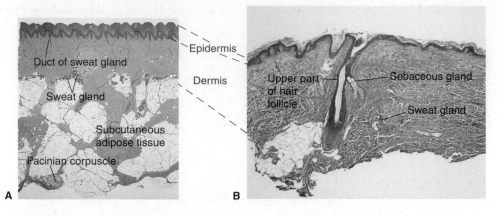

A   B

Plate 12-1
Thick skin (*A*) compared with thin skin (*B*), under very low power. The superficial stratum corneum on the epidermis is substantially thicker in *A* than in *B*.

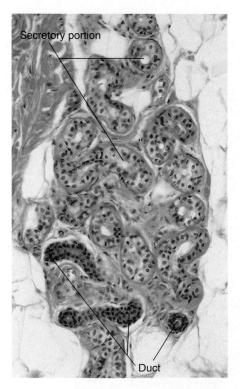

Plate 12-2
Eccrine sweat gland, showing the characteristic appearance of its secretory portion and duct.

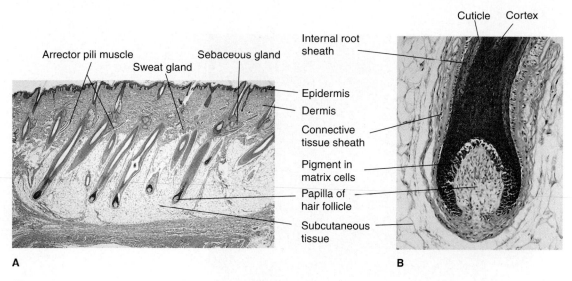

A

B

Plate 12-3

(*A*) Scalp, showing hair follicles and their associated appendages (very low power). (*B*) Base of a hair follicle, showing the dermal papilla and sheaths around the base of the hair (medium power).

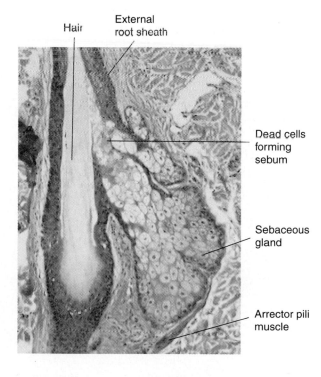

Plate 12-4

Upper part of a hair follicle, showing its associated sebaceous gland.

Chapter 13

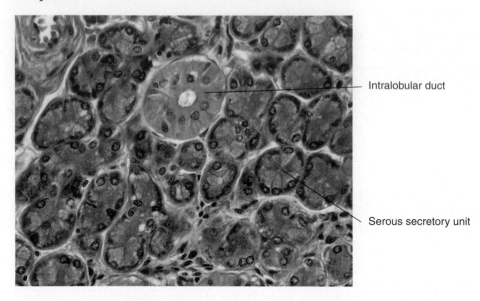

Intralobular duct

Serous secretory unit

Plate 13-1
Parotid gland, showing its serous secretory units and an intralobular duct (medium power).

Muscularis
mucosae   Submucosa   Epithelium

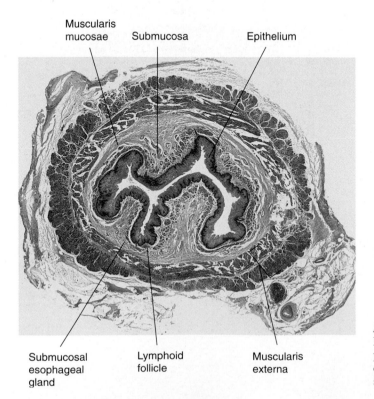

Submucosal
esophageal
gland

Lymphoid
follicle

Muscularis
externa

Plate 13-2
Esophagus (middle third, very low power). The muscularis externa contains skeletal muscle with some smooth muscle.

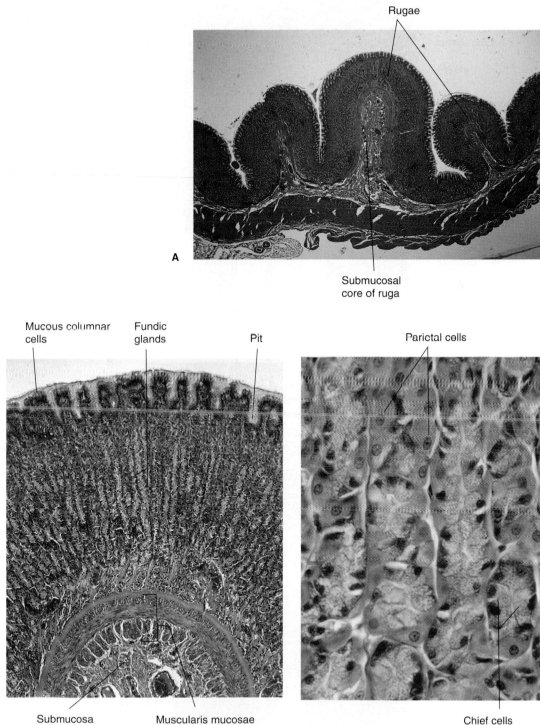

Rugae

Submucosal
core of ruga

Mucous columnar
cells

Fundic
glands

Pit

Parietal cells

A

B

Submucosa

Muscularis mucosae

Chief cells

C

Plate 13-3
Stomach (fundic region). (*A*) Full thickness of wall, showing the internal rugae (very low power).
(*B*) Mucosal epithelium, pits, and fundic glands (low power). (*C*) Fundic glands (high power).

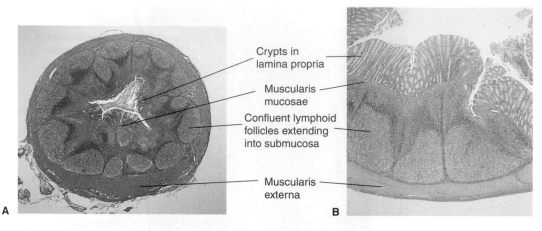

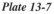

Crypts in
lamina propria

Muscularis
mucosae

Confluent lymphoid
follicles extending
into submucosa

Muscularis
externa

A

B

Plate 13-7
Appendix. (*A*) Very low power view. (*B*) Representative part of the wall (low power).

Interlobular septum   Acinus

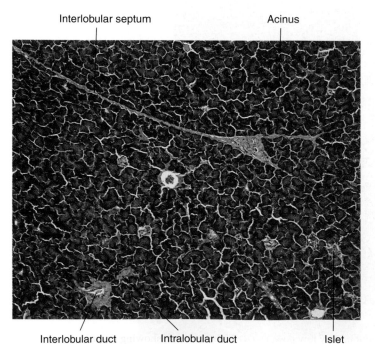

Interlobular duct   Intralobular duct   Islet

Plate 13-8
Pancreas, showing general
features (low power). Pancreatic
intralobular ducts are
inconspicuous.

Centroacinar cell nuclei

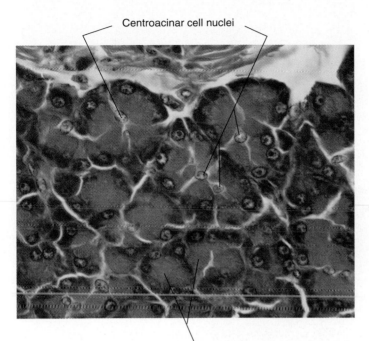

Plate 13-9
Pancreatic acini, showing nuclei of pancreatic centroacinar cells (oil immersion).

Acinar cells

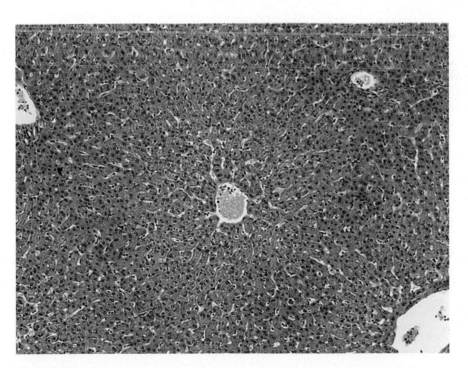

Plate 13-10
Liver, showing its general appearance (low power).

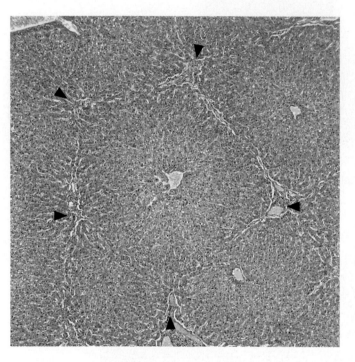

Plate 13-11
Classic liver lobule boundaries
(human liver). Arrowheads indicate
the position of portal areas. A central
vein may be recognized in the middle
of the lobule. It is evident from
observing Plates 13-10 and 13-11 that
normal human liver *lacks*
conspicuous interlobular fibrous
septa.

Chapter 14

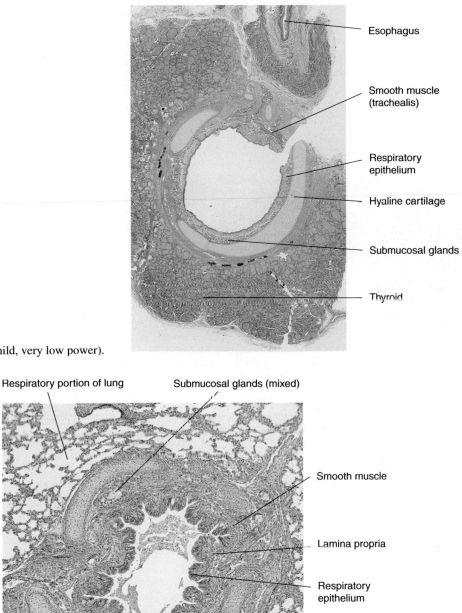

Esophagus

Smooth muscle
(trachealis)

Respiratory
epithelium

Hyaline cartilage

Submucosal glands

Thyroid

Plate 14-1
Trachea (of child, very low power).

Respiratory portion of lung   Submucosal glands (mixed)

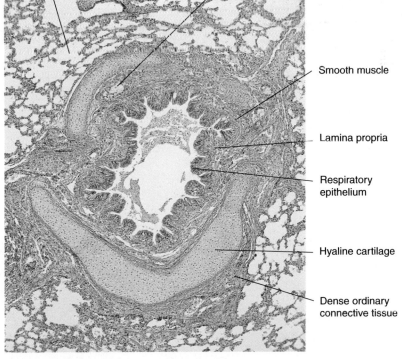

Smooth muscle

Lamina propria

Respiratory
epithelium

Hyaline cartilage

Dense ordinary
connective tissue

Plate 14-2
Intrapulmonary bronchus (in child's lung).

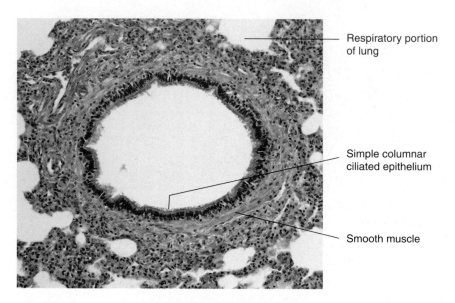

Respiratory portion
of lung

Simple columnar
ciliated epithelium

Smooth muscle

Plate 14-3
Bronchiole (in child's lung). Smooth muscle is fairly evident in this comparatively large
bronchiole.

Chapter 15

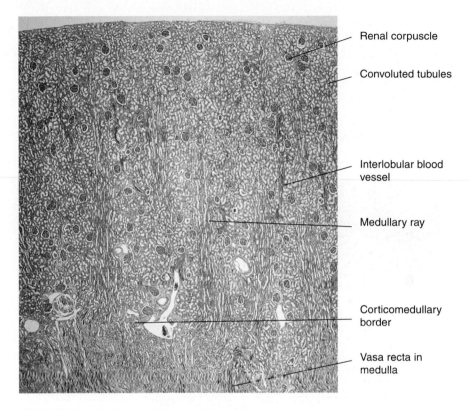

Renal corpuscle

Convoluted tubules

Interlobular blood vessel

Medullary ray

Corticomedullary border

Vasa recta in medulla

Plate 15-1
General features of the kidney cortex, showing renal corpuscles, medullary rays, and the position of the corticomedullary border (very low power).

Tubular pole of renal corpuscle

Distal convoluted tubule

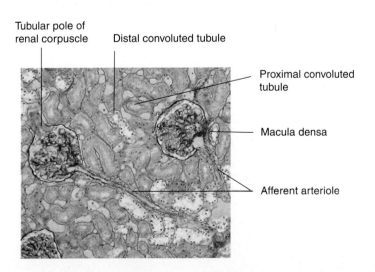

Proximal convoluted tubule

Macula densa

Afferent arteriole

Plate 15-2
Renal corpuscles, showing the arteriolar blood supply and adjacent kidney tubules (kidney; PAS stain).

Transitional epithelium

Lamina propria

Smooth muscle (longitudinal)

Smooth muscle (circular)

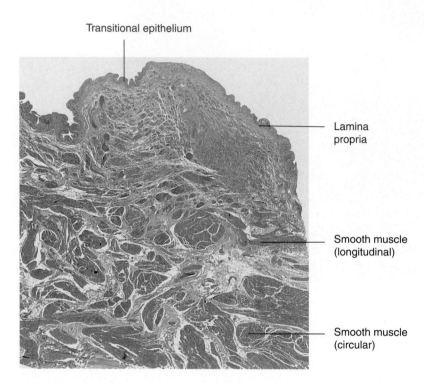

Plate 15-3
Urinary bladder, showing the arrangement of smooth muscle in its walls (very low power).

Chapter 16

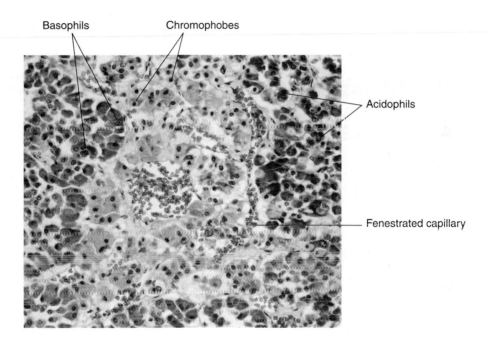

Basophils   Chromophobes

Acidophils

Fenestrated capillary

Plate 16-1
Anterior pituitary (Gomori stain, medium power).

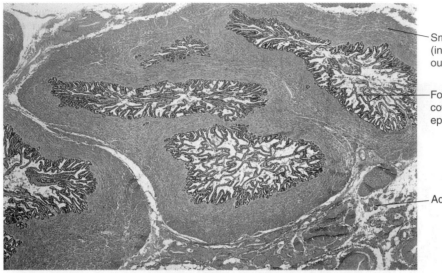

Smooth muscle (inner circular and outer longitudinal)

Folds of lamina propria covered with secretory epithelium

Adventitia

Plate 18-3
Seminal vesicle (very low power).

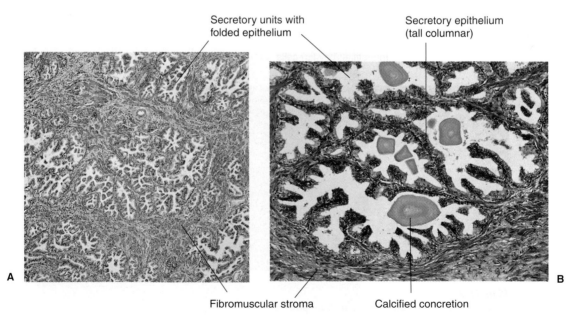

Secretory units with folded epithelium

Secretory epithelium (tall columnar)

Fibromuscular stroma

Calcified concretion

A

B

Plate 18-4
Prostate. (*A*) Low-power view. (*B*) Concretions may be found in prostatic secretory units (medium power).

Chapter 19

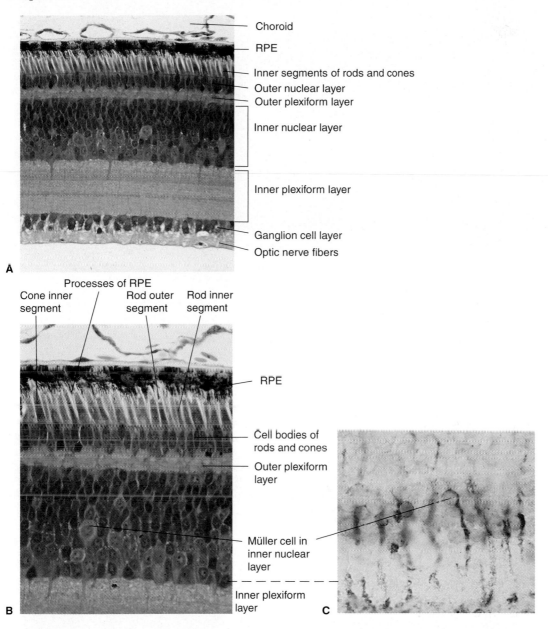

Plate 19-1

Retina (high power). (*A* and *B*) Semithin sections stained with toluidine blue (20-day chick). (*C*) Frozen section stained using a histochemical reaction for glial fibrillary acidic protein (GFAP; adult rat retina). The component layers of the retina are identified in (*A*). Details of the retinal pigment epithelium (RPE), photoreceptors, and inner nuclear layer are discernible in *B*. In *C*, the cell bodies of Müller cells are demonstrated in the inner nuclear layer by histochemical staining for GFAP.

CHAPTER 9

Nervous Tissue and Nervous System

OBJECTIVES

This chapter contains information that should enable you to do the following:

* Recognize neurons in H&E-stained sections and interpret their histological features
* Summarize the key differences between an axon and a dendrite
* State the key differences between gray matter and white matter and describe their respective histological compositions
* Name four types of neuroglia and specify their distinctive functions
* Discuss the production and functional importance of myelin
* Describe the LM appearance of nerves and various ganglia in the peripheral nervous system

Neurons (nerve cells) are specialized nondividing cells in which irritability and conductivity are highly developed. In response to effective stimuli, the electrically excitable cell membrane generates and transmits waves of excitation (nerve impulses) that rapidly pass along the nerve fibers. Nervous tissue, where neurons are uniquely found, is generally described in the functional context of the nervous system, made up of organs and structures collectively responsible for nervous function (Table 9-1). Impulses arising in constituent neurons of neural pathways in the nervous system influence whether other neurons contacting them at sites called **synapses** (Gk., Connections) generate impulses of their own. The impulses may trigger or inhibit generation of further impulses, depending on whether the transmitting synapses are *excitatory* or *inhibitory*. A two-neuron pathway permits extrinsic stimuli to elicit contraction of muscle cells. The first neuron is described as **afferent** (L. *ad*, to; *ferre*, to carry) because it carries **afferent (sensory) impulses** to the central nervous system. The second neuron is described as **efferent** (L. *ex*, out of) because it carries **efferent (motor) impulses** out of the central nervous system. The two neurons constitute a **simple reflex arc** (see Fig. 9-20). Because the body is made up of a number of segments, each with afferent and efferent neurons, abundant **interneurons (association neurons)**, constituting almost all of the brain, are necessary to process the impulse-coded information and to coordinate neural activities in the different segments. Each body segment includes the adjacent halves of contiguous vertebrae. The spinal nerve supply of the segmental tissues emerges bilaterally from the spinal cord through intervertebral foramina.

TABLE 9-1

NERVOUS TISSUE ORGANIZATION

CNS

Gray matter

White matter

PNS

Ganglia
   Cranial
   Spinal
   Autonomic

Peripheral nerves

Nerve endings
   Afferent
   Efferent

The axial part of the nervous system developing from the neural tube is the **central nervous system (CNS)**. It forms the **brain** and **spinal cord**, major roles of which are 1) to integrate sensory information and 2) to initiate and coordinate efferent responses. The brain also carries out the higher mental functions of thinking, learning, and remembering.

The **peripheral nervous system (PNS)** is a functional and anatomical extension of the CNS. It is primarily represented by **cranial nerves** from the brain, **spinal nerves** from the spinal cord, and nodules known as **ganglia** that house the associated neuronal cell bodies. The PNS develops primarily from neural crest (see later). Certain parts of afferent and efferent neurons, and all interneurons, lie within the CNS. The remaining parts of afferent and efferent neurons lie within the PNS.

STRUCTURAL BASIS OF NEURAL PATHWAYS

Neurons

Extending from the **cell body (perikaryon)** of each neuron are **nerve fibers** of two types (Fig. 9-1). Most are tapering **dendrites** (Gk. *dendron*, tree) with many fine branches. Generally not as long as the axon, dendrites branch dichotomously at acute angles (see Fig. 9-1*C*). They constitute a major site where impulses are *received* by the cell, their several orders of branching providing an extensive area for this purpose. Dendrites conduct impulses *toward* the cell body.

The other type of nerve fiber is single, not multiple as is the case in typical dendrites. Known as the **axon** (Gk., Axis), it follows a straighter course and does not taper (Fig. 9-2). The axon transmits impulses to its distal end, in most cases in a direction *away* from the cell body. Branching of the axon is limited to the distal end, except that in a few cases auxiliary side branches (**axon collaterals**) emerge from the axon more or less perpendicularly at intervals along its length.

Neurons with an axon and a single dendrite are described as **bipolar** (see Fig. 9-1*A*). In the development of many such cells, however, the proximal portions of the two neurites (neuronal processes) approximate closely and then fuse to form a single common proximal segment (see Fig. 9-1*B*). This kind of neuron is therefore often described as **pseudounipolar**. **Multipolar** neurons, the most common kind, have an axon and numerous dendrites (see Fig. 9-1*C*). Because they can receive impulses from a multitude of other neurons, they greatly expand the functional capacity of the nervous system. In H&E-stained sections, their cell bodies may appear fairly round (autonomic ganglion cells), star-shaped (anterior horn cells of the spinal cord), pyramidal (upper motor neurons of

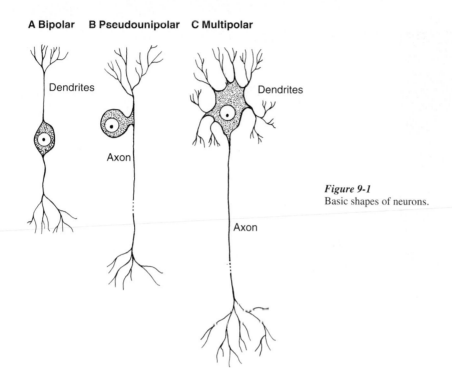

A Bipolar   B Pseudounipolar   C Multipolar

Dendrites

Axon

Dendrites

Axon

Figure 9-1
Basic shapes of neurons.

the motor cortex), or flask-shaped (Purkinje cells of the cerebellum). The nucleus, which generally lies near the middle of the cell body, is pale-staining with a conspicuous central round nucleolus, making it look like an owl's eye (Plate 9-1). This somewhat striking appearance of the nucleus is a helpful feature for recognizing neurons in sections. Another characteristic of neurons is that their cell body and major dendritic processes may exhibit intensely basophilic regions known as **Nissl bodies** representing ribosome-rich sites of active protein synthesis. The cell body houses numerous mitochondria, reflecting its substantial energy requirements. Golgi stacks and patches of rER further characterize this part of the cell. Microtubules and intermediate filaments maintain the neuron's highly asymmetrical shape (Fig. 9-3). Pigments, too, may be present since ageing neurons accumulate the wear-and-tear pigment **lipofuscin**, and neurons with cell bodies in the substantia nigra of the midbrain produce **melanin**. The larger dendrites contain most of the organelles represented in the cell body.

The longest nerve fiber in most kinds of neurons is the **axon**, the diameter of which ranges from 0.2 μm to 20 μm, depending on the class of neuron. The attachment site of the axon is sometimes recognizable as a pale-staining **axon hillock** on the cell body. The covering cell membrane of the axon is known as the **axolemma**; the internal cytoplasm of the axon is **axoplasm**. Investing the axolemma of a **myelinated axon** is a segmented **myelin sheath** interrupted at regular intervals by myelin-free gaps called **nodes (of Ranvier)**. This sheath will be described when we consider the PNS. The axolemma of **unmyelinated axons** is invested by astrocytic processes in the CNS and surface troughs of Schwann cells in the PNS. The axoplasm contains mitochondria, membranous vesicles, and a number of microtubules and neurofilaments (intermediate filaments). It is nevertheless virtually devoid of ribosomes, making the axon entirely dependent on the cell body for maintenance. Proteins and many other macromolecular constituents that become depleted by synaptic or metabolic activity are synthesized exclusively in the cell body. Together with certain organelles, they need to be conveyed on a continuous basis to the axon terminals, that is, in an anterograde direction.

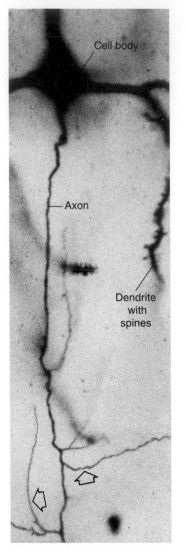

Figure 9-2
Multipolar neuron (cat pyramidal cell, modified Golgi stain), showing its axon, collaterals (*arrows*), and a dendrite.

Axonal (axoplasmic) transport has two main components. A **slow stream** travels a few millimeters each day, carrying cytosolic and cytoskeletal proteins (primarily enzymes, actin, and myosin) along the axon and maintaining the axon terminals. A **fast stream** carries axoplasmic vesicles in the anterograde direction at about 100 times this speed. The vesicles supply the various constituents needed by the axon terminals for replacing macromolecules expended during neurotransmission, including the enzymes, proteins, and phospholipids involved in local synaptic vesicle production. Anterograde movement of mitochondria is more intermittent and it occurs at an intermediate speed. At the same time, **retrograde flow** occurs in the reverse direction, that is, toward the cell body. About half as rapid as the fast anterograde stream, it returns unused or recycled constituents, along with materials (even infective virus particles) taken up by endocytosis, to the cell body. Substantial evidence indicates that the *anterograde* motor protein responsible for fast axonal transport is **kinesin**. Attached to the cytosolic surface of axoplasmic vesicles, this microtubule-activated ATPase drives the vesicles along the microtubule in the direction of its distal (**plus**) end. The *retrograde* motor protein driving membranous organelles back along microtubules (i.e., toward the cell body) is the microtubule-associated enzyme **cytoplasmic dynein**.

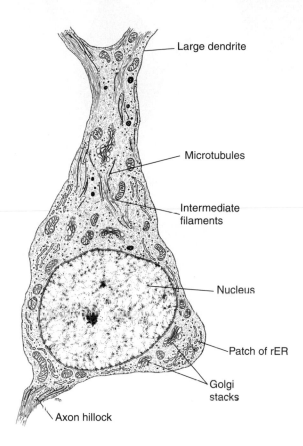

Large dendrite

Microtubules

Intermediate
filaments

Nucleus

Patch of rER

Golgi
stacks

Axon hillock

Figure 9-3
Multipolar neuron, showing major structural features
discernible in the cell body at the EM level (pyramidal
cell of motor cortex).

Synapses

Synapses are the special surface contact sites where neurotransmission occurs between neurons. The common type of synapse transmits impulses unidirectionally through the action of one or more **neurotransmitters** and is therefore termed a **chemical synapse**. The much rarer **electrical synapse** is a gap junction through which ions can freely pass and hence nerve impulses are directly conducted (see Fig. 9-5*D*). The mixed **conjoint synapse** is a combination of the two. The part of the synapse that delivers impulses, known as the **presynaptic terminal**, is commonly, but not always, an axon terminal (Fig. 9-4). The part of the synapse that receives impulses is the **postsynaptic terminal**, and the narrow intercellular space between the **pre-** and **post-synaptic membranes** is the **synaptic cleft**. If an axon synapses with a dendrite (see Fig. 9-4*A*) or lateral dendritic protrusion (**dendritic spine**), the synapse is described as **axodendritic** (see Figs. 9-2 and 9-4*B*). If the axon synapses with a nerve cell body, the synapse is **axosomatic** (see Fig. 9-4*A*), and if the axon synapses with another axon the synapse is **axoaxonic** (see Fig. 9-4*C*). An axon can synapse with a myelinated axon only at a site that is not insulated by myelin. Other synaptic arrangements exist but are more rare. For example, a dendrite can be postsynaptic to a nerve cell body, or even presynaptic to another dendrite, and nerve cell bodies can synapse with each other. The synapses found in muscle tissue (neuromuscular junctions) are described in Chapter 10.

Features that permit the presynaptic terminal of chemical synapses to be recognized in electron micrographs are 1) accumulations of **synaptic vesicles** containing neurotransmitter and 2) presence of **mitochondria** supplying energy for synaptic activity (Figs. 9-5 and 9-6). The presynaptic membrane of **directed synapses** is characterized by having a grid-like arrangement of interconnected

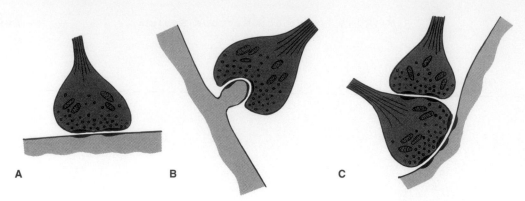

Figure 9-4
An axon terminal may synapse with a neuronal cell body or dendrite (*A*), a dendritic spine (*B*), or another axon terminal (*C*).

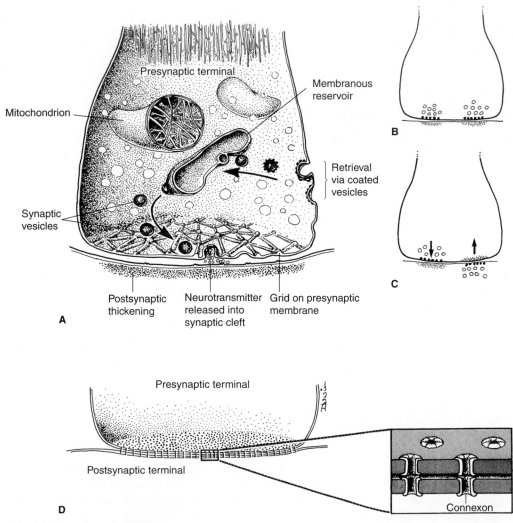

Figure 9-5
Membrane specializations at chemical and electrical synapses. (*A*) Directed chemical synapse with extensive postsynaptic thickening. (*B*) Directed chemical synapse with patchy postsynaptic thickening. (*C*) Directed reciprocal dendrodendritic chemical synapse with postsynaptic thickenings lying in the complementary (reciprocal) positions. Along with an excitatory synapse is an inhibitory synapse transmitting in the opposite direction. (*D*) Electrical synapse showing the gap junctional connexons responsible for direct electrical conduction.

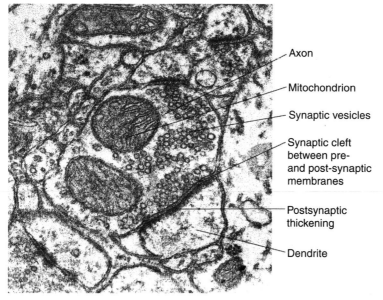

Axon

Mitochondrion

Synaptic vesicles

Synaptic cleft
between pre-
and post-synaptic
membranes

Postsynaptic
thickening

Dendrite

Figure 9-6
Electron micrograph of a chemical axodendritic synapse (rat occipital cortex, × 41,000).

electron-dense projections on its cytoplasmic surface. The gaps between the projections are of suitable dimensions to direct the synaptic vesicles into fusing with active zones in the presynaptic membrane when impulses arrive at the terminal (see Fig. 9-5A). The postsynaptic membrane also has electron-dense material adhering to its cytoplasmic surface, and in one type of chemical synapse this postsynaptic thickening is more conspicuous than the dense projections on the presynaptic membrane (see Fig. 9-6).

Nerve impulses are transient waves of depolarization that sweep rapidly across the nerve cell membrane. Each impulse is swiftly followed by a return to the electrically polarized resting state of the membrane. Impulses arriving at a presynaptic membrane open its calcium channels for a brief period. The ensuing influx of calcium ions causes stored synaptic vesicles to fuse with the membrane and results in the regulated discharge of neurotransmitter into the synaptic cleft. Interaction between the neurotransmitter and its receptors in the postsynaptic membrane then brings about an electrical change in the postsynaptic membrane. At some synapses, the interaction triggers **depolarization** of the postsynaptic membrane. These synapses are **excitatory**, because in this case the neurotransmission acts to *promote* generation of further impulses by the postsynaptic neuron. At other synapses, the interaction **hyperpolarizes** (additionally polarizes) the postsynaptic membrane. These synapses are **inhibitory**, because in this case the neurotransmission acts to *suppress* generation of additional impulses by the postsynaptic neuron. Summation of received excitatory and inhibitory impulses determines whether postsynaptic neurons generate impulses of their own.

During bursts of synaptic activity, fusing synaptic vesicles add supplemental amounts of membrane constituents to the presynaptic membrane. A local recycling mechanism retrieves the excess and even recovers some norepinephrine for reuse in producing more synaptic vesicles. The accumulating membrane constituents are retrieved from the periphery of the presynaptic terminal through active formation of coated vesicles. They are incorporated into a smooth-surfaced membranous reservoir from which further synaptic vesicles are produced (see Fig. 9-5A). In some cases, the neurotransmitter is synthesized locally within the reservoir, using precursors and enzymes brought to it by fast axonal transport.

CENTRAL NERVOUS SYSTEM

The central nervous system (CNS) develops from the **neural plate**, which originates axially from the mid-dorsal ectoderm of the embryo (Fig. 9-7A). This plate indents along its midline, forming the

spinal ganglion cells. Lipofuscin deposits may be present in the cytoplasm (see Fig. 3-27). A layer of flat **capsule cells** invests the cell body. Like the ganglion cells that they surround, the capsule cells are derived from neural crest neuroectoderm. They represent peripheral counterparts of the CNS neuroglia. The ganglion cells and their capsule cells are supported by a connective tissue framework, the counterpart of the connective tissue wrappings of peripheral nerves.

In sections, the cell body of a spinal ganglion cell appears rounded because the cell's two nerve fibers take origin from a single site that generally is missed in the plane of section. Close to the cell body, the proximal process divides at a T-shaped junction into two branches that extend in opposite directions (see Fig. 9-1*B*). The longer branch extends along a peripheral nerve and terminates at a sensory ending (see Fig. 9-21), whereas the shorter branch enters the spinal cord and synapses in the gray matter (Fig. 9-20). The entire length of the afferent fiber, except for a small receptive (dendritic) region at its sensory peripheral ending, actively transmits nerve impulses and has the structure of an axon. So in this special case, the peripheral and central afferent fibers are *both* considered to be part of the axon, with the cell body lying to one side of it.

Spinal ganglion cells are initially bipolar cells with two separate processes (see Fig. 9-1*A*). These processes, however, approach each other like the hands of a clock and then fuse, forming a single proximal segment common to both fibers (see Fig. 9-1*B*). They are accordingly often described as **pseudounipolar**.

Peripheral Nerves

In contrast to the CNS, the interior of which is soft and mushy, peripheral nerves are strong and resilient. This is due to a series of connective tissue sheaths that surround their nerve fibers. Thus, a fibrous sheath termed the **epineurium** invests each moderate- to large-sized nerve, surrounding it as a whole (Fig. 9-21). Internal to this, a more substantial sheath called the **perineurium** surrounds each fascicle (bundle) of nerve fibers. Then, within a fascicle, a delicate sheath of vascular loose

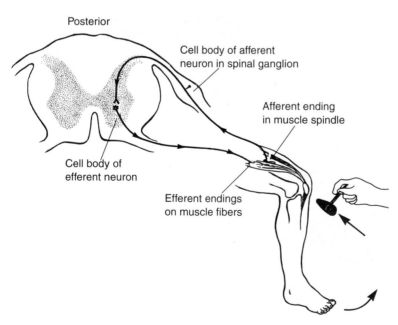

Figure 9-20
Neural basis of the stretch reflex, a simple reflex involving two neurons. The cell body of the afferent neuron lies in a spinal ganglion. The efferent neuron is an anterior horn cell (lower motor neuron) of the spinal cord.

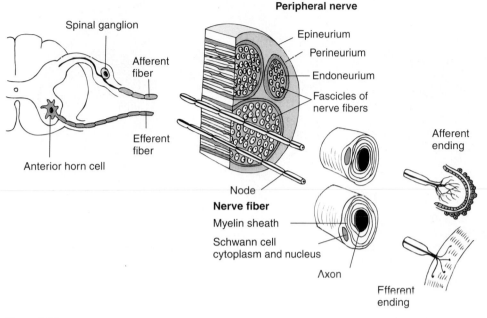

Figure 9-21
Peripheral nervous system (PNS) organization.

connective tissue known as the **endoneurium** invests each nerve fiber. Small peripheral nerves lack epineurium and have only perineurium and endoneurium (Plate 9-7).

Within the endoneurial sheath, each nerve fiber is also invested with a segmented cellular sheath termed the **sheath of Schwann** or **neurolemma (neurilemma)**. This sheath is made up of individual **Schwann cells**, which are peripheral counterparts of CNS neuroglia and in common with them are derived from neural crest neuroectoderm. In each segment of a **myelinated fiber**, two regions of the sheath are discernible at the LM level. A thin, outer layer of **Schwann cell cytoplasm** that contains the cell nucleus surrounds a thicker, inner nonstaining region that is part of the **myelin sheath** (see Fig. 9-21). The myelin of the PNS is all formed by Schwann cells. Each Schwann cell can myelinate only one segment of a single axon, however, so it takes a long series of Schwann cells to myelinate each axon. As in the CNS, the myelin sheath is interrupted by **nodes of Ranvier**, which lie between consecutive Schwann cells and are sites where myelinated axons may branch.

Peripheral Myelinated and Unmyelinated Nerve Fibers

When myelinating an axon segment, a Schwann cell accommodates the axon in a long groove (Fig. 9-22A). The cell produces a basement membrane along its connective tissue-associated surface (see Fig. 9-23), adheres to it, and begins to spread out. Its inner margin grows round and round the axon under the forming myelin (see Fig. 9-22B). In this manner, many layers of Schwann cell membrane are built up into a spiral (see Fig. 9-22C). The cytoplasm initially present between the apposed areas of cell membrane becomes squeezed back into the outer part of the Schwann cell, with the result that the apposed parts of this membrane come into contact and fuse. Accordingly, in the EM, a section of myelin sheath is characterized by a distinctive pattern of parallel electron-dense lines (Fig. 9-23). In peripheral myelin, this pattern corresponds to compacted double thicknesses of Schwann cell membrane. Small pockets of trapped cytoplasm create occasional discontinuities in the myelin of

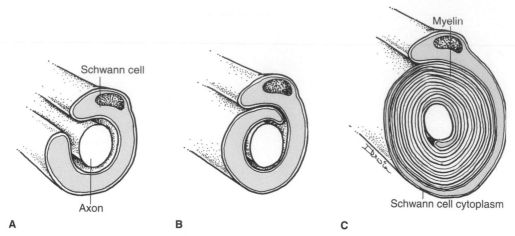

A   **B**   **C**

Figure 9-22
Axon myelination in the PNS. When the Schwann cell adheres to the basement membrane that lies at its periphery, the innermost cell margin keeps growing inward around the axon.

peripheral nerves. These discontinuities are termed **clefts of Schmidt-Lanterman**. The process of myelination in the CNS and PNS continues after birth and remains necessary during postnatal growth.

Along the internodal regions between consecutive nodes, myelin insulates the axolemma from tissue fluid. At the nodes, however, the axolemma is freely exposed to tissue fluid. This arrangement provides the basis for rapid impulse conduction by permitting local currents to flow in rapid succession. By passing through a local circuit of axoplasm and surrounding tissue fluid, current flows from each depolarized node to the next polarized one, depolarizing that node, and so on. Nerve impulses thus jump from node to node, resulting in a fast form of impulse conduction termed **saltatory conduction** (L. *saltare*, to jump).

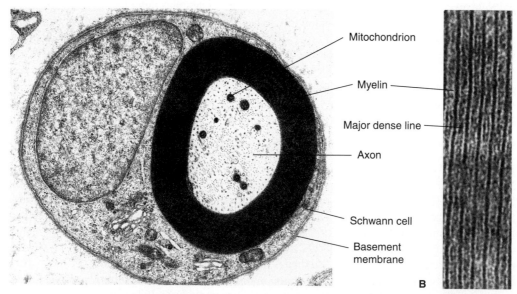

A   **B**

Figure 9-23
(*A*) Myelinated axon with its associated Schwann cell (peripheral nerve, electron micrograph). (*B*) Myelin in transverse section, showing its repetitive pattern of parallel electron-dense lines at higher magnification.

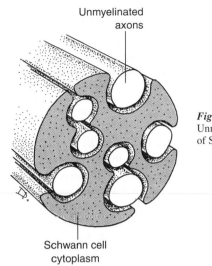

Figure 9-24
Unmyelinated axons in peripheral nerves are supported in superficial grooves of Schwann cells.

Some axons, however, are **unmyelinated**. When speed of conduction along the axon is less critical, the Schwann cells that constitute its neurolemma do not produce myelin. Moreover, in this case, each Schwann cell is able to accommodate a number of axons in individual troughs in its cytoplasm (Figs. 9-24 and 9-25), not just one as is the case in myelinated fibers. With such an arrangement, the Schwann cell cannot wrap around individual axons and myelin is not produced. Instead, long

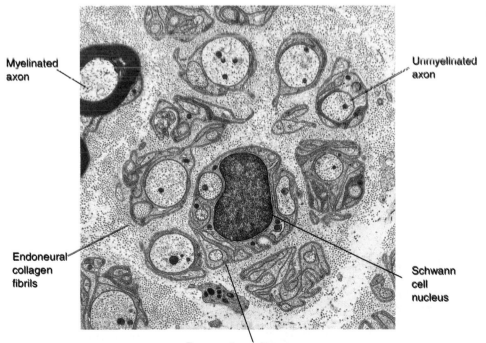

Figure 9-25
Electron micrograph of peripheral nerve, showing unmyelinated axons being supported by Schwann cells (compare with Fig. 9-22).

AUTONOMIC NERVOUS SYSTEM

Most physiological responses are subject to regulation by efferent nerve impulses, but only skeletal muscular contraction can be brought about at will. The responses that are normally beyond voluntary control are regulated automatically. The innervation of the circulatory system, smooth muscle, exocrine glands, and other viscera is accordingly called the **autonomic nervous system** (Gk. *autos*, self; *nomos*, law). The other part of the nervous system, concerned with the genesis of appropriate voluntary motor responses to afferent stimuli, is called the **somatic nervous system**. As in the somatic nervous system, afferent and efferent pathways exist for autonomic nerve impulses. When visceral afferent impulses reach the CNS from visceral receptors, they can trigger efferent impulses that pass along an autonomic two-neuron chain to visceral effectors.

Cardiac muscle, most smooth muscles, and exocrine glands are innervated by both anatomical divisions of the autonomic nervous system, which are known as its **sympathetic** and **parasympathetic divisions**, respectively. The functional responses elicited by neural activity in the one division are in many cases antagonistic to those elicited by the other. In each division, *two efferent neurons* are involved in carrying impulses from the CNS to the effector cells. The cell body of the first neuron of the efferent pathway lies in an intermediolateral column of gray matter of the spinal cord, whereas the cell body of the second neuron lies outside the CNS in an autonomic ganglion (Fig. 9-28). Because of this arrangement, the axon of the first neuron in the pathway is called the **preganglionic fiber**, and that of the second neuron is called the **postganglionic fiber**. From the CNS, preganglionic parasympathetic fibers emerge by way of certain cranial and sacral nerves, whereas preganglionic sympathetic fibers emerge by way of thoracic and lumbar nerves. In general, both kinds of preganglionic fibers are lightly myelinated whereas both kinds of postganglionic fibers are unmyelinated.

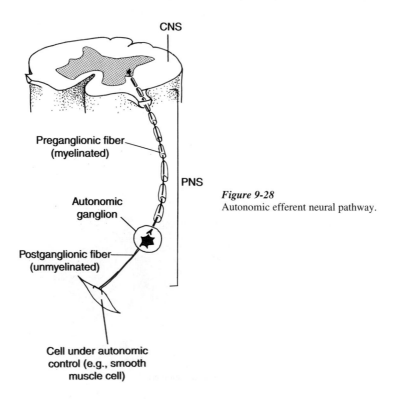

Figure 9-28
Autonomic efferent neural pathway.

Autonomic Ganglia

As in spinal ganglia, the **ganglion cells** and **capsule cells** of autonomic ganglia are 1) derived from neural crest and 2) supported by connective tissue. In autonomic ganglia, however, the ganglion cell margins are less distinct because the autonomic ganglion cells are multipolar. The capsule cell investment looks discontinuous because it is interrupted by the numerous dendrites of the ganglion cell (Fig. 9-29). Finally, it is more common to find the nucleus in an eccentric position in autonomic ganglion cells than is the case in spinal ganglion cells. A convenient site to observe autonomic ganglion cells is the **myenteric plexus**, which lies between the inner circular layer and the outer longitudinal layer of smooth muscle in the muscularis externa of the digestive tract (see Fig. 13-7). In sections of the digestive tract, this plexus appears as scattered groups of **parasympathetic ganglion cells** (Plate 9-8) interspersed with nerve fibers that include myelinated preganglionic parasympathetic fibers and unmyelinated postganglionic sympathetic fibers.

Autonomic Nerve Endings

Autonomic efferent endings are present in certain regions of the heart and in smooth muscle, exocrine glands, and adipose tissue. The autonomic endings on exocrine secretory cells resemble those on smooth muscle cells, described in Chapter 10. The terminations of postganglionic fibers are distended into a series of bulges (**varicosities**) associated with the cell membrane of the innervated cell and separated from it by a synaptic cleft. The varicosities contain mitochondria and numerous synaptic vesicles. The neurotransmitter released at these efferent endings is in some cases norepinephrine and in others, acetylcholine. Generally, norepinephrine is released at sympathetic endings, and acetylcholine is released at parasympathetic endings. The postganglionic sympathetic endings on

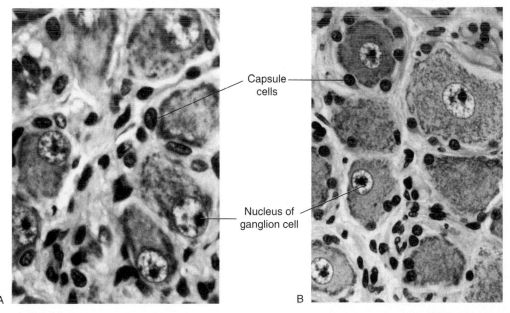

Capsule cells

Nucleus of ganglion cell

A   B

Figure 9-29
Ganglion and capsule cells of a parasympathetic autonomic ganglion (*A*) compared with the corresponding cells of a spinal ganglion (*B*). In *A*, nuclei commonly lie eccentrically in the cell body of ganglion cells, and the surrounding capsule cell layer has a more discontinuous appearance.

sweat glands, however, are an exception because they are cholinergic. The preganglionic fibers in each autonomic division are cholinergic.

Summary

For an outline of the general composition of nervous tissue, see Table 9-1. Neuronal cell bodies lie in the gray matter of the CNS and the ganglia of the PNS. The pseudounipolar cell bodies of most afferent neurons (conducting toward the CNS) lie in the spinal and cranial ganglia. The multipolar cell bodies of efferent neurons (conducting away from the CNS) are situated chiefly within the CNS, but some lie in autonomic ganglia.

The neuronal cell body has patchy cytoplasmic basophilia, indicating local concentrations of rER and free ribosomes. It also contains a large pale-staining nucleus with a prominent nucleolus, indicating active protein synthesis. It synthesizes proteins and other macromolecules needed by the axon, which in many cases is long, so the axon depends on the cell body for maintenance. Whereas constituents involved in synaptic transmission are transported by a fast stream, cytosolic proteins move in a slow stream. The anterograde motor is kinesin and the retrograde motor is cytoplasmic dynein. The axon commonly propagates impulses away from the cell body, and in many cases it is myelinated. Dendrites, which branch extensively and are unmyelinated, conduct impulses toward the cell body. Other parts of the neuron also can receive impulses. At most synapses, impulses are transmitted through release of a neurotransmitter. At electrical synapses, however, there is direct conduction. The presynaptic terminal of a chemical synapse is characterized by synaptic vesicles and mitochondria. The postsynaptic membrane, characterized by electron-dense thickening, depolarizes at excitatory synapses but hyperpolarizes at inhibitory synapses. Synaptic membranous constituents and certain neurotransmitters recycle in the presynaptic terminal.

Neuroglia arising mostly from neuroectoderm partly substitute for connective tissue that is minimal in the CNS but not the PNS. Included with neuroglia are microglia, resting macrophages that in adult life can arise from monocytes. The entirely neuroectoderm-derived, CNS-situated neuroglia are oligodendrocytes, which myelinate CNS axons; astrocytes, which are supportive and inductive cells; and ependymal cells, which line internal cavities of the CNS and cover the choroid plexuses.

Gray matter contains the cell bodies of neurons and neuroglia, capillaries, and nerve fibers, a large proportion of which are unmyelinated (neuropil). This component occupies an H-shaped central area in the spinal cord. Gray matter also constitutes the brain cortex, where it is organized as six layers in the cerebral cortex and three layers in the cerebellar cortex. Upper motor neurons of the cerebral cortex are pyramid-shaped, whereas Purkinje cells of the cerebellar cortex are flask-shaped with a vast dendritic tree. White matter contains myelinated axons arranged in tracts, neuroglia (mostly oligodendrocytes and fibrous astrocytes), and capillaries, but no cell bodies of neurons. Its position relative to gray matter is external in the spinal cord but internal in the brain. The structural basis of the blood–brain barrier is the presence of uninterrupted tight junctions between the endothelial cells of brain capillaries.

The CNS is protected by the fibrous dura, within which lies the arachnoid with its subarachnoid space filled with cerebrospinal fluid. Produced by the choroid plexuses, cerebrospinal fluid normally contains a few lymphocytes. Excess amounts are resorbed through arachnoid villi. The delicate innermost layer of the meninges (the pia mater) adheres to the surface of the brain and spinal cord. It is highly vascular.

Ganglia of the PNS consist of ganglion cells, peripheral neuroglia called capsule cells, and supporting connective tissue. Spinal ganglion cells are pseudounipolar, with a centrally located nucleus, and possess a uniform covering of capsule cells. In contrast, autonomic ganglion cells are multipolar, generally with an eccentric nucleus, and have a discontinuous covering of capsule cells.

In peripheral nerves, fascicles of myelinated or unmyelinated nerve fibers are surrounded by a strong perineurium and also, except in small nerves, an investing fibrous epineurium. Vascular loose connective tissue (endoneurium) lies between the individual nerve fibers. Peripheral neuroglia called Schwann cells invest axons either individually or as groups. The Schwann cell may wind around the axon, laying down thicknesses of cell membrane as myelin, or enclose several unmyelinated axons in its superficial troughs. Myelin is absent at nodes representing 1) borders between adjacent Schwann cells of the PNS or 2) borders between adjacent oligodendrocyte processes of the CNS. Because the axolemma is not insulated at nodes, internodes of myelinated axons depolarize consecutively (saltatory conduction). Myelinated and unmyelinated fibers regenerate readily in the PNS, but mature neurons do not divide. Equivalent satisfactory functional recovery does not occur in the CNS. Afferent nerve endings are intimately associated with sensory receptors. Efferent endings are found on muscle cells, secretory cells, and adipose tissue.

The autonomic nervous system consists of sympathetic and parasympathetic divisions, both of which are characterized by having two-neuron efferent pathways. In each case, the cell body of the second neuron lies in the autonomic ganglion. In contrast to the somatic nervous system, the autonomic nervous system is concerned with regulating involuntary responses.

Bibliography

Neurons, Neuroglia, Progenitors, and Stem Cells

Barres BA. New roles for glia. Neuroscience 11:3685, 1991.

Eriksson PS, Perfilieva E, Bjork-Eriksson T, et al. Neurogenesis in the adult human hippocampus. Nature Medicine 4(11):1313, 1998.

Graeber MB, Streit WJ. Perivascular microglia defined. Trends Neurosci 13:366, 1990.

Heuser JE, Reese TS. Structure of the synapse. In: Kandel ER, ed. Handbook of Physiology. The Nervous System, vol 1: Cellular Biology of Neurons. Baltimore, Williams & Wilkins, 1977, p 261.

Hollenbeck PJ. The transport and assembly of the axonal cytoskeleton. J Cell Biol 108:223, 1989.

Kempermann G, Gage FH. New nerve cells for the adult brain. Sci Am 280(5):48, 1999.

Kimelberg HK, Norenberg MD. Astrocytes. Sci Am 260(4):66, 1989.

Llinás RR. The cortex of the cerebellum. Sci Am 232(1):56, 1975.

Murphy S, ed. Astrocytes: Pharmacology and Function. San Diego, Academic Press, 1993.

Norton WT, ed. Oligodendroglia. Advances in Neurochemistry, vol 5. New York, Plenum, 1984.

Okabe S, Hirokawa N. Axonal transport. Curr Opin Cell Biol 1:91, 1989.

Peters A, Palay S, Webster H. The Fine Structure of the Nervous System: The Neurons and Supporting Cells, Philadelphia, WB Saunders, 1976.

Remahl S, Hildebrand C. Relation between axons and oligodendroglial cells during initial myelination: I. The glial unit. J Neurocytol 19:313, 1990.

Schnapp BJ, Reese TS. Dynein is the motor for retrograde axonal transport of organelles. Proc Natl Acad Sci USA 86:1548, 1989.

Schwartz JH. The transport of substances in nerve cells. Sci Am 242(4):152, 1980.

Sheetz MP, Steuer ER, Schroer TA. The mechanism and regulation of fast axonal transport. Trends Neurosci 12:474, 1989.

Thomas WE. Brain macrophages: evaluation of microglia and their functions. Brain Res Rev 17:61, 1992.

Travis J. Glia: the brain's other cells. Science 266:970, 1994.

Tropepe V, Coles BLK, Chiasson BJ et al. Retinal stem cells in the adult mammalian eye. Science 287(5460):2032, 2000.

Vale RD. Intracellular transport using microtubule-based motors. Annu Rev Cell Biol 3:347, 1987.

Vallee RB, Bloom GS. Mechanisms of fast and slow axonal transport. Annu Rev Neurosci 14:59, 1991.

Wilkin GP, Marriott DR, Cholewinski AJ. Astrocyte heterogeneity. Trends Neurosci 13:43, 1990.

Meninges, Cerebrospinal Fluid, and Blood–Brain Barrier

Abbott NJ. Glia and the blood–brain barrier. Nature 325:195, 1987.

Brightman MW, Reese TS. Junctions between intimated apposed cell membranes in the vertebrate brain. J Cell Biol 40:648, 1969.

Goldstein GW. Endothelial cell-astrocyte interactions: a cellular model of the blood–brain barrier. Ann NY Acad Sci 529:31, 1988.

Goldstein GW, Betz AL. The blood–brain barrier. Sci Am 255(3):74, 1986.

Janzer RC, Raff MC. Astrocytes induce blood–brain barrier properties in endothelial cells. Nature 325:253, 1987.

Kida S, Yamashima T, Kubota T, Ito H, Yamamoto S. A light and electron microscopic and immunohisto-chemical study of human arachnoid villi. J Neurosurg 69:429, 1988.

Nicholas DS, Weller RO. The fine anatomy of the human spinal meninges: a light and scanning electron microscopy study. J. Neurosurg 69:276, 1988.

Spector R, Johanson CE. The mammalian choroid plexus. Sci Am 261(5):68, 1989.

Stewart PA, Farrell CR, Coomber BL. Blood–brain barrier ultrastructure: beyond tight junctions. Ann NY Acad Sci 529:295, 1988.

Weed LH. Certain anatomical and physiological aspects of the meninges and cerebrospinal fluid. Brain 58:383, 1935.

Weed LH. Meninges and cerebrospinal fluid. J Anat 72:181, 1938.

Peripheral and Autonomic Nervous Systems

Boehm DH, Marks N. Myelin. In: Schwartz LM, Azar MM, eds. Advanced Cell Biology, New York, Van Nostrand Reinhold, 1981, p 163.

Bunge RP, Bunge MB, Bates M. Movements of the Schwann cell nucleus implicate progression of the inner (axon-related) Schwann cell process during myelination. J Cell Biol 109:273, 1989.

Chouchkov CV. Cutaneous receptors. In: Advances in Anatomy, Embryology, and Cell Biology, vol 54, fasc 5. Berlin, Springer-Verlag, 1978.

Halata Z. The mechanoreceptors of the mammalian skin. Ultrastructure and morphological classification. In: Advances in Anatomy, Embryology and Cell Biology, vol 50, fasc 5. Berlin, Springer-Verlag, 1975.

Iggo A. Cutaneous and subcutaneous sense organs. Br Med Bull 33:97, 1977.

Landon DN, ed. The Peripheral Nerve. London, Chapman & Hall, 1976.

Morell P, Norton WT. Myelin. Sci Am 242(5):88, 1980.

Rosenbluth J. Structure of the node of Ranvier. In: Chang DC, Tasaki I, Adelman WJ, Leuchtag HR, eds. Structure and Function in Excitable Cells. New York, Plenum, 1983, p 25.

Wilson-Pauwels L, Stewart PA, Akesson EJ. Autonomic Nerves. Hamilton, BC Decker, Inc., 1997.

Zagoren JC, Fedoroff S, eds. The Nodes of Ranvier. Orlando, FL, Academic Press, 1984.

CHAPTER 10

Muscle Tissue

OBJECTIVES

With the information in this chapter, you should be able to do the following:

- Depict how a sarcomere's filaments are arranged a) during relaxation and b) during contraction, relating muscle striations to the sarcomere
- Summarize the main similarities and differences between three different types of muscle
- Draw a labeled diagram of a motor end plate
- Explain how contraction is elicited in skeletal muscles
- Discuss why certain cell junctions exist between some muscle cells but not others
- Elaborate on which types of muscle can regenerate

Each kind of muscle in the body is made up of muscle cells and connective tissue. The muscle cells produce contractions; the connective tissue harnesses the pull. Connective tissue also conveys the extensive nerve fibers, blood vessels, and lymphatics characterizing muscle tissue.

Because muscle cells are narrow and long, they are known as **muscle fibers.** If the term *fiber* is used with reference to heart muscle, however, it means a linear series of cells joined end to end, of no fixed length.

Three histologically and functionally distinct types of muscle are recognized, each with particular characteristics. The first type described here is variously known as skeletal, voluntary, or striated muscle. It is called **skeletal** because its contractions generally move some part of the skeleton, and **voluntary** because its contractions generally occur at will. Microscopically, skeletal muscle exhibits dark and light transverse bands called **striations**, accounting for the rather outdated name **striated muscle.**

The next type of muscle considered in this chapter is called **cardiac** muscle because it constitutes the muscular walls of the heart (i.e., the **myocardium**). Cardiac muscle is similarly striated, but its contractile activity is not regulated at will. In other words, its contraction is **involuntary.** Cardiac muscle has several additional features that further justify its classification as a distinct type of muscle. For example, it is the only kind in which muscle cells are joined end to end by strong cell junctions.

The third type of muscle is not striated, so it is described as being **smooth.** Since its contraction cannot be controlled at will, it represents another kind of **involuntary** muscle. Smooth muscle is present in the walls of most blood vessels and hollow or tubular organs such as the intestine, and its degree of contraction regulates their luminal diameter.

Entire muscles are not always required to contract to their fullest extent. Except in the heart, partial contraction can be sustained over long periods (as, for example, in holding the head up). Sustained partial contraction of a muscle is commonly described as its **tonus**.

SKELETAL MUSCLE

Skeletal muscles were formerly more generally known as *striated muscles,* but since cardiac muscle also is striated this earlier name is now seldom used, mainly to avoid potential confusion.

The **connective tissue** components of skeletal muscles are arranged to facilitate transfer of contractile force to muscle attachments. The multiple connective tissue wrappings around the constituent muscle fibers are most easily recognized in transverse sections under very low power (Fig. 10-1). The muscle as a whole is enclosed by a dense connective tissue sheath called the **epimysium** (Gk. *epi*, upon; *mys*, muscle). From the epimysium, partitions extend inward and divide the interior of the muscle into fascicles (bundles) of muscle fibers. The partitions that surround the fascicles as fibrous sheaths are collectively known as the **perimysium** (Gk. *peri*, around). They convey blood vessels, lymphatics, and nerves inward from the epimysium. Lastly, delicate partitions of loose connective tissue extending from the perimysium into individual fascicles intimately ensheath each muscle fiber. These relatively thin, intrafascicular partitions contain capillaries and nerve fibers and they constitute the **endomysium** (Gk. *endon*, within). The collagen fibers of the multiple fibrous wrappings merge with those of the dense connective tissue structures on which the muscle pulls, commonly tendons, aponeuroses, or periosteum.

Skeletal Muscle Fibers

Skeletal muscle fibers are long and cylindrical with rounded ends. They extend the full length of short muscles but only partway along larger ones. Each fiber contains many nuclei, so skeletal muscle fibers are **multinucleated** cells. The relatively long nuclei occupy a peripheral position just under the cell surface (Plate 10-1).

Seen under high power in longitudinal sections, skeletal muscle fibers show a distinctive pattern of alternating dark- and light-staining transverse **bands** (Fig. 10-2). Under polarized light, the dark-staining bands are birefringent (anisotropic) whereas the light-staining bands are isotropic. The dark bands are therefore called **A** (for *anisotropic*) **bands**, and the light ones, **I** (for *isotropic*) **bands**. A dark line called the **Z line** bisects each I band. In relaxed fibers, a paler region termed the **H zone** is sometimes discernible in the middle of the A band.

Although it seems as if each band traverses the entire muscle fiber in a continuous manner, this is not the case. The cytoplasm of the cell, termed **sarcoplasm** (Gk. *sarkos*, flesh), contains striated cylindrical contractile elements called **myofibrils** that extend the full length of the fiber. The pattern of striation on these thread-like components, which are sometimes discernible under oil immersion (see Fig. 10-2), shows precise lateral registration. Hence, each so-called **band** of the muscle fiber is made up of closely approximated segments of numerous myofibrils.

Basis of Muscle Striation

The basic contractile unit of skeletal muscle is the **sarcomere** (Gk. *meros*, part), which is the part of a myofibril lying between consecutive Z lines. Thus, each myofibril represents a continuous series of sarcomeres joined at shared Z lines. The relaxed sarcomere, with a length of 2 to 3 μm, contracts

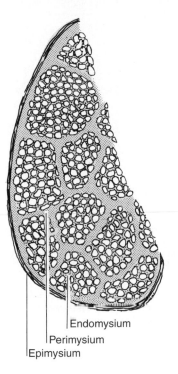

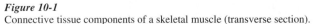

Figure 10-1
Connective tissue components of a skeletal muscle (transverse section).

Endomysium
Perimysium
Epimysium

to roughly half its resting length, pulling its two **Z** lines closer together. A sarcomere contains two sets of contractile filaments, namely, **actin**-containing **thin filaments** 1 μm long and 6 to 7 nm in diameter, and **myosin**-containing **thick filaments** 1.5 μm long and 12 to 15 nm in diameter. Both sets of filaments are longitudinally oriented in the myofibril. Half the thin filaments are attached to each Z line. Their free ends interdigitate with parallel thick filaments in the midregion of the sarcomere (Fig. 10-3). As originally proposed in Huxley's **sliding filament** theory, muscular contraction is the result of inward sliding of the thin filaments along the fixed thick ones until they nearly meet in the middle of the sarcomere (see Fig. 10-3*B*). This sliding action shortens the distance between Z lines. During relaxation, the two sets of thin filaments revert to their former position, restoring the resting length of the sarcomere (see Fig. 10-3*A*).

The light-staining I bands contain only thin filaments (Fig. 10-4), whereas the dark-staining A bands contain both types of filaments (see Fig. 10-15). The pale-staining H zone found in the middle of A bands of relaxed fibers (see Fig. 10-2) represents the part of the A band where only thick filaments are present (see Fig. 10-4*A*). When the fiber contracts, the H zone virtually disappears, becoming as dense as the remainder of the A band (see Fig. 10-4*B*). Finally, a dark-staining **M line** traversing the middle of the H zone is occasionally discernible. Fine transverse filaments interconnecting the thick filaments at the M line (see Figs. 10-4*A* and 10-15) contain the protein **myomesin** and the enzyme **creatine kinase.**

When the muscle contracts, its A bands do not alter in length, but its I bands shorten because the fine filaments slide farther into the A bands (compare *A* and *B* in Fig. 10-4). At the same time, the H zone virtually disappears (see Fig. 10-4*B*).

The thin filament attachments along either side of a Z line lie between the corresponding attachments on the other side, giving the Z line a characteristic zigzag appearance (see Fig. 10-4). The Z lines, which contain the protein α-**actinin**, interconnect sets of thin filaments that belong to adjacent sarcomeres, and they represent the structures on which these filaments pull.

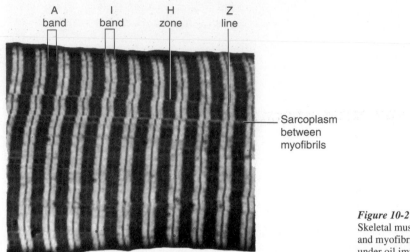

Figure 10-2
Skeletal muscle fiber, showing striations
and myofibrils (longitudinal section seen
under oil immersion, toluidine blue).

Besides possessing interdigitating sets of contractile filaments, sarcomeres are provided with fine longitudinal elastic filaments that contain the high molecular weight protein, **titin** (also known as **connectin**). Titin molecules are long enough to connect an M line to a Z line. At one end they have a domain that is incorporated into a thick filament, and at the other end they have a spring-like, elastic domain that connects the thick filament to a Z line. A **nebulin** molecule extending along each thin filament is believed to provide the template determining the length of the filament. Comparatively rigid lattices and ring-like arrangements of intermediate filaments provide further internal and external support for the sarcomere.

Red, White, and Intermediate Skeletal Muscle Fibers

Mitochondria supplying ATP for contraction and glycogen are plentiful in the sarcoplasm between myofibrils and peripheral cytoplasm of skeletal muscle fibers. In addition, the sarcoplasm contains a reddish brown protein called **myoglobin** that in several respects is similar to the red protein hemoglobin in erythrocytes. Myoglobin takes up oxygen from the blood and stores it in the sarcoplasm, hence oxygen too is available in the amounts generally required for energy production. A high content of myoglobin and abundant mitochondria are characteristic of dark-colored muscles, for example, the dark meat in chickens. The dark color is due to a preponderance of **red fibers,** which are so called because of the relative abundance of myoglobin and mitochondria. A substantial content of these two components enables red fibers to maintain contractions over long periods.

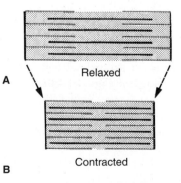

Figure 10-3
Basic organization of a sarcomere. (*A*) Thin filaments are anchored to the Z lines indicating ends of sarcomeres. (*B*)
Contraction pulls Z lines closer together.

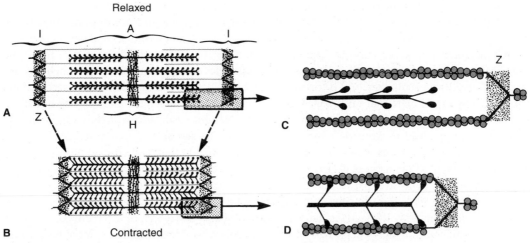

Figure 10-4
Structural components of the sarcomere that constitute the basis of muscle striations. The area indicated in *A* is shown in more detail in *C*; the area indicated in *B* is similarly shown in *D*. In *C*, cross bridges on the thick filaments are not interacting with actin in the thin filaments. In *D*, interaction of these cross bridges with actin produces a contraction.

There are other muscles, however, such as the white meat (pectoral muscles) in chickens, that contain a higher proportion of **white fibers,** so named because myoglobin and mitochondria are less abundant in them. Adapted for shorter bursts of more rapid contractile activity, these lighter-colored muscles fatigue more rapidly. Finally, **intermediate fibers** are structurally and functionally intermediate between red and white fibers. Most human muscles are made up of all three kinds of fibers.

Efferent Innervation of Skeletal Muscle

Each skeletal muscle fiber is provided with an **efferent nerve ending.** Individual lower motor neurons supply a number of muscle fibers widely distributed throughout the muscle, hence contractions involve the muscle as a whole, not just local regions of it. In certain skeletal muscles, as few as three to five muscle fibers are supplied by each motor neuron. The regulation of contraction in such muscles (e.g., the extrinsic ocular muscles responsible for delicate eye movements) is correspondingly precise.

When efferent impulses stimulate skeletal muscle fibers to contract, these always shorten to their fullest extent. Graded contractions of skeletal muscles depend on the number of muscle fibers stimulated to contract, not on partial contraction of individual fibers. A **motor unit** consists of one lower motor neuron and all the skeletal muscle fibers that it innervates. Efferent impulses from the neuron cause all the muscle fibers in the unit to contract fully, and unless this neuron produces the impulses, none of the fibers contracts at all. The strength of a skeletal muscle contraction is therefore a function of the number of motor units participating in the contraction.

Motor End Plate

Internal to the sheath-like delicate endomysium, and attached to it by a basement membrane, is the **sarcolemma** (cell membrane) of the muscle fiber (Gk. *lemma*, husk). During relaxation, the sarcolemma is electrically polarized. Contraction occurs when efferent impulses initiate a wave of **depolarization** that spreads quickly over the sarcolemma.

The site of the neuromuscular junction between a lower motor neuron and the skeletal muscle fiber that it innervates is indicated by a flat, branching plate termed a **motor end plate** (Fig. 10-5). Here, an excitatory synapse exists between the branching motor axon terminals and the shallow sarcolemmal grooves in which they lie. The myelin sheath of the axon extends almost as far as the branching presynaptic terminal (Fig. 10-6), beyond which level each terminal axon branch lies under a roof of Schwann cells (see Fig. 10-6*B* and *C*). Between the apposed axolemma and sarcolemma is a narrow **synaptic cleft,** and invaginated into the sarcoplasm beneath the cleft, sarcolemmal extensions called **junctional folds** increase the area of sarcolemma associated with the axolemma. Mitochondria are plentiful in the axon terminals and also in the sarcoplasm under the end plate, reflecting substantial energy demands in the end plate region. In addition, numerous **synaptic vesicles** containing the neurotransmitter **acetylcholine** are present within the axon terminals. The motor end plate is a directed chemical synapse where depolarization of the lower motor neuron causes synaptic vesicles to fuse with specific sites on the presynaptic terminal. Resulting exocytosis of acetylcholine into the synaptic cleft leads to depolarization of the apposed area of sarcolemma, initiating a wave of depolarization that sweeps over the entire sarcolemma. Meanwhile, acetylcholine released during neuromuscular transmission is broken down by the enzyme **acetylcholinesterase**, which is associated with the region of basement membrane in the synaptic cleft.

Depolarization of the axon terminal in efferent excitation leads to an influx of calcium ions that causes synaptic vesicles to make contact with the axolemma and discharge their content into the synaptic cleft. At this directed synapse, the sites where synaptic vesicles fuse with the axolemma are concentrated opposite the underlying slitlike openings of the junctional folds. The sarcolemmal acetylcholine receptors lie mostly along the openings of the junctional folds. Superfluous axolemmal membrane constituents resulting from intense synaptic activity are retrieved and recycled as described under Synapses in Chapter 9.

CLINICAL IMPLICATIONS: ACETYLCHOLINE RECEPTORS: MYASTHENIA GRAVIS

Myasthenia gravis (Gk. *mys*, muscle; *astheneia*, weakness) is a debilitating condition characterized by progressive weakness in certain muscles. Its essential basis is generally a deficiency of **acetylcholine receptors** in the end plate region of the sarcolemma. Motor impulses accordingly fail to elicit the contraction of enough muscle fibers to produce effective contractions. This condition is in most cases due to patients developing antibodies to their own acetylcholine receptor subunits. In approximately 20% of cases, however, antibodies to titin are formed.

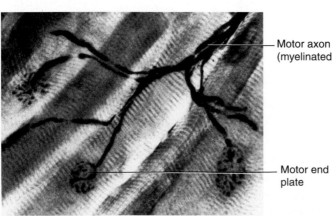

Motor axon
(myelinated)

Motor end
plate

Figure 10-5
Motor end plates of skeletal muscle fibers (gold chloride stain).

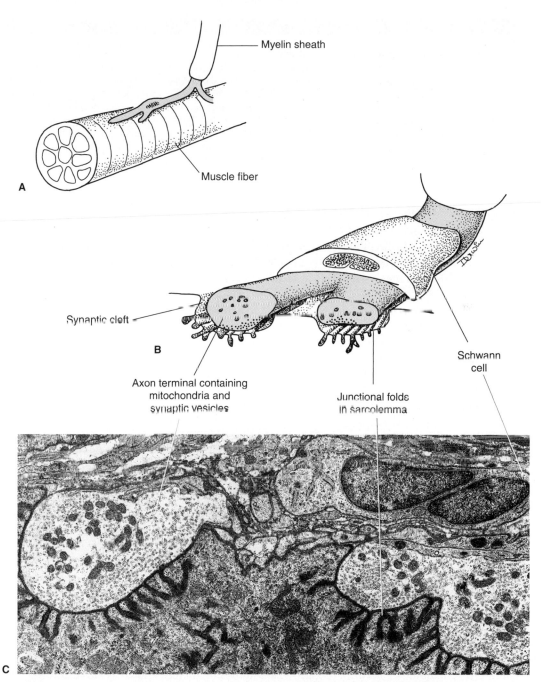

Myelin sheath

Muscle fiber

A

Synaptic cleft

B

Axon terminal containing
mitochondria and
synaptic vesicles

Junctional folds
in sarcolemma

Schwann
cell

C

Figure 10-6
Electron micrograph and explanatory diagrams showing the histological organization of a motor end plate.

CLINICAL IMPLICATIONS

Sarcolemmal Cytoskeleton: Muscular Dystrophy
Closely associated with the inner (cytoplasmic) surface of the sarcolemma is the **membrane cytoskeleton**
of the muscle cell, which contains the actin-binding protein **dystrophin**. In patients with **muscular dystrophy,** chronic degeneration of muscle fibers can lead to severe muscular weakness, which is potentially
fatal if it involves respiratory muscles or results in cardiac arrhythmia. In Duchenne muscular dystrophy,
the dystrophin is lacking, and in a milder form of the disease the dystrophin is altered, suggesting that this
protein plays a key role in attaching thin filaments to the sarcolemma and maintaining overall integrity in
muscle fibers. Present in neurons as well as all three types of muscle cells, dystrophin apparently reinforces
or stabilizes the cell membrane in some essential manner.

Transverse Tubules (T Tubules)

Branching tubular invaginations of the sarcolemma extend deep into the interior of the muscle fiber.
Called **transverse tubules (T tubules),** their role is to conduct waves of depolarization rapidly into
all parts of the fiber. In human skeletal muscle fibers, the T tubules lie at the junctions of A and I
bands (Fig. 10-7). In *amphibian* skeletal muscle fibers, however, where they were first characterized, they lie at the level of Z lines. These tubules are described as transverse (T) tubules because
they penetrate the fiber, and also branch within it, in a transverse plane. The branching T tubules that
encircle the fiber's myofibrils in that plane conduct depolarization to all of them simultaneously.

Because an intracellular regulatory compartment called the sarcoplasmic reticulum is involved
in mediating the contractile response, waves of depolarization do not stimulate the contraction of
myofibrils directly. The T tubules lie in intimate apposition with the limiting membrane of this regulatory compartment in an arrangement that liberates stored intracellular calcium ions when there is
a sarcolemmal depolarization, as described in the next section.

Sarcoplasmic Reticulum

Corresponding to the sER in other cell types, the **sarcoplasmic reticulum** of muscle cells is a separate cytoplasmic compartment consisting of flat cisternae and anastomosing tubules interconnected
as collar-like complexes around each myofibril. As shown in Figure 10-7 (see also Fig. 10-15A), two
pairs of closely associated **terminal cisternae** encircle each sarcomere. Each pair of terminal
cisternae lies at an A band–I band junction. The associated cisternae of each pair border on a branching T tubule that also encircles myofibrils at this level. A site where a transverse section of a terminal cisterna is seen on each side of a T-tubule is described as a **triad** (two triads may be recognized
in Fig. 10-7). Where the closely apposed terminal cisternae border on the associated T tubule, fast
calcium-release channels are present in the membrane of the sarcoplasmic reticulum. The position
of these channels may be seen in well-prepared EM sections as characteristic rows of uniformly
spaced, electron dense particles originally described as **junctional feet.** Thus, each sarcomere is en-
circled by two T tubules (one at each junction of the A and I bands), each T tubule is flanked by two
terminal cisternae, and there are four terminal cisternae per sarcomere. A second part of the sarcoplasmic reticulum is a network of narrow, anastomosing tubules known as **sarcotubules.** These
tubules interconnect cisternae that belong to adjacent pairs of terminal cisternae, but not the neighboring cisternae of each pair (see Figs. 10-7 and 10-15A). Sarcotubules extend more or less longitudinally, but in the midregion of the sarcomere they anastomose extensively. The resulting network
gives the sarcoplasmic reticulum the overall appearance of a lacy sleeve.

The primary function of the sarcoplasmic reticulum is to regulate the **calcium ion concentration** within the myofibrils, which in turn determines whether thin filaments interact with thick ones
and bring about a contraction. When the muscle fiber is relaxed, calcium ions are stored in the lu-

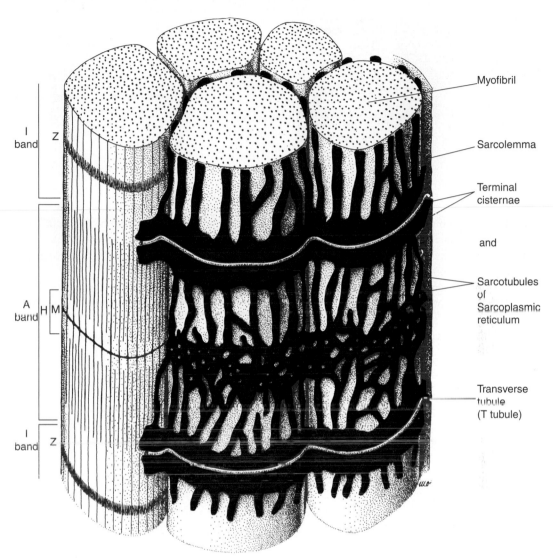

Figure 10-7
Diagram showing the sarcoplasmic reticulum and transverse tubules of a skeletal muscle fiber in relation to myofibrillar striations. The triple association where two terminal cisternae flank a transverse tubule is called a **triad**.

men of its sarcoplasmic reticulum. The moment the sarcolemmal lining of the T tubules depolarizes, the fast calcium-release channels in the sarcoplasmic reticulum membrane open and release membrane-segregated calcium ions. On entering myofibrils, liberated calcium ions enable thick filaments to interact with thin ones, as outlined below.

Basis of Skeletal Muscle Contraction

Extending from the **thick filaments,** composed primarily of **myosin**, are tiny projections termed **cross bridges** each representing a part of the myosin molecule (Fig. 10-8). The **thin filaments** of skeletal muscle fibers contain the proteins **actin, troponin,** and **tropomyosin** (Fig. 10-9). Unless stimulated, the muscle fiber remains relaxed because troponin and tropomyosin in the thin filaments

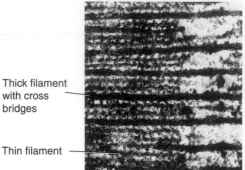

Thick filament
with cross
bridges

Thin filament

Figure 10-8
Electron micrograph of part of a sarcomere, showing the cross
bridges on thick filaments (extracted rabbit psoas muscle,
× 150,000).

prevent actin from interacting with myosin in the thick filaments. However, the block occurs only
when cytosolic calcium levels are low. Calcium ions released by the sarcoplasmic reticulum as a result of sarcolemmal depolarization temporarily remove the constraints imposed by troponin and
tropomyosin, enabling the two types of filaments to interact.

The orientation of myosin molecules in thick filaments permits the cross bridge part of the
molecule to oscillate back and forth by swiveling on the remainder (see Fig. 10-9*B*). Immediately
following efferent stimulation of the fiber and resulting release of stored calcium ions into its myofibrils, cross bridges latch onto actin in the thin filaments. Once attached, they alter their position
slightly, disconnect, and swivel back to their former position, ready to latch on for another cycle of

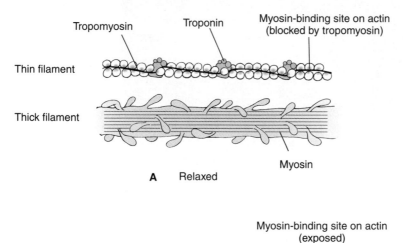

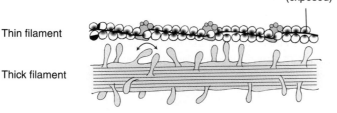

B   Contracting

Figure 10-9
During muscular contraction, the double globular head region of myosin in the thick filaments interacts with actin in the
thin filaments.

operation. This oscillation cycle occurs with extreme rapidity, pulling the thin filaments farther in between the thick ones in a single swift movement. The energy expended in contraction is obtained from ATP that becomes hydrolyzed through the actin-activated ATPase activity of myosin. A well-known consequence of ATP depletion at death is that it leaves actin and myosin tightly interlocked until autolysis allows the muscles to be stretched passively. The result is post-mortem **rigor mortis** (L, rigidity of death).

Afferent Innervation of Skeletal Muscle

In addition to efferent innervation, skeletal muscles are provided with **afferent nerve endings** sensitive to stretch. Groups of muscle fibers with these sensory nerve endings are distributed throughout the muscle. They are arranged in parallel with ordinary muscle fibers and lie within spindle-shaped structures called **muscle spindles.** The spindle fibers are of two distinct types. One type is characterized by having an expanded midregion that contains numerous nuclei (Fig. 10-10, *right*). Coiled around its wide midregion is an afferent nerve ending known as a **primary ending** or, due to

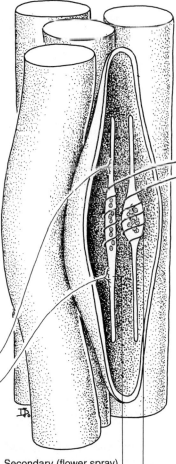

Figure 10-10
The two distinctive types of muscle fibers characterizing muscle spindles, with their afferent innervation (efferent innervation omitted). Both primary and secondary afferent endings respond to stretch.

Secondary (flower spray) endings

Primary (annulospiral) endings

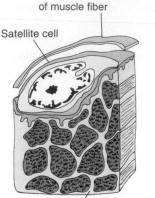

Basement membrane
of muscle fiber

Satellite cell

Figure 10-11
Satellite cells lie at the perimeter of skeletal muscle fibers, internal to their basement
membrane.

Skeletal muscle fiber

its shape, **annulospiral ending.** The other type of spindle fiber has a row of nuclei lined up along its
midregion. It is also supplied with a **primary (annulospiral) ending,** but in addition it has two **secondary (flower spray) endings,** one on each side of the primary ending (see Fig. 10-10, *left*). The
primary endings in both types of fibers respond to the amount and rate of stretch of the muscle,
whereas the secondary endings, confined to the second type of fiber, respond only to the amount of
stretch. The two kinds of afferent endings serve as stretch receptors, registering any differences between the length of the spindle fibers and the length of the muscle as a whole. The occurrence of
such discrepancies is signaled to the CNS through afferent nerve fibers. Lower motor neurons counteract any disparity by eliciting supplementary contraction of extrafusal (L. *extra*, outside; *fusus*,
spindle) fibers of the muscle (see Fig. 9-20).

Growth and Regeneration of Skeletal Muscle

Skeletal muscle fibers are highly specialized, multinucleated cells that cannot divide. On an individual basis, they can nevertheless be replaced by new skeletal muscle fibers derived from **satellite
(myosatellite) cells**, which are unipotential stem cells that lie in close association with skeletal muscle fibers, enclosed within the same basement membrane (Fig. 10-11). Satellite cells persist as a potential source of new **myoblasts** (muscle cell precursors) capable of fusing with one another to form
new skeletal muscle fibers if these are needed. Furthermore, during postnatal growth, their myoblast
progeny lengthen existing skeletal muscle fibers by fusing with them. The number of new skeletal
muscle fibers produced postnatally is nevertheless insufficient to compensate for major muscle degeneration or trauma. Instead of becoming effectively restored through regeneration, massively
damaged skeletal muscle is essentially replaced by a disorganized mixture of new muscle cells and
fibrous scar tissue. Hence, skeletal muscle has only *limited* potential for regeneration. A recent finding that circulating cells derived from bone marrow produce new skeletal muscle fibers if muscle
damage is severe suggests that supplementary measures can compensate for severe depletion of
satellite cells.

Skeletal muscles generally respond to repetitive strenuous exercise by enlarging. Their additional growth is brought about by **hypertrophy** (enlargement) of the existing muscle fibers, not formation of supplementary new muscle fibers. Increased numbers and significant lengthening of the
myofibrils in the pre-existing muscle fibers greatly augment the functional efficiency of the muscle
mass.

CARDIAC MUSCLE

Cardiac muscle, which although **striated** is **involuntary**, constitutes the muscular walls of the heart. Some cardiac muscle is also present in the walls of the pulmonary vein and superior vena cava. A histological feature of cardiac muscle fibers is that they branch and anastomose. Furthermore, the nuclei lie centrally in the fibers (Plate 10-2). The **endomysium** appearing as slit-like regions between the muscle fibers is a very vascular loose connective tissue profusely supplied with capillaries and lymphatics. Cardiac muscle fibers are attached to the endomysium by their surrounding basement membrane.

Cardiac Muscle Fibers

Cardiac muscle fibers are basically branching chains of cardiac muscle cells joined end to end by three kinds of cell junctions. These fibers have the same general pattern of striations as skeletal muscle fibers, but in addition they are traversed by **intercalated disks**, structures that are unique to cardiac muscle fibers. In longitudinal LM sections, intercalated disks appear as darkly stained irregular lines, some of which extend across the fiber in a step-like pattern (as illustrated in the inset of Fig. 10-12 and also on the left of Fig. 10-13A). These irregular transverse structures indicate the positions of apposed borders of contiguous muscle cells. Most cardiac muscle cells have a single nucleus, but a few of them contain two. Occupying a central position in the muscle cell, the nucleus is relatively large and pale-staining (see Figs. 10-13 and 10-14). If found along with intercalated disks and a branching pattern of the fibers, a central position and such an appearance of the nucleus confirm the histological distinction between cardiac and skeletal muscle.

Involuntary contraction of cardiac muscle is brought about through filament sliding, as described earlier in the chapter. In cardiac muscle, however, contraction is **myogenic**, meaning that it is a spontaneous, intrinsic rhythmic activity of the muscle cells themselves. Because rhythmic contractile activity is an inherent property of cardiac muscle cells, only the rate of contraction (the **heart rate**) is regulated by autonomic nerve impulses.

The fine structure of cardiac muscle is essentially similar to that of skeletal muscle. In cardiac muscle, however, the myofibrils vary in diameter and anastomose instead of being uniformly

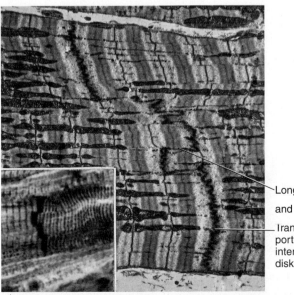

Longitudinal and Transverse portions of intercalated disk

Figure 10-12
Electron micrograph of part of a cardiac muscle fiber, showing an intercalated disk (canine ventricular cardiac muscle, × 5100). (*Inset*) Comparable intercalated disk (same source) seen with the LM.

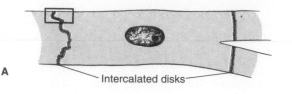

A

Intercalated disks

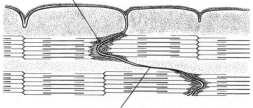

Transverse portion (myofibrillar junctions,
desmosomes, and gap junctions)

B

Longitudinal portion (contains large
gap junctions)

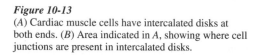

Figure 10-13

(*A*) Cardiac muscle cells have intercalated disks at both ends. (*B*) Area indicated in *A*, showing where cell junctions are present in intercalated disks.

cylindrical and separate (see Fig. 10-14). Between the myofibrils and at the poles of the nucleus lie numerous mitochondria, their large size and relative abundance reflecting the unremitting energy requirements of this type of muscle.

Also concentrated at the poles of the nucleus in the atrial cardiac muscle cells are electron-dense **atrial granules**. These secretory granules contain the precursor of a peptide hormone called **atrial natriuretic peptide** (ANP) that is liberated in response to atrial distention. ANP is involved in regulating blood pressure and blood volume through direct and indirect effects on renal excretion, blood vessel tonus, aldosterone secretion, and certain regulatory centers in the brain. An important action of ANP is that it lowers blood pressure.

The T tubules of cardiac muscle are wider but less numerous than those of skeletal muscle. They lie at the Z line level, not at junctions of A bands and I bands. Thus there is only one level of T tubule

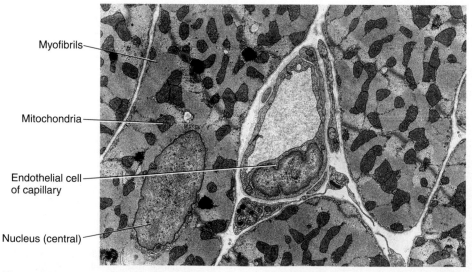

Myofibrils

Mitochondria

Endothelial cell
of capillary

Nucleus (central)

Figure 10-14

Electron micrograph of cardiac muscle, showing several cardiac muscle fibers and an endomysial capillary (cat ventricular papillary muscle, transverse section).

entry per sarcomere. The sarcoplasmic reticulum is a somewhat smaller and less elaborate compartment, consisting of interconnected longitudinal sarcotubules without the large collar-like terminal cisternae that are present in skeletal muscle fibers (Fig. 10-15). Because a smaller proportion of the calcium required for contraction can be stored in the sarcoplasmic reticulum, cardiac muscle cells are extremely dependent on **extracellular calcium ions**, which enter by way of the sarcolemma and wider T tubules. Such an influx of extracellular calcium triggers the release of internal calcium ions stored within the sarcoplasmic reticulum, and these enter the myofibrils and elicit contraction. As in skeletal muscle, relaxation occurs when calcium is pumped back into the sarcoplasmic reticulum. Hence extracellular calcium as well as intracellular calcium is necessary for cardiac contraction. When the heart beats, all its muscle cells participate in each contraction. The force with which they contract, however, is calcium-dependent and can be modulated, so that during exercise, for example, the force of cardiac contraction is increased.

Intercalated Disks

The EM shows that at intercalated disks, the cell membranes of contiguous cardiac muscle cells interdigitate extensively and are interconnected by three different kinds of cell junctions (see Chap. 4). Intercalated disks traverse the fibers at the level of Z lines even when they follow a stepwise course. Thus **transverse portions** of the disk seen at the level of different Z lines are interconnected by **longitudinal portions** (see Figs. 10-12 and 10-13B).

The transverse portions of the disk are provided with three kinds of cell junctions. **Fascia adherens junctions**, which are patch-shaped adhering (anchoring) junctions where electron-dense material attaches the thin filaments to the sarcolemma (see Fig. 10-13B), interconnect individual myofibrils that belong to adjoining cells. Expanded **desmosomes**, the second kind of junction, are sites

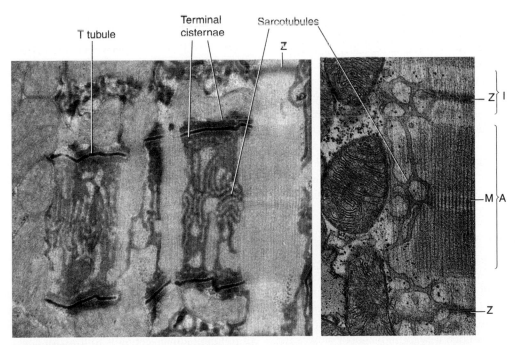

Figure 10-15
Electron micrographs showing distribution of the sarcoplasmic reticulum in relation to myofibrils and striations in (*A*) skeletal muscle and (*B*) cardiac muscle.

of strong adhesion that minimize separation of the contiguous muscle cells when they contract. Small **gap junctions**, the third kind of transverse junction, provide direct electrical communication between contiguous muscle cells by being freely permeable to ions. Larger gap junctions, the only kind of junction found in the longitudinal parts of the disk, further facilitate this electrical conduction. Thus intercalated disks transmit pull, provide strong intercellular attachment, and provide direct electrical continuity between individual cardiac muscle cells so that waves of depolarization can spread rapidly over the entire heart muscle by passing from cell to cell. The heart even possesses its own special impulse-conducting system, made up of extra-large cardiac muscle cells linked together in this manner and microscopically recognizable on either side of the interventricular septum as **Purkinje fibers**, described in Chapter 11 under Impulse-Conducting System of the Heart.

Growth and Local Replacement of Cardiac Muscle

As in skeletal muscles, the cardiac response to increased functional demands is muscle fiber enlargement, that is, **hypertrophy** of existing cardiac muscle cells. Cardiac muscle cells that *die* are not replaced because 1) cardiac muscle cells do not divide, and 2) cardiac muscle has no counterpart of the satellite (myosatellite) cell present in skeletal muscle, and is therefore not equipped to produce more muscle cells. Cardiac muscle is accordingly regarded as having *negligible inherent potential* for regeneration. If a portion of the myocardium dies, it becomes replaced locally by fibrous, noncontractile scar tissue.

SMOOTH MUSCLE

Where smooth muscle is present in the walls of tubes and other hollow viscera, it is commonly arranged as layers. Within these layers, bundles of smooth muscle fibers are surrounded by sheaths of loose connective tissue (Plate 10-3) that convey capillaries and autonomic efferent nerve fibers to the muscle fibers. Contraction of smooth muscle is involuntary, as in cardiac muscle. Furthermore, smooth muscle cells are individually capable of energy-efficient **partial contraction** and are able to maintain tonus more or less indefinitely. Hence smooth muscle has the important role of regulating the luminal diameters of hollow organs and most tubes in the body. In addition, the smooth muscle of the digestive tract, ureters, and uterine tubes undergoes slow rhythmic contractions, with resulting successive waves of contraction, known as **peristaltic waves**, that sweep along these tubes and propel their contents along. Contraction is nevertheless a comparatively slow process in most smooth muscles. In the walls of arteries and other blood vessels, smooth muscle not only regulates luminal diameter but also can revert to a **synthetic state** in which it produces interstitial matrix components of the vessel wall, notably **elastin** but also collagen and proteoglycans. Smooth muscle cells are attached to this matrix by their surrounding basement membrane.

Smooth Muscle Fibers

When used in the context of smooth muscle, the term *fiber* denotes a single cell, as in skeletal muscle. Each fiber is elongated and tapered (see Figs. 10-17A and 10-18) with a central rod-shaped nucleus, and it lacks striations (hence its name). The relaxed length of the fiber depends on where it is situated. Thus, the smooth muscle fibers in small blood vessels are shorter than those in the uterine wall during a pregnancy. The rod-shaped nucleus is so long that it becomes pleated when the cell shortens, so one way to find smooth muscle fibers cut in longitudinal section is to look for snake-like nuclei (Fig. 10-16). This aid to recognition, however, is reliable only if muscle fibers can be found in a contracted state.

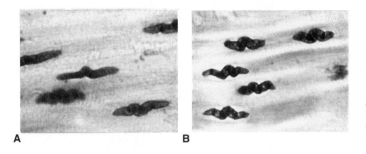

A   B

Figure 10-16
Pleated nuclei are a characteristic feature
of contracted smooth muscle fibers
(high power).

Basis of Smooth Muscle Contraction

Well-prepared electron micrographs reveal **thin** (6 to 8 nm), **thick** (14 to 16 nm), and **intermediate** (10 nm) **filaments** in smooth muscle fibers. The contractile filaments, however, are not arranged in the same recognizable pattern as those in sarcomeres of skeletal or cardiac muscle, nor are Z lines present. Smooth muscle cells shorten because of a somewhat different arrangement of the filaments. Thin filaments and intermediate filaments are attached to **dense bodies**, electron-dense structures containing α-actinin that are considered counterparts of Z lines. Dense bodies are distributed throughout the cytoplasm, but some adhere to the cell membrane. Bundles of intermediate filaments extend from one dense body to another, forming an interconnecting cable-like system that harnesses pull generated by thin filaments sliding between thick ones. These filament bundles also transmit the pull to the dense bodies attached to the cell membrane. When superficial dense bodies are pulled inward, regions of cell membrane balloon out between them (Figs. 10-17C and 10-18). The overall resulting change in cell shape shortens the long axis of the fiber, bringing about a contraction.

The thin filaments contain actin and tropomyosin, but *lack troponin*. Smooth muscle cells respond to variations in cytosolic calcium levels through the action of a different protein called **calmodulin**. Myosin light-chain kinase, an enzyme that these cells produce only when sufficient calcium is present, phosphorylates myosin, promoting its assembly into thick filaments as well as its subsequent interaction with actin.

Mitochondria and stored glycogen lie mostly near the poles of the nucleus in the cytosol of smooth muscle cells. The sarcoplasmic reticulum is only minimally represented, consisting of

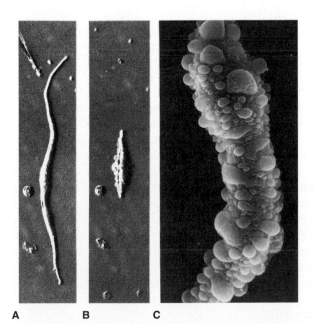

A   B   C

Figure 10-17
Contraction in smooth muscle cells. (*A*) Living muscle fiber, relaxed. (*B*) Same muscle fiber, fully contracted. (*C*) Scanning electron micrograph of a fully contracted smooth muscle fiber (compare this with Fig. 10-16, *right*).

Intermediate filament bundles
attached to dense bodies

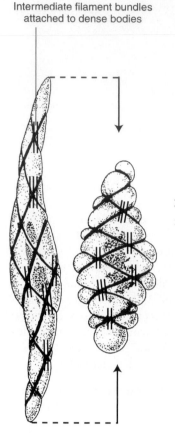

Figure 10-18
The contractile force generated by a smooth muscle fiber is transmitted to the cell
membrane by bundles of attached intermediate filaments.

narrow sarcotubules with no terminal cisternae. There are no transverse (T) tubules, but rows of sub-surface vesicles termed **caveolae** opening onto the cell surface are considered probable counterparts of T tubules.

Efferent Innervation of Smooth Muscle

Smooth muscles have two distinct patterns of efferent innervation. In **visceral smooth muscles** (e.g., those in tubular walls and hollow viscera), which are able to maintain prolonged partial contractions (tonus) and in some cases produce peristaltic waves, only a few of the muscle fibers have their own neuromuscular junction. Excitation spreads from the few stimulated fibers to all the others by way of **gap junctions** between the muscle fibers, as in cardiac muscle. This kind of muscle is character-ized by a certain amount of spontaneous contractile activity, and nonneural stimuli such as stretch, histamine, and oxytocin can also bring about its contraction.

In **multiunit smooth muscles** (e.g., the pupillary sphincter of the eye), contraction is more pre-cisely regulated and also faster. For this degree of control, every muscle fiber needs to be individu-ally innervated, and gap junctions are generally also present. The pattern of innervation found in multiunit smooth muscles resembles that of skeletal muscles, but the innervated muscle fibers are less widely distributed. Many smooth muscles have an intermediate arrangement in which up to one half of the muscle fibers are supplied with their own neuromuscular junction, and the remainder is stimulated indirectly by means of gap junctions.

TABLE 10-1

SKELETAL, CARDIAC, AND SMOOTH MUSCLE: COMPARATIVE FEATURES

Structural Features	Skeletal Muscle	Cardiac Muscle	Smooth Muscle
Site	Skeleton-associated	Heart and certain associated vessels	Vessels, organs, and viscera; arranged as layers
Connective tissue component	Epi-, peri-, and endomysium	Endomysium	Sheaths around fiber bundles
Fibers	Single large cells	Branching chains of cells	Single cells
Striations	Present	Present	Absent
Nucleus	Many per cell, peripheral	1 or 2 per cell, central	1 per cell, central; pleats during contraction
T tubules	At A band–I band junctions	At Z lines; wider but fewer	Absent; caveolae instead
Cell junctions	Absent	Gap and fascia adherens junctions, desmosomes	Gap junctions
Other distinctive features	Elaborate sarcoplasmic reticulum; afferent nerve endings in muscle spindles; more myoglobin and mitochondria in red fibers than in white fibers	Intercalated disks; atrial granules containing ANP	Can synthesize elastin and other matrix constituents; sarcomeres indistinguishable

Functional Characteristics

Contractile regulation	Voluntary	Involuntary	Involuntary
Characteristics of contraction	All-or-nothing in each fiber; graded contractions involve fewer motors units; white fibers contract and fatigue faster than red fibers	Force and rate of contraction can be modulated; contraction is spontaneous and rhythmic; requires external calcium; all fibers contract during heartbeat	Comparatively slow; can be partial in each fiber; spontaneous in visceral muscles; faster and more precise in multiunit muscles
Efferent Regulation	Somatic efferent, by way of motor end plate of lower motor neuron; motor units can have many or few muscle fibers	Autonomic efferent, by way of sinoatrial and atrioventricular nodes	Autonomic efferent, by way of neuromuscular junctions on some or all muscle fibers (visceral versus multiunit muscles)

Growth and Regeneration

Response to increased demands	Hypertrophy	Hypertrophy	Hypertrophy and hyperplasia
Proliferative potential of mature muscle cells	None	None	Marked
Regenerative potential	Limited, through satellite cells and their myoblast progeny	None	Extensive; both direct and through pericytes

Postganglionic autonomic axons branch repeatedly near the smooth muscle fibers that they supply. Each branch extends across a number of smooth muscle fibers, bulging to form a string of nondirected en passant **autonomic neuromuscular junctions.** Such junctions are a series of distentions (varicosities) of the postganglionic fiber that fit into corresponding shallow depressions on the muscle fiber. A **synaptic cleft** lies between the axolemma and the cell membrane of the muscle cell, and the associated axoplasm contains local accumulations of mitochondria and synaptic vesicles. These vesicles are filled with **acetylcholine** in parasympathetic fibers or **norepinephrine** in sympathetic fibers. Smooth muscle cells have two distinct (α and β) adrenergic receptors for norepinephrine and certain other chemically related neurotransmitters. Axolemmal impulses elicit a broad-based, nondirected release of the neurotransmitter. On entering the synaptic cleft, the neurotransmitter causes depolarization of the cell membrane, with resulting muscle fiber contraction. Such nondirected discharge of the neurotransmitter is often referred to as **volume transmission**.

Growth and Regeneration of Smooth Muscle

As in the other two types of muscle, one response of smooth muscle to increased demands is **hypertrophy** of its existing fibers. This is not its only response, however. Smooth muscle cells retain the capacity for mitosis and therefore can increase in number (which is referred to as **hyperplasia**) as well as enlarge. Moreover, new smooth muscle cells can be generated at any time from incompletely differentiated cells called **pericytes** (described in Chap. 5) that lie scattered along certain small blood vessels. Hence smooth muscle has a remarkable potential for regeneration that far exceeds the regenerative capacity of the other two types of muscle.

Summary

Distinctive features of the three types of muscle tissue are compared in Table 10-1.

In a skeletal muscle fiber, contraction is elicited by somatic efferent impulses arriving at its motor end plate and bringing about a release of acetylcholine that rapidly depolarizes the sarcolemma under the end plate. The resulting wave of depolarization enters T tubules and triggers a release of stored calcium ions from the sarcoplasmic reticulum. Through interaction with regulatory proteins in the thin filaments, the intracellularly released calcium ions enable actin in these filaments to interact with myosin in the thick filaments. Contraction, which requires ATP as an energy source, is a result of thin filaments sliding farther in between thick ones and pulling Z lines of sarcomeres closer together. This causes I bands to shorten but leaves the length of A bands unchanged. During relaxation, calcium ions are pumped back into the sarcoplasmic reticulum ready for the next contraction.

Special features of cardiac and smooth muscle are indicated in Table 10-1 and discussed in the text.

Bibliography

Skeletal Muscle and Its Contraction

Byers TJ, Kunkel LM, Watkins SC. The subcellular distribution of dystrophin in mouse skeletal, cardiac, and smooth muscle. J Cell Biol 115:411, 1991.

Campion DR. The muscle satellite cell: a review. Int Rev Cytol 87:225, 1984.

Carlson BM. The regeneration of skeletal muscle: a review. Am J Anat 137:119, 1973.

Cohen C. The protein switch of muscle contraction. Sci Am 233(5):36, 1975.

Couteaux R. Motor end plate structure. In: Bourne GH, ed. The Structure and Function of Muscle, vol 1. New York, Academic Press, 1960, p 337.

Drachman DB. Myasthenia gravis. N Engl J Med 298:136, 186, 1978.

Ervasti JM, Campbell KP. Membrane organization of the dystrophin-glycoprotein complex. Cell 66:1121, 1991.

Lester HA. The response to acetylcholine. Sci Am 236(2):106, 1977.

Franzini-Armstrong C, Peachey LD. Striated muscle: contractile and control mechanisms. J Cell Biol 91:166S, 1981.

Fulton AB, Isaacs WB. Titin, a huge elastic sarcomeric protein with a probable role in morphogenesis. BioEssays 13:157, 1991.

Huxley HE. Sliding filaments and molecular motile systems. J Biol Chem 265:8347, 1990.

Huxley HE. A personal view of muscle and motility mechanisms. Annu Rev Physiol 58:1, 1996.

Ishikawa H. Fine structure of skeletal muscle. In: Dowben RM, Shay JW, eds. Cell and Muscle Motility, vol 4. New York, Plenum, 1983, p 1.

Keller T. Structure and function of titin and nebulin. Current Opin Cell Biol 7:32, 1995.

Landon DN. Skeletal muscle: normal morphology, development and innervation. In: Mastaglia FL, Walton J, eds. Skeletal Muscle Pathology. Edinburgh, Churchill-Livingstone, 1982, p 1.

Miyatake M, Miike T, Zhao J-E, Yoshioka K, Uchino M, Usuku G. Dystrophin: localization and presumed function. Muscle Nerve 14:113, 1991.

Monaco AP. Dystrophin, the protein product of the Duchenne/Becker muscular dystrophy gene. Trends Biochem Sci 14:412, 1989.

Moore JC. The Golgi tendon organ and the muscle spindle. Am J Occup Ther 28:415, 1974.

Murray JM, Weber A. The cooperative action of muscle proteins. Sci Am 230(2):59, 1974

Pasternak C, Wong S, Elson EL. Mechanical function of dystrophin in muscle cells. J Cell Biol 128:355, 1995.

Patten RM, Ovalle WK. Muscle spindle ultrastructure revealed by conventional and high-resolution scanning electron microscopy. Anat Rec 230:183, 1991.

Petrof BJ, Shrager JB, Stedman HH, Kelly AM, Sweeny HL. Dystrophin protects the sarcolemma from stresses developed during muscle contraction. Proc Natl Acad Sci USA 90:3710, 1993.

Trinick J. Elastic filaments and giant proteins in muscle. Curr Opin Cell Biol 3:112, 1991.

Zubrzycka-Gaarn EE, Hutter OF, Karpati G, et al. Dystrophin is tightly associated with the sarcolemma of mammalian skeletal muscle fibers. Exp Cell Res 192:278, 1991.

Cardiac Muscle

Cantin M, Genest J. The heart as an endocrine gland. Sci Am 254(2):76, 1986.

Challice CE, Virágh S, eds. Ultrastructure of the Mammalian Heart. Ultrastructure in Biological Systems, vol 6. New York, Academic Press, 1973.

Fawcett DW, McNutt NS. The ultrastructure of the cat myocardium: I. Ventricular papillary muscle. J Cell Biol 42:1, 1969.

Forbes MS, Sperelakis N. The membrane systems and cytoskeletal elements of mammalian myocardial cells. Cell and Muscle Motility 3:89, 1983.

Forssmann WG, Girardier L. A study of the T-system in rat heart. J Cell Biol 44:1, 1970.

Hoyt RH, Cohen ML, Saffitz JE. Distribution and three-dimensional structure of intercellular junctions in canine myocardium. Circ Res 64:563, 1989.

McNutt NS, Fawcett DW. The ultrastructure of the cat myocardium. II. Atrial Muscle. J Cell Biol 42:46, 1969.

Morgan JP, Perreault DL, Morgan KG. The cellular basis of contraction and relaxation in cardiac muscle and vascular smooth muscle. Am Heart J 121:961, 1991.

Ogata T, Yamasaki Y. High-resolution scanning electron microscopic studies on the three-dimensional structure of the transverse-axial tubular system, sarcoplasmic reticulum and intercalated disc of the rat myocardium. Anat Rec 228:277, 1990.

Sever NJ. The cardiac gap junction and intercalated disk. Int J Cardiol 26:137, 1990.

Sommer JR, Johnson EA. Ultrastructure of cardiac muscle. In: Berne RM, Sperelakis N, Geiger SR, eds. Handbook of Physiology, sect 2: The Cardiovascular System, vol I. The Heart, Bethesda, MD, American Physiological Society, 1979, p 113.

Sommer JR, Waugh RA. The ultrastructure of the mammalian cardiac muscle cell—with special emphasis on the tubular membrane systems: a review. Am J Pathol 82:192, 1976.

Tunwell REA, Wickenden C, Bertran BMA, Shevchenko VI et al. The human cardiac muscle ryanodine receptor-calcium relase channel: identification, primary structure and topological analysis. Biochem J 318:477, 1996.

Smooth Muscle

Devine CE. Vascular smooth muscle, morphology and ultrastructure. In: Kaley G, Altura BM, eds. Microcirculation, vol 2. Baltimore, University Park Press, 1978.

Devine CE, Somlyo AP. Thick filaments in vascular smooth muscle. J Cell Biol 49:636, 1971.

Draeger A, Amos WB, Ikebe M, Small JV. The cytoskeleton and contractile apparatus of smooth muscle. J Cell Biol 111:2463, 1990.

Fay FS, Delise CM. Contraction of isolated smooth muscle cells: structural changes. Proc Natl Acad Sci USA 70:641, 1973.

Gabella G. Fine structure of smooth muscle. Proc Trans R Soc Lond [Biol], 265:7, 1973.

Gabella G. Smooth muscle cell junctions and structural aspects of contraction. Br Med Bull 35(3):213, 1979.

Lehman W, Moody C, Craig R. Caldesmon and the structure of vertebrate smooth muscle thin filaments: a minireview. Ann NY Acad Sci 599:75, 1990.

Motta PM, ed. Ultrastructure of Smooth Muscle. Boston, Kluwer Academic Publishers, 1990.

Rhodin JAG. Vascular smooth muscle. In: Bohr DF, Somlyo AP, Sparks HV Jr, Geiger SR (executive ed), eds. Handbook of Physiology, sect 2: The Cardiovascular System. Bethesda, MD, American Physiological Society, 1980, p 1.

Somlyo AP, Somlyo AV. Ultrastructural aspects of activation and contraction of vascular smooth muscle. Fed Proc 35:1288, 1976.

Somlyo AP, Somlyo AV, Ashton FT, Vallières J. Vertebrate smooth muscle: ultrastructure and function. In: Goldman R, Pollard T, Rosenbaum J, eds. Cell Motility. Book A: Motility, Muscle and Non-Muscle Cells. Cold Spring Harbor Conference on Cell Proliferation. Cold Spring Harbor, NY, Cold Spring Harbor Laboratory, 1976, p 165.

Trybus KM. Regulation of smooth muscle myosin. Cell Motil Cytoskeleton 18:81, 1991.

CHAPTER 11

Circulatory System

OBJECTIVES

On studying this chapter, you should be able to do the following:

- Describe the tissue layers and histological features of the heart
- Trace the series of events leading to effective heartbeats
- Recognize live kinds of blood vessels in routine sections
- Summarize the essential differences between the various kinds of arteries and veins
- Relate the histological structure of three kinds of capillaries to their respective functions
- Draw a schematic diagram of the blood vessel arrangement in a terminal vascular bed

In this and each subsequent chapter we consider a *system*, which is a group of organs and other body parts that collectively carries out some special function for the body as a whole. Two parts of the circulatory system function in parallel. The **cardiovascular** or **blood circulatory system** distributes blood throughout the body, and the **lymphatic system** collects surplus tissue fluid as lymph.

CARDIOVASCULAR SYSTEM

Essential requirements such as oxygen and nutrients are distributed in the blood, which the heart pumps through the body's blood vessels. The heart is a dual combination of circulation pumps belonging to separate circuits and arranged side by side as depicted in Figure 11-1. The left side of the heart receives blood from the lungs and pumps it through the remainder of the body, maintaining the **systemic circulation**. The right side of the heart pumps blood through the lungs, maintaining the **pulmonary circulation**. Both sides of the heart have an **atrium** that collects blood and a **ventricle** that ejects it. The coordinated action of all four chambers enables the heart to maintain these two circulations concurrently.

Blood ejected by the heart under substantial hydrostatic pressure is distributed by a branched system of thick-walled **arteries**, the finest branches of which (**arterioles**) have a proportionately narrow lumen. Mainly because blood acts as a viscous fluid, the relatively narrow lumen of arterioles reduces the hydrostatic pressure of blood entering open **capillaries**. The thin fragile walls of capillaries facilitate exchange of oxygen, nutrients, waste products, and other substances between

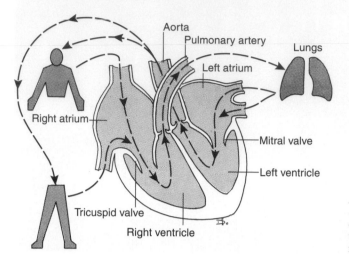

Figure 11-1
Simple schematic diagram of the blood circulation (systemic circulation shown on the left; pulmonary circulation shown on the right).

blood plasma and tissue fluid. Capillaries also produce and can resorb tissue fluid (as described in Chapter 5), and they facilitate oxygen uptake and carbon dioxide clearance from the lungs, nutrient absorption from the intestine, and toxic waste excretion from the kidneys. Blood flow through capillaries is regulated by arterioles and also by intermediate vessels called **metarterioles**, which open into thin-walled **thoroughfare channels** that act as rapid bypass channels. Blood from capillaries and thoroughfare channels passes into thin-walled **venules**, which resemble wide capillaries. In the acute inflammatory reaction, venules produce characteristic plasma and leukocytic exudates. Venules lead into small **veins**, which open into larger veins, and so on. The largest veins return deoxygenated blood to the heart. In contrast, the arteries of the systemic circulation distribute oxygenated blood, whereas the pulmonary artery takes deoxygenated blood to the lungs where it becomes reoxygenated.

The histological organization of the various components of the circulatory system conforms to a single general plan, outlined in the next section.

Blood Vessel and Heart Walls: General Organization

The walls of the blood vessels, heart, and lymphatics are conventionally regarded as being constructed of three concentric coats or **tunicae**, as follows.

Tunica Intima

The innermost coat is known as the **tunica intima** or **intima**. In blood vessels, it consists of 1) a lining membrane termed the **endothelium**, 2) an underlying **basement membrane**, 3) a variable amount of subendothelial **connective tissue**, and 4) an **internal elastic lamina** (layer of elastin), which is not present in some small vessels. The tunica intima of the heart is its lining, the **endocardium**, which is made up primarily of **endothelium** and **connective tissue** of various kinds (see later).

Tunica Media

The middle coat, termed the **tunica media** or **media**, generally includes two components arranged as concentric layers: 1) **muscle fibers**, which are smooth muscle fibers in most blood vessels but cardiac muscle fibers in the heart and certain of its large associated vessels, and 2) **elastin**. Some small vessels, however, lack muscle fibers and elastic laminae in their media. In the heart, this middle coat is highly developed as the **myocardium**, the substantial muscular layer of the heart wall.

Tunica Adventitia

The outermost coat, called the **tunica adventitia** or **adventitia**, is predominantly **loose connective tissue**, together with some **smooth muscle** in certain large vessels. It is supplied by tiny blood vessels of its own called **vasa vasorum** (L, vessels of the vessels), which in some cases supply the outer part of the media also. The tunica adventitia of the heart is called the **epicardium**, meaning the covering of the heart, and it consists of **connective tissue** and a **mesothelium**.

Heart

The walls of the heart are made up chiefly of myocardium and endocardium. The epicardium is commonly regarded as part of the pericardium.

Myocardium

The muscular walls of the heart, representing the tunica media, are primarily constructed of cardiac muscle fibers. The endomysial loose connective tissue that lies between the muscle fibers supplies them with abundant capillaries (see Fig. 10-14) and also with lymphatics. As explained under Cardiac Muscle in Chapter 10, cardiac muscle fibers are branching chains made up of cardiac muscle cells joined end to end by intercalated disks. These disks are sites of adhering (anchoring) junctions and gap junctions (see Fig. 10-13). The adhering junctions counteract cell separation as a result of repeated contractions, and the gap junctions provide direct electrical continuity, ensuring that each wave of excitation spreads through the entire myocardium.

Endocardium

The cardiac equivalent of the tunica intima is the endocardium, which lines the heart chambers and covers heart valves. Endothelium, with its underlying basement membrane and adjacent loose connective tissue, lies at the luminal surface of the endocardium. Deep to the loose connective tissue lies a layer of dense ordinary connective tissue, and beneath this some fat cells are generally present (see Fig. 11-4A). Merging with the endomysium of the myocardium, the fat-containing layer contains branches of the special impulse-conducting system of the heart.

Epicardium

Corresponding to the tunica adventitia, the epicardium is made up of 1) a layer of fibroelastic connective tissue, with blood vessels, lymphatics, nerve fibers, and a certain amount of fat tissue, that merges with the endomysium of the myocardium, and 2) a superficial mesothelial membrane consisting of squamous epithelial cells.

Anatomical Association of Pericardium and Epicardium

The heart is enclosed by a two-layered connective tissue sac called the **pericardium**, made up of a tough fibroelastic external layer, the **fibrous pericardium**, and a delicate mesothelial serous lining, the **serous pericardium** (Fig. 11-2). The developing heart invaginates into the serous pericardium and thus becomes covered by a visceral layer of it. Hence, at the roots of the great vessels associated with the heart, the investing **visceral layer** of serous pericardium is continuous with the **parietal layer** of serous pericardium on the inner aspect of the fibrous pericardium. The narrow potential space enclosed by the serous pericardium, known as the **pericardial cavity**, contains a thin film of serous fluid that facilitates the pumping action of the heart. Accordingly,

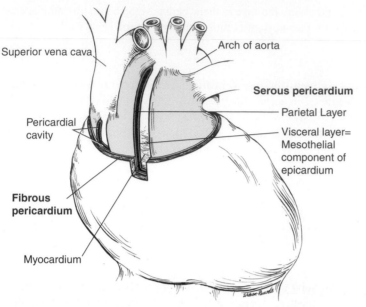

Superior vena cava

Arch of aorta

Serous pericardium

Parietal Layer

Visceral layer=
Mesothelial
component of
epicardium

Pericardial
cavity

**Fibrous
pericardium**

Myocardium

Figure 11-2
Anatomical relations of the heart to
serous and fibrous pericardium
(anterior view, serous pericardium
shown in color).

the superficial mesothelial membrane belonging to the epicardium represents the visceral layer of serous peri-cardium covering the heart, and it is a part of the serous lining of the pericardial cavity.

Pumping Action of the Heart

The sac-like atria accommodate only a small volume of the blood returning to the heart between ventricular ejections. A large part of the venous return carries on through the open atrioventricular (AV) valves and enters the relaxed ventricles below. The AV valves remain open while the atria contract, but when the ventricles begin to contract a moment later, the AV valves close owing to the increase in intraventricular pressure. Rising right ventricular hydrostatic pressure opens the valve at the base of the pulmonary artery (see Fig. 11-1) and blood enters the pulmonary circulation. Rising left ventricular hydrostatic pressure opens the aortic valve and blood enters the systemic circulation. Following ventricular ejection, the pulmonary and aortic valves both close owing to back-pressure developing beyond them. The AV valves then open and blood flows from the atria to the ventricles.

Impulse-Conducting System of the Heart

For efficient pumping of the heart and to ensure that systemic and pulmonary circulations flow concurrently, the events outlined earlier must occur in the correct sequence and synchronously on the left and right sides of the heart. A specialized impulse-conducting system plays a key role in coordinating cardiac contraction (Fig. 11-3). It is a conduction pathway that consists entirely of cardiac muscle cells, some specialized for initiating the impulses for contraction and others adapted for conducting these impulses rapidly throughout the heart, as next described.

SINOATRIAL NODE

The sinoatrial (SA) node is a small mass of specialized cardiac muscle fibers and associated fibro-elastic connective tissue. It lies in the wall of the superior vena cava, close to the site where this borders on the right atrium (see Fig. 11-3). The SA node is supplied with efferent postganglionic fibers from both divisions of the autonomic nervous system, as well as having its own individual blood

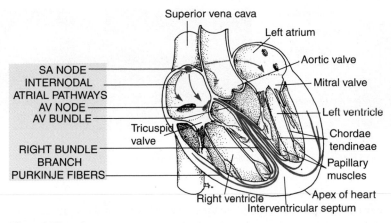

Figure 11-3
Coronary impulse-conducting system (coronal plane).

supply. Each wave of excitation eliciting a heartbeat originates as a spontaneous depolarization of cardiac muscle **pacemaker cells** in the SA node. The SA node is accordingly often referred to as the pacemaker of the heart. The frequency of SA nodal depolarization depends on which of the autonomic divisions is supplying efferent impulses. **Sympathetic** stimulation **accelerates** the heart rate and **increases** the force of cardiac contraction. **Parasympathetic** stimulation **lowers** the heart rate. Each wave of depolarization that originates in the SA node is conducted by way of gap junctions along **internodal atrial pathways** and spreads through ordinary atrial muscle fibers, triggering their contraction. The muscle fibers of the SA node are somewhat narrower than ordinary atrial fibers, and since their role is to initiate and conduct impulses, not to undergo strong contractions, they contain fewer myofibrils.

ATRIOVENTRICULAR NODE AND AV BUNDLE

The next part of the impulse-conducting system to become depolarized is the AV node. It lies in the interatrial septum (see Fig. 11-3), near the opening of the coronary sinus. When the wave of depolarization reaches this node from the internodal atrial pathways, it is momentarily delayed by the nodal cells and then conducted to the ventricles. Like the SA node, the AV node has its own artery and is supplied with efferent postganglionic nerve fibers from both autonomic divisions. Also, it resembles the SA node in its histological organization.

From the AV node, the wave of depolarization is conducted along a bundle of specialized conducting cardiac muscle fibers known as the **AV bundle** or **bundle of His**. This part of the conduction path extends anteriorly from the AV node, penetrates the fibrous partition lying between atrial and ventricular muscle, and enters the interventricular septum, where it divides into left and right branches (see Fig. 11-3). Roughly halfway down the septum, its two branches become bundles of typical **Purkinje fibers**.

PURKINJE FIBERS

Purkinje fibers of the heart lie in the deepest layer of the endocardium. These specialized conducting fibers are particularly large and easy to recognize in the sheep's heart (Fig. 11-4A). Wider than ordinary ventricular fibers, Purkinje fibers contain fewer myofibrils, and these have a peripheral arrangement around the fiber's central sarcoplasmic core. This wide central core contains abundant glycogen, giving the fiber a pale, empty look except for central nuclei (see Fig. 11-4B). Purkinje

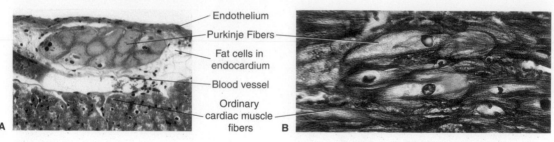

Labels (left to right, top to bottom):
Endothelium
Purkinje Fibers
Fat cells in endocardium
Blood vessel
Ordinary cardiac muscle fibers

A   B

Figure 11-4
Purkinje fibers in the endocardium. (*A*) Transverse section (sheep's heart). (*B*) Longitudinal section (human heart).

fibers extend down the interventricular septum and continue up the lateral walls of the ventricles, but before they reach the lateral ventricular myocardium, they supply the **papillary muscles** of the heart (see Fig. 11-3). This conduction sequence ensures that the papillary muscles are the first parts of the ventricular musculature to depolarize and hence contract. Purkinje fibers conduct the wave of depolarization to the anteroseptal region of the ventricular myocardium before it reaches the posterobasal region, so ventricular contraction begins at the apex of the heart and then spreads up the lateral ventricular walls.

Cardiac Valves
Each ventricle has inlet and outlet valves, both of the flap (**leaflet**) type. The **heart valve leaflet** is an intimal sheet with a core of irregular dense ordinary connective tissue that is mostly avascular. Elastic fibers are distributed asymmetrically in the leaflet, and endothelium covers its entire surface. The base of the fibrous core is attached to a supporting ring that constitutes part of the fibrous skeleton of the heart.

The AV (inlet) valve of the right ventricle has three leaflets (**cusps**) and is therefore called the **tricuspid valve**, whereas that of the left ventricle has two leaflets and because of its resemblance to a bishop's miter (tall cap) is called the **mitral valve**. The tricuspid and mitral valves need to withstand substantial back pressures during ventricular contraction, and without necessary measures would be blown inside out like umbrellas on windy days. Excessive excursion of the valve leaflets is resisted by the **chordae tendineae** (see Fig. 11-3), which are tendon-like cords extending from papillary muscles to fibrous cores of valve leaflets. Because papillary muscles are the initial parts of the ventricular myocardium to undergo a contraction, they pull on the chordae tendineae and stop the valve leaflets from being blown up into the atria.

The outlet valve of the right ventricle is often described as being **semilunar** (L. *semi*, half; *luna*, moon) because it is made up of three almost half-moon-shaped leaflets. Because it is situated at the origin of the pulmonary artery, it is known as the **pulmonary valve**. Located in the proximal end of the aorta is the **aortic valve**, the outlet valve of the left ventricle, also with three semilunar valve leaflets (see Figs. 11-3 and 11-5). The leaflets of both valves have a similar general construction (fibrous sheets covered with endothelium; Fig. 11-6) to those of AV valves, except that they are thinner and lack chordae tendineae. Arteries other than the pulmonary artery and aorta are not provided with valves.

The origins of the pulmonary artery and aorta (from the right and left ventricles, respectively) are supported by rings of fibrous tissue. Similar rings support the AV orifices at roughly the same level. The strong fibrous rings surrounding these four major orifices resist dilatation when blood is being ejected through them. Furthermore, the fibrous rings merge with the membranous part of the interventricular septum. This central mass of interconnected fibrous tissue provides support and at-

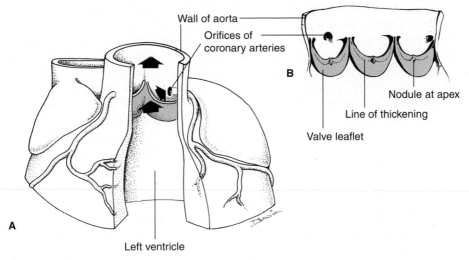

Wall of aorta
Orifices of
coronary arteries
B
Nodule at apex
Line of thickening
Valve leaflet
Left ventricle
A

Figure 11-5
Aortic valve. (*A*) Valve leaflets at the base of the ascending aorta. (*B*) Aortic valve leaflets (aortic wall spread out flat).

tachment for free ends of myocardial muscle fibers, so it is sometimes referred to as the **skeleton** of the heart.

Arteries and Arterioles

The branching arteries that conduct blood from the heart and distribute it throughout the body are classified as elastic arteries, muscular arteries (known also as distributing arteries), and arterioles. Before describing their histological structure, it is helpful to consider their respective roles because their detailed structure and respective functions are interdependent.

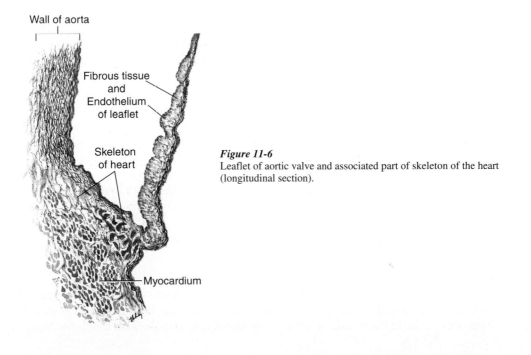

Wall of aorta

Fibrous tissue
and
Endothelium
of leaflet

Skeleton
of heart

Myocardium

Figure 11-6
Leaflet of aortic valve and associated part of skeleton of the heart
(longitudinal section).

The hydrostatic pressure of arterial blood is greatest during the ventricular ejection phase, but adequate pressure must also be maintained between ventricular contractions. The narrow caliber of terminal branches of the arterial tree (i.e., arterioles) resists viscous blood flow, and the resulting back pressure causes the ventricular output to stretch the walls of arteries. Stretch is maximal in the aorta and pulmonary artery, i.e., both of the great arteries conveying blood from the heart. This is because their walls consist primarily of **elastin**. Their substantial capacity for stretch accommodates some of the blood ejected by the ventricles. Elastic recoil of their stretched walls then maintains arterial blood pressure between ventricular ejections. These two great arteries are accordingly termed **elastic arteries**. The arterial hydrostatic pressure resulting from ventricular contraction is called **systolic blood pressure** (Gk. *systolē*, contraction), whereas the interim pressure maintained by the elastic arteries is called **diastolic blood pressure** (Gk. *diastolē*, dilatation).

The essential roles of **muscular arteries** are to distribute appropriate volumes of blood to the various parts of the body and to ensure that at any given moment the local blood flow matches the requirements. The walls of muscular arteries consist primarily of **smooth muscle**, together with some **elastin**. Blood flow is regulated by the luminal diameter of these arteries. The smooth muscle tonus on which their diameter depends is regulated by certain hormones and other factors as well as the sympathetic division of the autonomic nervous system, postganglionic fibers of which innervate vascular smooth muscle.

Large and medium-sized blood vessels present in sections are generally arteries or veins. These vessels are usually distinguishable by observing 1) wall thickness and 2) size and general shape of the lumen. As may be seen in Plate 11-1, arteries are thick-walled. This is because they are required to withstand arterial blood pressure. The arterial lumen looks more or less round because there is only a minor tendency for such thick-walled vessels to collapse at death. In contrast, veins have relatively thin walls because they have only to accommodate blood under venous blood pressure. The relatively wide venous lumen tends to flatten at death, when veins collapse because the venous blood pressure drops.

The three coats of the blood vessel wall are not always discernible, but they are clearly recognizable in muscular arteries so we shall begin with these.

Muscular (Distributing) Arteries

The thin intima of muscular arteries (see Plate 11-1) has an **endothelium** on its luminal border and a substantial fenestrated layer of elastin called the **internal elastic lamina** at its outer border. In H&E-stained sections, the internal elastic lamina is generally seen as a conspicuous wavy pink refractile line, duplicated in some arteries. The basement membrane of the endothelium lies in close apposition with this elastic lamina. The thick **media** consists of a so-called circular layer of smooth muscle, made up of many layers of smooth muscle cells that lie in a helical arrangement along the vessel. Interposed between the smooth muscle cells is an interstitial matrix, predominantly elastin, which was formed by these vascular smooth muscle cells when they were in the synthetic state. The outer border of the media is indicated by the **external elastic lamina**, which is a somewhat less conspicuous fenestrated layer of elastin. The thickness of the adventitia varies, but in many cases it is comparable to the thickness of the media. The adventitia consists chiefly of elastic fibers, together with some collagen. It is provided with vasa vasorum that commonly extend into the periphery of the media and supply this as well. Lymphatics, too, are present in the adventitia.

Elastic Arteries

The **intima** of elastic arteries is substantially thicker than that seen in muscular arteries (compare Plate 11-2 with Plate 11-1). Indeed, the intima of the aorta accounts for about one quarter of the thickness of the whole wall. In H&E-stained sections, the intima appears paler than the media. Many fenestrated elastic laminae and elastic fibers are present in the so-called **subendothelial layer** between the endothelium and the internal elastic lamina. The intimal cells are mostly smooth muscle cells that produced the interstitial matrix of the vessel, but some fibroblasts also are present. The internal elastic lamina that delineates the periphery of the intima is less conspicuous than in muscular arteries and seldom can be distinguished from the other elastic laminae in the walls. The thick media constitutes the major part of the aortic wall. It consists primarily of a great many fenestrated elastic laminae that become increasingly numerous with age. Between these laminae lie the smooth muscle cells that produced the elastin and the other matrix constituents of the media. Whereas the outer half to two thirds of the media is supplied by vasa vasorum, the inner third or so of the media, and all of the intima, depend on diffusion of oxygen and nutrients from the lumen. An indistinct external elastic lamina indicates the outermost limit of the media. The thin adventitia consists largely of elastic and collagen fibers. It is provided with lymphatic capillaries as well as vasa vasorum.

CLINICAL IMPLICATIONS

Atherosclerotic Plaques

Atherosclerosis is a potentially life-threatening disease in which arteries of either type develop characteristic lesions known as **atheromatous (atherosclerotic) plaques** (Fig. 11-7). Widely viewed as an interactive, multistaged tissue response to repeated focal damage of the arterial endothelium, this condition appears to result from local dysfunction and minor disruption of the intimal endothelial cell barrier in arteries. Such damage sets in motion a highly complex, extended series of interrelated events that includes 1) focal adhesion and subendothelial invasion of monocytes that transform into proliferating macrophages that accumulate lipids, becoming lipid-laden **foam cells**; 2) migration of smooth muscle cells from the media into the intima at the affected site; 3) intense growth factor—elicited proliferative and secretory responses in smooth muscle cells that have entered the intima; 4) intracellular deposition of LDL–derived cholesterol in the intimal macrophages and smooth muscle cells, making both appear as foam cells; 5) extracellular deposition of LDL–derived cholesterol in the newly produced intimal interstitial matrix; and 6) local calcification, accompanied by hardening of the plaque and further weakening of the arterial wall. The contribution of invading **T cells** (CD4$^+$ cells together with CD8$^+$ cells) in the developing lesion has not been fully elucidated. A further complication is that platelets may aggregate on collagen that becomes exposed at denuded surfaces of lesions. The ensuing release reaction liberates platelet-derived growth factor, a chemoattractant and additional potent promoter of proliferation for smooth muscle cells. Furthermore, platelet aggregation may lead to formation of a thrombus that may become large enough to occlude the entire arterial lumen. An additional danger is that the thrombus, or part of it, may detach and obstruct an important artery elsewhere (**thromboembolism**). Critical occlusion of a coronary artery as a result of intimal thickening, thrombotic involvement, or thromboembolism may result in a **myocardial infarct** (necrosis of a part of the myocardium), manifested as a **heart attack**. Critical occlusion of a cerebral artery may result in a **cerebral infarct** (regional necrosis of the cerebrum) that may be manifested as a **stroke**.

Arterioles

Arterial vessels with an overall diameter of 100 μm or less are called **arterioles**. In distinguishing these vessels from small muscular arteries, it is helpful to remember that the wall of an arteriole is thick relative to the diameter of the lumen and appears almost as wide as the lumen (Plate 11-3). The **intima** of an arteriole consists of the endothelium and its basement membrane with an apposed internal elastic lamina. The media is represented by only one or two layers of smooth muscle cells (the easiest way to recognize an arteriole), together with an inconspicuous external elastic lamina. The adventitia contains a few elastic and collagen fibers. Internal and external elastic laminae are lacking in the smallest arterioles supplying blood to capillaries.

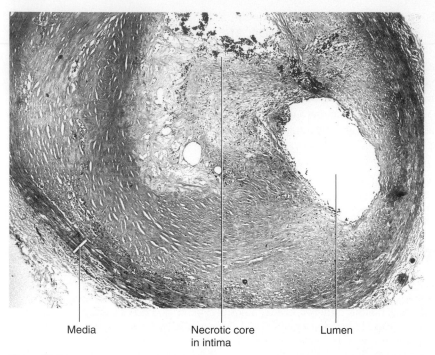

Media   Necrotic core   Lumen
                 in intima

Figure 11-7
The lumen of this coronary artery is significantly occluded by the intimal thickening associated with an atherosclerotic plaque.

CLINICAL IMPLICATIONS

Arteriolar Involvement in Hypertension
Because **arterioles** are relatively small vessels with proportionately thick muscular walls and a correspondingly narrow lumen, they have the important role of reducing the hydrostatic pressure of blood before it enters capillaries. A clinically important consequence of such an arrangement is that the tonus in arterioles has a profound effect on blood pressure. Indeed, the degree of partial contraction of the smooth muscle in the media of these vessels is the main factor that determines peripheral resistance to blood flow, and if the overall tonus in arterioles becomes extreme, it leads to the development of high blood pressure (**hypertension**).

Capillaries and Sinusoids

Blood capillaries are small, thin-walled vessels with a luminal diameter of 8 to 10 μm. Because they are only slightly wider than erythrocytes, these flow along them in single file. Capillaries do not exist singly but in networks, constituting **capillary beds** that provide tissue fluid, oxygen, and nutrients for the body tissues. These tiny vessels may be seen to advantage in transverse sections of skeletal muscle, where they mostly appear as pale-staining or empty rings barely larger than an erythrocyte. The nucleus of an endothelial cell, or a luminal erythrocyte or leukocyte, may also be seen (Fig. 11-8). Without precautions for keeping tissue capillaries distended when they are fixed, endothelial cell nuclei tend to bulge into the lumen of the vessel.

Even though individual endothelial cells generally extend all the way around a capillary lumen, in electron micrographs it is common to see parts of more than one endothelial cell in any given transverse section (Fig. 11-9). Lying external to the endothelium is the endothelial basement

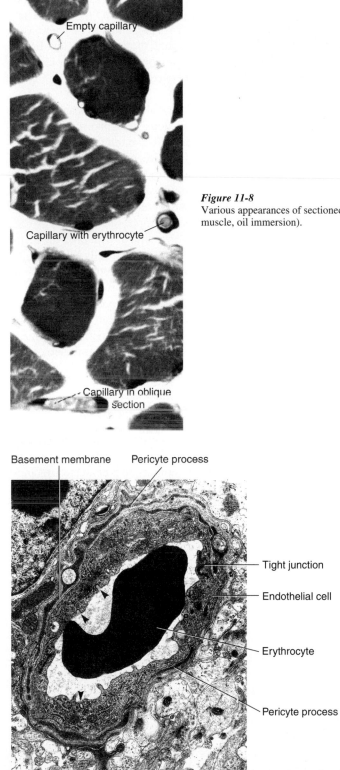

Figure 11-8
Various appearances of sectioned capillaries (transverse section of skeletal muscle, oil immersion).

Figure 11-9
Continuous capillary in an electron micrograph of an immature chick brain. Arrowheads indicate coated pits. Pericyte processes and the lamina densa of the surrounding basement membrane are also discernible.

membrane. Besides having the usual organelles, the endothelial cells of most capillaries contain many endocytotic pits and vesicles (some of these are indicated by arrowheads in Fig. 11-9). These invaginations form along the internal and external cell borders and are presumed to fuse with each other from time to time, producing tortuous transient channels through the cytoplasm that briefly interconnect the two cell borders. Sporadic development of these tiny open transcellular channels permits intermittent bidirectional exchange of macromolecules between blood plasma and tissue fluid.

In capillaries of most parts of the body, the lateral margins of the endothelial cells are interconnected by tight junctions that are band shaped (**fascia occludens** junctions, see Chap. 4 and also Fig. 5-9A). Because these junctions do not occupy entire cell perimeters, slit-like intercellular clefts exist between them through which tissue fluid and small molecules can freely pass. In capillaries of most parts of the brain, however, tight junctions of the continuous (**zonula occludens**) type extend around entire endothelial cell perimeters and constitute the structural basis of the blood—brain barrier (see Chap. 9). For an explanation of the role that capillaries play in tissue fluid production and resorption, see Figure 5-6 and Chapter 5, under Interstitial Fluid and Lymphatic Drainage.

The capillary wall is supported by the endothelial basement membrane. Scattered along the course of the capillary are **pericytes** (see Fig. 11-9). These poorly characterized cells are widely regarded as being phagocytic and potentially or marginally contractile. More importantly, they can give rise to smooth muscle cells and fibroblasts if the need arises for a vessel such as an arteriole, metarteriole, or muscular venule to develop from a preexisting capillary. In common with smooth muscle cells, pericytes are surrounded by a basement membrane, and they are so intimately apposed to the endothelium that they are often described as being insinuated into the basement membrane of the capillary (see Figs. 11-9 and 5-9). The endothelium, pericytes, and basement membrane constitute the intima of the vessel. Capillaries have no media at all and scarcely any traces of connective tissue in their adventitia.

Continuous and Fenestrated Capillaries

There are two subtypes of blood capillaries, termed continuous and fenestrated. **Continuous capillaries** are continuous in the sense that the cytoplasm of their endothelial cells constitutes an uninterrupted (i.e., unfenestrated) lining. This is the common type of capillary that characterizes most body tissues. **Fenestrated capillaries** (Fig. 11-10) are typical of most endocrine organs and the connective tissue layer of the absorptive intestinal lining. Capillaries of this type are more permeable because the endothelial cell cytoplasm is perforated by circular fenestrations. These **fenestrae** (L. windows) are individually covered over with thin diaphragms (see Fig. 11-10A) in all fenestrated capillaries except the glomerular capillaries producing urinary filtrate, where they represent true openings that facilitate filtration. The endothelial lining cells of liver sinusoids also have freely permeable, open fenestrae. Fenestral diaphragms are marginally thinner than a single cell membrane but slightly thicker centrally. They remain incompletely characterized.

Sinusoids

Sinusoids are thin-walled, capillary-like venous blood vessels that have an unusually wide lumen and an associated population of macrophages. They are described in connection with myeloid tissue and the spleen in Chapter 7 and under Liver in Chapter 13.

Metarterioles, Venules, and Arteriovenous Anastomoses

Studies of blood flow in living tissues show that other kinds of blood vessels, less easy to identify in histological sections, are additional important components of the microcirculation.

Diaphragm
of fenestra

Fenestra

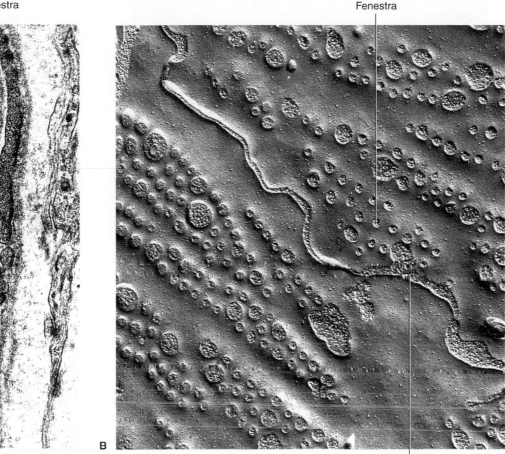

A

B

Basement
membrane

Border between
endothelial cells

Figure 11-10
Electron micrographs showing fenestrated capillaries seen in (*A*) longitudinal section and (*B*) surface view (freeze-fracture replica of the luminal surface).

Metarterioles

Not all the capillaries in capillary beds are supplied directly by arterioles. Many capillaries are supplied by vessels known as **metarterioles** (Gk. *meta*, after), which resemble wide capillaries except that in addition to endothelial cells, their walls contain a discontinuous layer of smooth muscle cells (shown as black semicircles in Fig. 11-11). Moreover, the distal portion of a metarteriole, the part of it known as a **thoroughfare channel**, empties into a venule. Because this extension from the metarteriole has a comparatively wide caliber, it can channel blood past the network of capillaries and into a venule much as a throughway can take traffic off city streets. The origin of a capillary from an arteriole or a metarteriole is guarded by smooth muscle cells, the tonus of which regulates the diameter of the aperture that they surround. When these muscle cells contract fully, the **precapillary sphincter** that they constitute so constricts the origin of the capillary that no blood can enter it, and as a result blood is diverted through a thoroughfare channel instead.

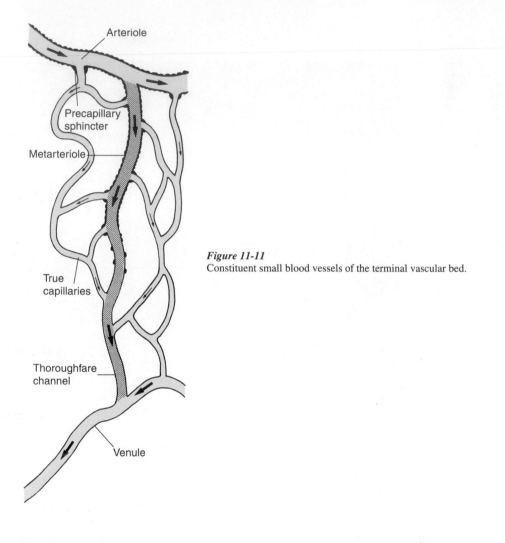

Figure 11-11
Constituent small blood vessels of the terminal vascular bed.

Venules

Capillaries and thoroughfare channels open into slightly wider thin-walled blood vessels called **venules** (see Plate 11-3). These are vessels from which plasma and leukocytes escape during the acute inflammatory reaction. Both components pass through intercellular slits that open up between fascia occludens junctions along endothelial cell perimeters. External to the endothelium (but included in the intima) is the endothelial basement membrane (Fig. 11-12), which in small venules encloses scattered pericytes as well. Small venules lack a media but possess a minimal adventitia represented by a few collagen fibers and occasional fibroblasts. Larger venules have a media that contains smooth muscle cells, but not always a complete layer of them, and an adventitia only slightly thicker than that seen in small venules.

Arteriovenous Anastomoses

In some parts of the body, appropriate amounts of blood pass directly from the arterial to the venous side of the circulation without entering the terminal vascular bed. Vessels called **arteriovenous anastomoses** or **A-V shunts** are interposed so that they may shunt blood directly from arteries to veins or, more commonly, from arterioles to venules. These shunts have thick muscular walls prox-

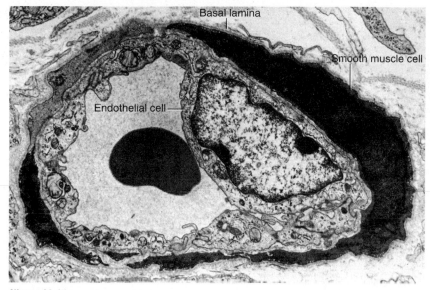

Figure 11-12
Electron micrograph showing a partly collapsed venule. A smooth muscle cell in the media and the surrounding basement membrane (basal lamina) are indicated.

imally but a wider lumen distally, and some are coiled or convoluted. Shunts in the dermis enable the body to conserve heat by diverting blood away from superficial dermal capillaries.

Veins

Veins are thinner walled than their companion arteries, with a wide lumen that generally appears flattened in sections (see Plate 11-1). Although the internal and external elastic laminae are fairly substantial in arteries, they are poorly represented and hence inconspicuous in veins. The wall structure of veins varies in the following respects with regard to the caliber of the vessel.

Small and Medium-Sized Veins

The thin intima of small and medium-sized veins (see Plate 11-1) consists of an endothelium, its thin basement membrane, and only a trace of underlying connective tissue with a very meager internal elastic lamina. Medium-sized veins also possess intimal flap **valves** arranged as paired semilunar leaflets that permit venous blood flow toward the heart but not away from it. Each leaflet is essentially an endothelium-covered intimal fold with a central core of elastin-containing connective tissue reinforcing it. The media of veins is much thinner than that of their companion arteries. In most veins, the media consists of a few circular layers of smooth muscle interspersed with collagen and elastic fibers. However, cerebral, dural, and certain other veins lack smooth muscle cells in their media. In contrast, certain veins of the limbs, notably the superficial veins of the legs, have a thick muscular media that resists the distention resulting from venous return against gravity. This is particularly true of the great saphenous veins, which due to their superficial positions are poorly supported by subcutaneous adipose tissue. These veins have inner longitudinal and outer circular layers of smooth muscle in their media (Fig. 11-13). In general, however, the thickest coat of veins is their adventitia, made up of wide collagen fibers, elastic fibers, fibroblasts, and smooth muscle cells (see Plate 11-1).

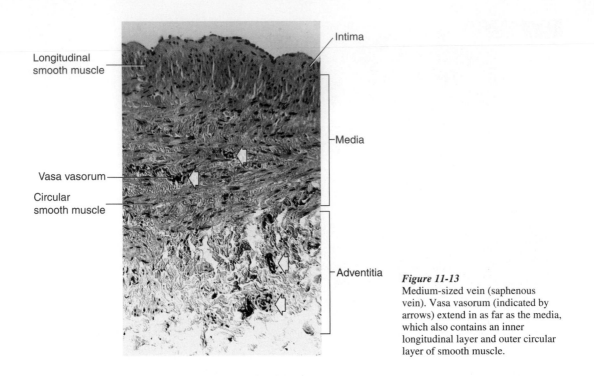

Figure 11-13
Medium-sized vein (saphenous vein). Vasa vasorum (indicated by arrows) extend in as far as the media, which also contains an inner longitudinal layer and outer circular layer of smooth muscle.

Large Veins

The intima of large veins is similar to that of other veins, with an incomplete internal elastic lamina. The media contains a few circular layers of smooth muscle but in general is poorly developed (Plate 11-4). The adventitia, by far the thickest coat, contains longitudinal bundles of collagen fibers along with some elastic fibers, smooth muscle cells, and fibroblasts. Major longitudinal bundles of smooth muscle characterize the exceptionally well-developed adventitia of the **inferior vena cava** (see Plate 11-4).

Vasa Vasorum and Lymphatics of Veins

Vasa vasorum are more extensive in veins than in arteries. These thin-walled nutrient vessels may be seen to advantage in the walls of a medium-sized vein such as a saphenous vein (see Fig. 11-13, *arrows*). Supplying the adventitia and permeating deep into the media, they have the essential function of providing the venous walls with oxygen, since the luminal blood in veins (except the pulmonary vein) has a low oxygen tension. In addition, the walls of veins are liberally supplied with lymphatic capillaries.

CLINICAL IMPLICATIONS

Venous Valves
An unfortunate consequence of aging is that the valves in veins may become incompetent due to dilatation of the venous walls. Furthermore, once the walls of a superficial or unsupported vein have lost some of their elasticity and become generally weakened, the entire vein tends to dilate under the strain of supporting a column of blood against gravity. This becomes aggravated by failure of the valves to close tightly and prevent retrograde blood flow. Veins (e.g., those of the legs) that become lengthened, tortuous, and irregularly dilated as a result of increasing incompetence of their valves are termed **varicose veins**.

LYMPHATIC SYSTEM

The lymphatic system is considered a separate part of the circulatory system. It consists of a body-wide network of vessels known as **lymphatics** with closely associated masses of encapsulated lymphoid tissue called **lymph nodes** (described in Chapter 7). The role of the lymphatic system is to withdraw excess tissue fluid from the body's interstitial (intercellular) fluid compartment as **lymph**, filter this through lymph nodes, and then return it to the bloodstream. Tissue fluid, suspended particulate matter, and interstitial macromolecules collect in **lymphatic capillaries**, which are thin-walled small tributaries of the lymphatic system. The collected lymph is pumped through lymphatic vessels of various sizes and then empties into the blood circulatory system by way of two main ducts, the **thoracic duct** and the **right lymphatic duct**, which open at the junction of the subclavian and internal jugular veins on the left and right sides of the body, respectively.

Lymphatic Capillaries

Lymphatic capillaries (Fig. 11-14) resemble continuous blood capillaries, yet differ from them in the following respects. First, because their basement membrane is either incomplete or lacking, it does not impede luminal access of interstitial macromolecules such as antigens and other proteins. Secondly, one end of a lymphatic capillary ends blindly, whereas both ends of a blood capillary join other vessels. Thirdly, unlike blood capillaries, lymphatic capillaries lack closely associated pericytes. Lymphatic capillaries can also be very much wider than blood capillaries. The last difference is that tiny bundles of so-called **anchoring filaments**, some of which appear to contain collagen, anchor the outer surface of lymphatic capillaries to interstitial matrix fibers in the surrounding

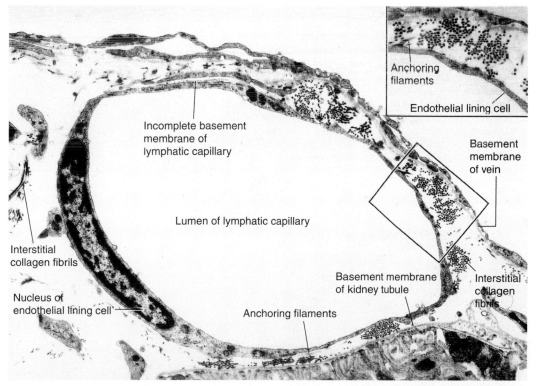

Figure 11-14
Electron micrograph of a lymphatic capillary (rat kidney, × 10,000). (*Inset*) Details in area indicated by box.

connective tissue. Like guy-wires, these fine extracellular filaments hold the thin-walled vessels open under conditions of edema in which interstitial hydrostatic pressure in the surrounding tissue might otherwise cause their collapse.

Lymphatic Vessels

In sections, lymphatic vessels (lymphatics) are not easy to distinguish from small or medium-sized veins. Sometimes the only reliable clue is an absence of blood cells, other than a few lymphocytes, from the lumen of the vessel. Commonly, only an area of pale pink staining (due to lymph proteins) is observed in the lumen of an artifact-free section of a lymphatic (Fig. 11-15). Small lymphatics consist of an endothelium and an extremely thin external coat of loose connective tissue. Medium-sized and large lymphatics are regarded as having the conventional three coats, but these layers are hard to discern even in large lymphatics. The intima consists of an endothelium and a few elastic fibers, and the media and adventitia are both made up of smooth muscle cells and connective tissue fibers. The larger lymphatics have paired apposing valve leaflets, but the consecutive valves are not as widely spaced as they are in veins. A distended lymphatic therefore has a beaded appearance due to dilatation of the short segments between the valves. Each valve leaflet is an intimal fold with a central thin core of delicate connective tissue covered by endothelium. Lymph is propelled along lymphatics by peristaltic contraction of the smooth muscle cells in their walls. Also, external compression caused by pulsation of adjacent blood vessels and the movement of adjacent body parts can augment the pumping action of individual lymphatic segments, aiding lymph propulsion.

CLINICAL IMPLICATIONS

Lymphatic Involvement in Disease Processes
Because lymphatics continually withdraw excess tissue fluid and protein from the interstitial space, a persisting regional **edema (lymphedema)** may be an indication that certain lymphatics have become chronically obstructed. Possible causes of such swelling include trauma, surgical excision of lymphatics (intentional or otherwise), blockage of lymphatics by cancer cells that have spread from a malignant tumor, and lymphatic obstruction by certain kinds of parasites. Even more important is that lymphatic vessels provide open channels that almost invite the spread of infectious agents, inflammatory mediators, and cancer cells. Any neoplastic cells that invade the lumen of a lymphatic from a malignant tumor and then break loose may become disseminated through the body by way of the lymph or by way of the lymph return to the venous side of the blood circulation (**metastatic** spread).

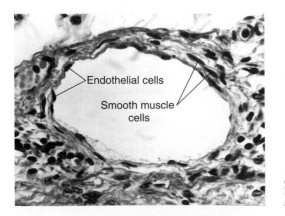

Figure 11-15
Lymphatic vessel. Wall layers are indistinct and blood cells are absent from the lumen.

Table 11-1

CIRCULATORY SYSTEM: MAJOR DISTINGUISHING FEATURES OF COMPONENTS

Component	Principal Functions	Thickness of Wall (Overall)	Intima	Media	Adventitia
Cardiovascular System					
Heart	Pumps blood through systemic and pulmonary circulations; generates systolic blood pressure	Thick	Endocardium = thin lining of heart chambers and covering of heart valves. Endothelium, basement membrane, supporting connective tissue, and Purkinje fibers	Myocardium = thick contractile walls of heart. Cardiac muscle fibers and endomysium	Epicardium = thin covering of heart. Mesothelium (= visceral layer of serous pericardium) and supporting connective tissue
Elastic arteries (e.g., aorta)	Convey blood under arterial pressure from the heart; maintain diastolic blood pressure	Thick	Relatively thick and elastic. Endothelium and basement membrane; elastic laminae; inconspicuous internal elastic lamina; smooth muscle cells; fibroblasts	Extremely thick and elastic. Numerous elastic laminae; interposed smooth muscle cells; indistinct external elastic lamina: vasa vasorum in outer half	Thin. Elastic and collagen fibers; vasa vasorum and lymphatics present
Muscular (distributing) arteries	Distribute appropriate volumes of blood under arterial pressure to body parts	Thick	Thin. Endothelium, basement membrane, and conspicuous internal elastic lamina	Thick, contractile, and elastic. Many circular layers of smooth muscle, interspersed with elastin, etc.; inconspicuous external elastic lamina: peripheral vasa vasorum	Thick, strong, and elastic. Elastic and collagen fibers; vasa vasorum and lymphatics present
Arterioles	Reduce arterial blood pressure to that of terminal vascular bed; regulate blood flow through capillary beds	Thick relative to lumen	Thin. Endothelium, basement membrane, and internal elastic lamina (absent in smallest arterioles)	Thickest in large arterioles; one or two smooth muscle layers; inconspicuous external elastic lamina (absent in smallest arterioles)	Thin. Elastic and collagen fibers

(continued)

Table 11-1

CIRCULATORY SYSTEM: MAJOR DISTINGUISHING FEATURES OF COMPONENTS *(CONTINUED)*

Component	Principal Functions	Thickness of Wall (Overall)	Intima	Media	Adventitia
Metarterioles	Regulate blood flow through capillary beds; conduct blood into bypass channels	Thin	Very thin. Endothelium and basement membrane	Thin and contractile. Single discontinuous layer of smooth muscle proximally	Extremely thin. Only traces of connective tissue
Capillaries (continuous and fenestrated)	Facilitate exchanges between blood and tissue fluid; produce and resorb tissue fluid; produce urinary filtrate in the kidneys	Thin	Very thin for efficient diffusion. Endothelium, basement membrane, and pericytes	Absent	Extremely thin. Only traces of connective tissue
Venules	Accept capillary blood; produce fluid and leukocytic exudates in acute inflammation	Thin	Thin. Endothelium, basement membrane, and pericytes (small venules)	Absent in small venules. Thin in large venules; usually a single smooth muscle layer	Very thin. Collagen fibers
Small and medium-sized veins	Carry blood under low hydrostatic pressure back to the heart	Thin	Thin. Endothelium, basement membrane, and traces of connective tissue: unrecognizable internal elastic lamina; valves present	Thin and contractile, Smooth muscle, interposed collagen and elastic fibers; indistinct external elastic lamina; exceptionally, smooth muscle is either prominent or absent; vasa vasorum and lymphatics present	Moderately thick, strong, and supportive. Collagen and elastic fibers, fibroblasts, smooth muscle cells; vasa vasorum and lymphatics present

(continued)

Table 11-1

CIRCULATORY SYSTEM: MAJOR DISTINGUISHING FEATURES OF COMPONENTS *(CONTINUED)*					
Component	Principal Functions	Thickness of Wall (Overall)	Intima	Media	Adventitia
Large veins (e.g., vena cava)	Return blood under low hydrostatic pressure to the heart	Thin	Thin. Endothelium, basement membrane, and traces of connective tissue; incomplete internal elastic lamina	Thin. Few layers of smooth muscle; indistinct external elastic lamina; vasa vasorum and lymphatics present	Thick and contractile. Longitudinal smooth muscle, collagen, elastic fibers, and fibroblasts; vasa vasorum and lymphatics present
Lymphatic System					
Lymphatic capillaries	Collect surplus tissue fluid and interstitial macromolecules (e.g., antigens, other proteins)	Thin	Very thin, facilitating lymph access. Endothelium with absent or discontinuous basement membrane: pericytes absent	Absent	Very thin. Traces of connective tissue; associated anchoring filaments
Large lymphatics	Carry lymph to lymphatic ducts, which empty it into the bloodstream	Thin	Thin. Endothelium and elastic fibers; valves present	Thin. Smooth muscle and connective tissue fibers	Moderate. Smooth muscle and connective tissue fibers

Summary

The chief distinguishing features of the various parts of the circulatory system are summarized in Table 11-1. Additionally, it should be remembered that coordination of the heartbeat involves conduction of waves of excitation through the impulse-conducting system of the heart. Each cardiac depolarization arises spontaneously in the SA node. The frequency of depolarization is regulated by autonomic efferent nerve impulses. Each wave of excitation spreads via atrial pathways to the AV node, from which it passes through AV bundle and Purkinje fibers to papillary muscles and then on to the remaining ventricular myocardium. Ventricular contraction accordingly follows atrial contraction, beginning in the papillary muscles and the apex of the heart.

Bibliography

Cardiac Conduction System

Fitzgerald D, Lazzara R. Functional anatomy of the conduction system. Hosp Pract 23(6):81, 1988.

Virágh S, Challice CE. The impulse generation and conduction system of the heart. In Challice CE, Virágh S (eds). Ultrastructure of the Human Heart. New York, Academic Press, 1973.

Wellens HJJ, Lie KI, Janse MJ, eds. The Conduction System of the Heart. Structure, Function and Clinical Implications. Leiden, Stenfert Kroese, 1976.

Blood Vessels and Atherosclerosis

Basha BJ, Sowers JR. Atherosclerosis: an update. Am Heart J 131:1192, 1996.

Bearer EL, Orci L, Sors P. Endothelial fenestral diaphragms: a quick-freeze, deep-etch study. Cell Biol 100:418, 1985.

Kaley G, Altura BM, eds. Microcirculation, vols 1—3. Baltimore, University Park Press, 1977 to 1978.

Lindsay J, Hurst JW, eds. The Aorta. New York, Grune & Stratton, 1979.

Rhodin JAG. Ultrastructure of mammalian venous capillaries, venules and small collecting veins. J Ultrastr Res 25:452, 1968.

Rhodin JAG. Architecture of the vessel wall. In: Bohr DF, Somlyo AP, Sparks HV, eds. Handbook of Physiology, sect 2: The Cardiovascular System, vol 2. Vascular Smooth Muscle. Bethesda, American Physiological Society, 1980, p 1.

Ross R. Atherosclerosis: a problem of the biology of arterial wall cells and their interactions with blood cell components. Arteriosclerosis 1:293, 1981.

Ross R. The pathogenesis of atherosclerosis—An update. N Engl J Med 314:488, 1986.

Ross R. The vessel wall. In: Fozzard HA, Haber E, Jennings RB, Katz AM, Morgan HE, eds. The Heart and Cardiovascular System: Scientific Foundations, ed 2, vol 1. New York, Raven Pess, 1992, p 163.

Simionescu M, Simionescu N. Ultrastructure of the microvascular wall: functional correlations. In: Hamilton WF, Dow P, eds. Handbook of Physiology, sect 2, vol. 4. Bethesda, MD, American Physiological Society, 1984, p 41.

Simionescu M, Simionescu N. Endothelial transport of macromolecules: transcytosis and endocytosis. A look from cell biology. Cell Biol Rev 25:1, 1991.

Stary HC, Chandler AB, Disnmore RE, Fuster V et al. A definition of advanced types of atherosclerotic lesions and a histological classification of atherosclerosis: a report from the Committee on Vascular Lesions of the Council on Atherosclerosis, American Heart Association. Circulation 92:1355, 1995.

Stary HC, Chandler AB, Glasgov S, Guyton JR et al. A definition of initial, fatty streak, and intermediate lesions of atherosclerosis: a report from the Committee on Vascular Lesions of the Council on Atherosclerosis, American Heart Association. Circulation 89:2462, 1994.

Wissler RW. Update on the pathogenesis of atherosclerosis. Am J Med 91(Suppl 1B):3S, 1991.

Woolf N. Pathology of atherosclerosis. Br Med Bull 46:960, 1990.

Lymphatic System

Gerli R, Ibba L, Fruschelli C. A fibrillar elastic apparatus around human lymph capillaries. Anat Embryol 181:281, 1990.

Johnston MG, ed. Experimental Biology of the Lymphatic Circulation. Research Monographs in Cell and Tissue Physiology, vol 9. Amsterdam, Elsevier, 1985.

Leak LV. Electron microscopic observations on lymphatic capillaries and the structural components of the connective tissue—lymph interface. Microvasc Res 2:391, 1970.

Ryan TJ. Structure and function of lymphatics. J Invest Dermatol 93(Suppl):18S, 1989.

CHAPTER 12

Integumentary System

OBJECTIVES

This chapter should enable you to do the following:

- Recognize five epidermal layers in a section of thick skin and explain their functional significance
- Summarize the essential differences between thick skin and thin skin
- Outline the cellular basis of skin pigmentation
- Draw a labeled diagram of a hair follicle with its associated skin components
- Recognize two different types of glands in a section of thin skin
- Explain briefly how skin lacerations heal

The skin and various accessory structures that cover and protect the external surface of the body (Table 12-1) constitute the **integumentary system** (L. *integumentum*, covering). Representing the body's most massive organ, the **skin** is made up of two main components—an ectoderm-derived layer of stratified squamous keratinizing epithelium called the **epidermis** (Gk. *epi*, upon), and an underlying mesoderm-derived layer of connective tissue called the **dermis** (Gk., skin). In common with other epithelia, the epidermis is devoid of blood vessels. Its nourishment is dependent on diffusion from capillaries in the dermal connective tissue (see Fig. 4-1). Nourishment sustains only deep layers of the epidermis, however, so by the time more superficial cells reach the body surface, they are nothing more than dead flakes of keratin. Closely associated with the skin are various accessory structures known as **skin appendages**. This term is applied to the **hair** and **nails** as well as three types of cutaneous **glands** that release secretions onto the skin surface (listed in Table 12-1). Exclusively ectodermal in origin, the skin appendages develop as epidermal downgrowths into the dermis (see Fig. 4-8). The bases of hair follicles and most sweat glands descend even farther than this, with the result that their deepest parts lie in the **subcutaneous tissue (hypodermis)** below the skin (Plate 12-1). The subcutaneous layer, also known as **superficial fascia**, is essentially loose connective tissue with a variable proportion of adipose tissue. In some parts of the body, irregular dense ordinary connective tissue lies in this position. Substantial collagen bundles anchor the dermis to the subcutaneous tissue in a manner that allows most regions of skin to be shifted over deeper tissues.

TABLE 12-1

INTEGUMENTARY SYSTEM COMPONENTS

Skin (Thick, Thin)
   Epidermis
   Dermis
   Hypodermis (subcutaneous tissue)

Skin Appendages
   Hairs (growing in hair follicles)
   Nails (growing in nail grooves)
   Eccrine sweat glands (opening on the skin surface)
   Sebaceous glands (opening into hair follicles)
   Apocrine sweat glands (opening into hair follicles)

Two distinct types of skin are recognized—thick skin and thin skin. These names refer only to the proportional thickness of the epidermis, not total dermal thickness. The **thick skin** covering palms of the hands and soles of the feet is characterized by a substantial epidermis with a thick keratinous surface layer (see Plate 12-1A). The **thin skin** covering the remainder of the body has a thinner epidermis with a relatively thin keratinous surface layer, yet the total thickness of thin skin exceeds that of thick skin (compare Plate 12-1B with Plate 12-1A).

CUTANEOUS FUNCTIONS

The epidermis undergoes continual cell turnover and constitutes an endlessly renewing and self-repairing barrier to the outside world. As well as being highly resistant to abrasion and infection, its superficial layers are virtually waterproof, guarding against desiccation and also water uptake across the external body surface. Another role of the epidermis is to produce melanin, the light-scattering effect of which protects underlying tissues from the damaging effects of ultraviolet light. Moderate exposure to light energy of this wavelength is nevertheless beneficial since it enables the skin to synthesize the precursor of vitamin D_3 (cholecalciferol) from 7-dehydrocholesterol, a cholesterol derivative from the liver. By producing sweat, the skin also plays a key role in regulating body temperature, and it serves as an ancillary excretory organ. Lastly, the skin plays an essential role in the perception of our environment, since it covers the body surface and it is profusely provided with sensory receptors.

THICK SKIN

The **thick skin** present on the palmar surface of the hands and fingers and the plantar surface of the feet and toes exhibits a distinctive pattern of whorled surface **friction ridges**. These ridges are visible even with the unaided eye, and they are helpful in identifying individual persons because their detailed configuration (**dermatoglyphic pattern**) is unique in each person. Known as **primary epidermal ridges**, the surface ridges overlie **primary dermal ridges** (Fig. 12-1A). Each primary dermal ridge, however, is subdivided into two **secondary dermal ridges** by downgrowth of epidermis along its crest (see Fig. 12-1B). Projecting from the crest of each secondary dermal ridge are several rows of tall conical projections, up to 0.2 mm high, known as **dermal papillae** (Figs. 12-2A and 12-3). The epidermal downgrowth that creates the secondary dermal ridges is called an **interpapillary peg**, even though it is really a ridge-shaped structure.

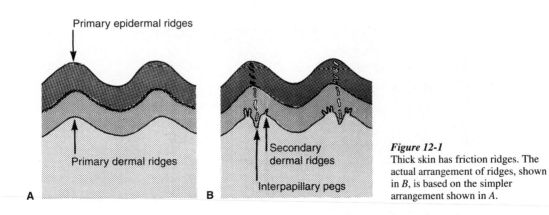

Figure 12-1
Thick skin has friction ridges. The actual arrangement of ridges, shown in *B*, is based on the simpler arrangement shown in *A*.

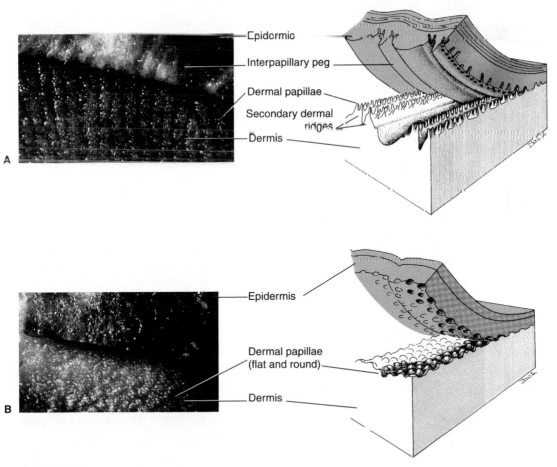

Figure 12-2
Whole preparations with explanatory drawings showing the dermal–epidermal border in thick skin (*A*) compared with that in thin skin (*B*). Epidermis was peeled away to expose dermal ridges and papillae.

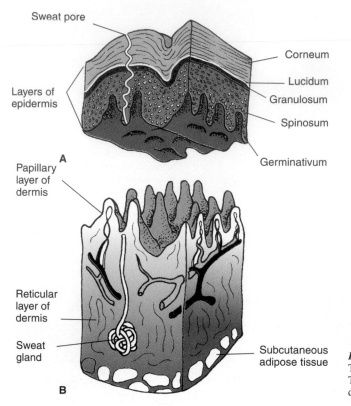

Figure 12-3
The various layers constituting thick skin. The epidermal layers indicated in *B* are depicted in *A*.

Epidermal Layers

The outer region of the epidermis is made up of tiny scales of soft keratin derived from cells called **keratinocytes**. Arising at the base of the epidermis, these committed cells undergo gradual transformation into keratin scales when they become displaced toward the surface. Thus, the keratin layer is replaced from below as fast as it is worn away from the surface. As keratinocytes make their 4-week journey to the skin surface, they mature and undergo consecutive changes in their histological appearance. Because of these changes, the epidermis of thick skin exhibits five recognizable layers, named according to the level of maturation of the keratinocytes in the layer. The five layers appear as follows.

Stratum Germinativum

The deepest layer of the epidermis is a single layer of low columnar cells (see Fig. 12-3). It is known as the stratum germinativum because it gives rise to new keratinocytes, so mitotic figures are occasionally found in this layer. **Hemidesmosomes** (see Fig. 4-4*F*) anchor cells of the stratum germinativum to the basement membrane that attaches the epidermis to the dermis. **Desmosomes** strongly attach these cells to each other and to cells in the stratum spinosum.

Stratum Spinosum

In contrast to the stratum germinativum, the stratum spinosum is several cells thick. When seen in routine LM sections, its polyhedral cells commonly look as if they were joined by spine-like processes, so they are sometimes referred to as **prickle cells** (Fig. 12-4*A*). With the EM, it may be seen

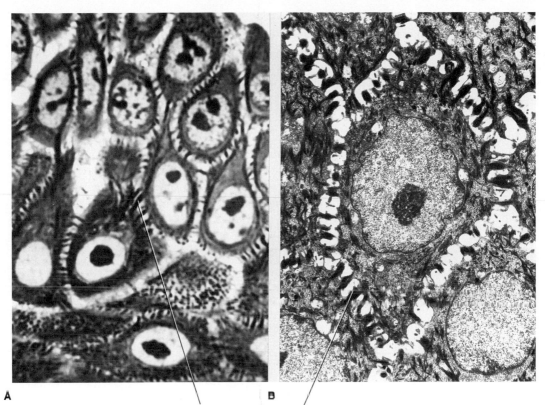

Tonofibrils (tonofilament bundles)
anchored to desmosome

Figure 12-4
Prickle cells in the stratum spinosum. (*A*) Oil-immersion view. (*B*) Electron micrograph. The characteristic spiked shape of prickle cells is a result of shrinkage artifact.

that each spine is a site where a **desmosome** bonds contiguous cell membranes together and that the characteristic scalloped outline of each cell is attributable to shrinkage artifact (see Fig. 12-4*B*). As described in Chapter 4 under Adhering (Anchoring) Junctions, cable-like bundles of **tonofilaments** anchored to the plaques of desmosomes (see Figs. 4-4*D* and 4-7) distribute tensile stresses from cell to cell, enabling the epidermis to withstand rough treatment. The cable-like intermediate filament bundles (originally termed **tonofibrils**) are just discernible with the LM. Lipid-containing **lamellar granules** are present in the uppermost cells of the stratum spinosum.

Stratum Granulosum
The stratum granulosum (see Fig. 12-3) is only a few cells thick. It consists of rather flattened cells that contain characteristic basophilic granules. These **keratohyalin granules** are considered the source of the amorphous protein component of **soft keratin**, the form of keratin that characterizes skin. With the EM, keratohyalin granules appear as angular lumpy masses of electron-dense material. Lipid derived from previously formed lamellar granules becomes released into intercellular spaces in this layer.

Stratum Lucidum

A barely distinguishable, thin transparent layer lies just superficial to the stratum granulosum (see Fig. 12-3). This **stratum lucidum** is difficult to recognize in routine LM sections. Its tightly packed cells are dead, and their nuclei are well on the way to vanishing through karyolysis. The flattened cells now consist essentially of a cell membrane that envelops closely packed keratin filaments complexed with amorphous protein.

Stratum Corneum

By the time keratinocytes reach the stratum corneum, that is, the compact layer of soft keratin at the surface of the epidermis, their organelles and nuclei have disappeared. The cells have been transformed into flat scales of the resistant protein keratin, and they remain strongly attached to one another and to the rest of the epidermis by desmosomes. Lipid present in the intercellular spaces also contributes to the highly waterproof properties of this layer.

CLINICAL IMPLICATIONS

Accelerated Keratinocyte Turnover in Psoriasis
Dysregulated turnover of keratinocytes can result in **psoriasis**, a chronic skin disorder characterized by dark red circumscribed lesions with obvious silvery white superficial scales. Mitosis occurs in more than just the stratum germinativum, involving the three deepest layers of cells in the epidermis, and overproduced keratinocytes reach the skin surface in less than 1 week. This time interval is too short for adequate maturation to occur in newly formed keratinocytes, so the stratum corneum fails to become a strongly cohesive, compact layer of soft keratin.

Dermis

The dermis of both thick and thin skin is made up of a superficial layer of loose connective tissue that merges with an underlying layer of irregular dense ordinary connective tissue. The superficial layer is richly supplied with capillaries and extends up into the epidermis as small projections called **dermal papillae**. It is accordingly known as the **papillary layer** of dermis (see Fig. 12-3). The tall conical papillae of thick skin (see Fig. 12-2A) provide the large surface area required to nourish living cells in the thick epidermis of this kind of skin. They also contribute significantly to the strength of epidermal adhesion. The underlying tough fibrous layer is called the **reticular layer** of dermis (see Fig. 12-3) because it contains substantial bundles of collagen woven into a coarse network. The reticular layer is not as vascular as the papillary layer except where glands and hair follicles extend through it. In addition to collagen, the dermis contains numerous elastic fibers and scattered fibroblasts, macrophages, and fat cells.

CLINICAL IMPLICATIONS

Skin Healing
As every youngster soon discovers, skin has a substantial potential for regeneration. Generally it is only a matter of weeks before abrasions, lacerations, or surgical incisions heal over, provided they are properly managed and do not become infected. To promote healing and to minimize scarring, the edges of any deep cuts need to be approximated with sutures. This measure enables cut edges of the epidermis to grow toward each other fairly readily, beneath the scab, until the dermis is again fully covered by epidermis. Meanwhile, new fibroblasts, many of which arise from pericytes associated with subcutaneous capillaries and venules, lay down new collagen fibers under the site of damage, and the restored dermis regains its former strength.

(continued)

The extensive regenerative potential of skin facilitates skin grafting from one region of the body surface to another. During healing at the donor site, new epidermal cells from parts of the hair follicles in thin skin and parts of sweat glands that are still intact in the deep dermis and subcutaneous tissue supplement epidermal regrowth at the periphery of the site.

ECCRINE SWEAT GLANDS

Thick skin is profusely supplied with eccrine sweat glands, the only skin appendages present in thick skin. These are simple tubular glands with an irregularly coiled **secretory portion (unit)** and a slightly helical **duct** that conveys sweat to the skin surface. The secretory portion is generally situated just below the dermis in the subcutaneous tissue (see Plate 12-1A). This part of the gland may be recognizable in sections as a cluster of small rings each representing a transverse or oblique section through one turn of the coil (Plate 12-2). Most of the secretory cells are low columnar with relatively pale-staining cytoplasm. Long, thin myoepithelial cells, adapted for contraction but representing specialized epidermal cells, are arranged helically around the periphery of the secretory portion, lying between the secretory cells and their investing basement membrane. Myoepithelial cell contraction contributes to sweat expulsion under conditions of extreme fear, stress, or anxiety (sweaty palms). In H&E-stained sections, the sweat gland duct appears somewhat darker than the secretory portion (see Plate 12-2). This is chiefly because in the walls of the duct there are two layers of cells, whereas in the secretory portion there is only a single layer. Because the duct cells are smaller than the secretory cells, darkly stained nuclei are more plentiful in the duct wall. Hence, in sweat glands, lighter-staining regions correspond to the secretory unit and darker-staining regions correspond to the duct. Another unusual feature of sweat glands is that the lumen of the secretory unit is generally a little wider than the lumen of the duct. The duct pursues a slightly helical course through the dermis, enters an interpapillary peg (cells of which serve as its walls), and opens onto the crest of an epidermal ridge at a sweat pore (see Fig. 12-3). Sweat is a clear fluid containing water, electrolytes (sodium, potassium, and chloride), and waste products (urea, ammonia, and lactic acid). Secreted sodium and chloride can be resorbed by the duct cells. Aldosterone, a hormone produced in the outer region of the adrenal cortex, increases the amount of sodium they resorb.

THIN SKIN

Areas of body surface not adapted for as much wear and tear have a less substantial epidermis with a relatively thin surface layer of keratin. However, the name **thin skin** is in a sense misleading, since the total thickness of thin skin is greater than that of thick skin (see Plate 12-1). The fact that the dermis of thin skin, although variable in thickness, is more substantial than the dermis of thick skin makes thin skin the easier kind to suture. Furthermore, thin skin lacks friction ridges and has a less dense distribution of **eccrine sweat glands** (see Plate 12-1B). Thin skin also possesses certain appendages not found in thick skin—**hairs** that grow out of **hair follicles, sebaceous glands,** and sweat glands of another type called **apocrine sweat glands**. Hair follicles and their associated sebaceous glands are distributed profusely over the scalp and certain other parts of the body surface. They are distributed less densely over most other areas of thin skin. In contrast, apocrine sweat glands have a limited distribution (see later).

Fewer epidermal layers are distinguishable in thin skin than in thick skin (Fig. 12-5). The stratum germinativum looks the same, but the stratum spinosum is significantly thinner. The stratum granulosum is sometimes indistinct or discontinuous, and the stratum lucidum is absent. The stratum corneum is not very thick (see Plate 12-1 and Fig. 12-5).

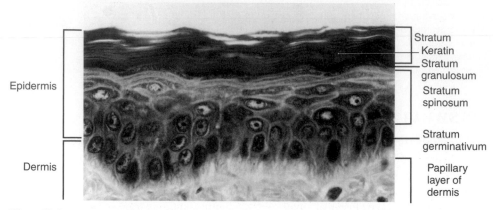

Epidermis

Dermis

Stratum
Keratin
Stratum
granulosum
Stratum
spinosum

Stratum
germinativum

Papillary
layer of
dermis

Figure 12-5
Epidermis of thin skin, showing its constituent layers (monkey's ear).

The dermal papillae of thin skin are fewer, lower, and broader than those of thick skin (compare Fig. 12-2*B* with Fig. 12-2*A*). The body surface shows no external indication as to where these papillae lie. The dermis of thin skin resembles that of thick skin but it is thicker.

SKIN PIGMENTATION

Variations of skin color in persons of different races, and varying depths of suntan (or freckles) developing after exposure to sunlight, may be attributed to differences in the concentration and distribution of **melanin** in the epidermis. Regardless of race or overexposure to the elements, some cutaneous melanin is normally found in everyone except **albinos**, who because of an inherent defect cannot produce this pigment.

Melanocytes are melanin-synthesizing cells that develop from neural crest cells and migrate to the dermal-epidermal border, where they take up a position below and between the cells of the stratum germinativum (Fig. 12-6). They accordingly lie on the epidermal side of the basement membrane delineating this border. The ability of melanocytes to synthesize melanin depends on production of the enzyme **tyrosinase**, which converts tyrosine (through an intermediate called 3,4-dihydroxyphenylalanine) into a melanin precursor. Tyrosinase is synthesized by the rER and routed by way of the Golgi apparatus to membranous vesicles called **premelanosomes**. Melanin is subsequently synthesized in these vesicles, which then become **melanosomes (melanin granules)**. At the EM level, a lamellar or grid-like internal scaffolding seen in melanosomes early in melanin deposition becomes progressively obscured by melanin. Melanocytes possess long cytoplasmic extensions that ramify between keratinocytes deep in the epidermis (see Fig. 12-6). The melanin granules that melanocytes produce subsequently become transferred to keratinocytes by phagocytosis. In light-skinned races, melanin is mostly concentrated deep in the epidermis, particularly in cells of the stratum germinativum (Fig. 12-7). This pigment shields DNA of dividing cells of the epidermis and superficial underlying tissues from damaging, potentially carcinogenic (cancer-causing) ultraviolet radiation. The predominant skin color in different races depends more on extent of melanization, size, and degree of aggregation of melanosomes in epidermal cells than on inherent differences in the proportion of melanocytes in the epidermal cell population.

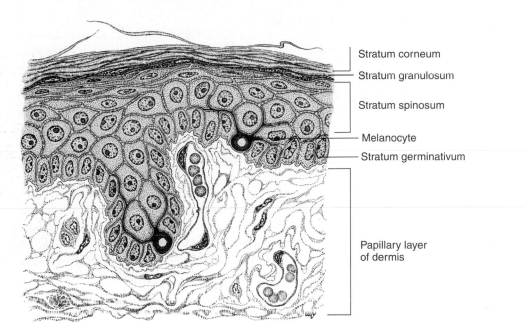

Figure 12-6
Melanocytes in the stratum germinativum possess branching processes that ramify between keratinocytes.

In addition to the melanin found in the epidermis, cells that have acquired melanin through phagocytosis may be found in the dermis. In infants of the Mongol race, such melanin-containing cells may accumulate deep in the dermis of the sacral region, where they are visible through the overlying tissues as a circumscribed bluish-gray to brown patch known as a **mongolian spot**. Such spots are harmless and usually disappear spontaneously in the early years of life.

In addition to numerous melanocytes and abundant keratinocytes, the epidermis contains some specialized basal cells with intimately associated afferent nerve endings (Merkel cells, described under Cutaneous Sensory Receptors). As described in the next section, there is also a scattered population of dendritic cells of myeloid descent (Langerhans cells) that are involved in cutaneous immune responses.

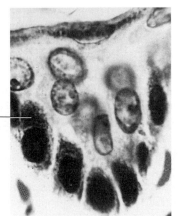

Figure 12-7
Thin skin, showing melanin-containing cells in the stratum germinativum (high power).

CUTANEOUS IMMUNE RESPONSES

Langerhans cells are irregularly shaped dendritic cells, without keratin filaments or melanosomes, that lie interposed between cells of the stratum germinativum and scattered through the other keratinocyte layers. The nucleus of these cells is irregularly indented. The cytoplasm contains distinctive granules (**Langerhans cell granules** or **Birbeck granules**), most of which are shaped like a cupped disk and have a central linear density that may be seen in certain planes of section. Some granules have a vesicular membranous expansion at one end of the linear density, which makes them look like tiny tennis racquets. The origin and functional significance of these rather extraordinary granules remains speculative. It has been suggested that they may participate in the endocytic pathway through which macromolecules are internalized by the cell.

Langerhans cells are also found in wet stratified squamous epithelia and regional lymph nodes involved in dermal lymphatic drainage, suggesting that either they or their precursors are motile. Representing the skin's chief **antigen-presenting cells**, they play a key role in facilitating cutaneous contact hypersensitivity reactions (i.e., **allergic contact dermatitis**). Whereas **Langerhans cells** act as antigen-presenting cells for helper T cells, **keratinocytes** constitute a rich source of interleukin-1 (see Chapter 7 and Table 7-2) and may also promote functional maturation of skin-localizing T lymphocytes.

HAIR FOLLICLES AND HAIR GROWTH

Hair follicles are tubular invaginations of the epidermis that produce hairs. Like sweat glands, they develop as downgrowths of epidermis into dermis and subcutaneous tissue. The growing region of most hairs accordingly lies in the subcutaneous tissue below the dermis. Two different forms of keratin are associated with hair follicles. **Soft keratin**, the form that characterizes the epidermis, is present both as the inner root sheath and also as the soft center within most kinds of hairs. **Hard keratin**, a stronger form of keratin with a higher content of disulfide bonds, constitutes the substance of hair. Hair follicles are so long that there is little chance of finding a longitudinal section of the entire structure in any given section. To see all the features described in the following, it is necessary to examine many follicles cut at different levels. The usual practice is to study scalp sections, since density of hair follicles in the scalp is higher than at any other site (Plate 12-3*A*).

The walls of hair follicles are made up of 1) the **external root sheath**, which is a tubular invagination of the epidermis, and 2) the **internal root sheath**, its sleeve-like lining made of soft keratin (Fig. 12-8 and Plate 12-3*B*). Investing each hair follicle is a **connective tissue sheath**. Deep within the follicle, epidermal cells produce the hair and its internal root sheath. At the base of the follicle is the **hair matrix**, a mass of proliferating cells that fits over a nutritive **papilla** of loose connective tissue. When progeny of matrix cells become displaced from below, they mature and begin forming keratin. The cells destined to form soft keratin of the internal root sheath produce acidophilic **trichohyalin granules**, but equivalent granules are lacking in cells destined to form hard keratin. The transition zone between maturing epidermal cells and hard keratin is called the **keratogenous zone** of the hair. Hence, each hair is produced through proliferation of matrix cells at the base of the follicle and subsequent transformation of progeny cells into hard keratin in the lower part of the follicle.

Hairs generally have a narrow **medulla** (central core) of soft keratin, but in certain cases they lack such a core. Surrounding the medulla (if this is present) is the hair **cortex**. The outermost layer of the hair is called the hair **cuticle** (see Fig. 12-8). It consists of shingle-like scales that by interlocking with complementary scales on the innermost surface of the internal root sheath anchor the hair in its follicle. Both the cortex and the cuticle of the hair are composed of hard keratin. The soft downy hairs typical of the general body surface are referred to as **vellus**, whereas the comparatively

CHAPTER 13

Digestive System

OBJECTIVES

After reading the contents of this chapter, you should be able to:

- Outline the general wall structure of the gastrointestinal tract
- Draw a detailed, labeled diagram of a tooth in its socket
- Recognize histological sections of five different regions of the gastrointestinal tract
- State three structural adaptations in the gastrointestinal tract that facilitate absorption
- Summarize the principal histological differences between the stomach, small intestine, and large intestine
- State the chief similarities and differences between the various salivary glands and the pancreas
- Explain why the liver requires its portal areas
- Discuss the differences between a liver acinus and a classic liver lobule

The **digestive system** (Fig. 13-1) develops from embryonic endoderm. Its major parts, listed in Table 13-1, are essentially the **gut (gastrointestinal tract)** and **accessory digestive glands**. Its various components are collectively responsible for processing, digesting, and absorbing ingested food and eliminating the residue. The liver and pancreas, representing large accessory digestive glands, lie outside the gastrointestinal wall and deliver their secretions through ducts to the gut lumen. Numerous small glands situated in the gut wall further facilitate the digestive process. Key roles of the digestive system are 1) the **digestion** of food and 2) the **absorption** of digestive products across the epithelial lining. The absorptive process involves blood capillaries in most cases, but the more circuitous route of lymphatic drainage in the case of digested fats. Within the gut lumen, food becomes degraded into simple compounds (e.g., proteins are broken down to amino acids, fats to free fatty acids, polysaccharides to simple sugars) through the catalytic action of **digestive enzymes** produced primarily by the accessory digestive glands. Blood delivers these simple compounds to the body tissues, where they are used for cell maintenance, growth, and proliferation. The upper part of the digestive tract (from oral cavity to esophagus) accepts food, prepares it for digestion, and conveys it to the stomach. Here, addition of gastric juice starts the digestive process. Digestion of food continues in the small intestine, and many useful products are absorbed there. Absorption is then completed in the large intestine. Also, water is withdrawn and the semisolid residue becomes compacted.

TABLE 13-1

DIGESTIVE SYSTEM COMPONENTS

Oral Cavity and Pharynx
    Tongue and lingual tonsil
    Teeth, gingiva, and periodontal tissues
    Salivary glands
    Palate and palatine tonsils

Esophagus

Stomach
    Cardiac region
    Fundic region
    Pyloric region

Small Intestine
    Duodenum
    Jejunum
    Ileum

Large Intestine
    Cecum
    Appendix
    Colon
    Rectum
    Anal canal

Major Accessory Glands
    Pancreas
    Liver and gallbladder

Several features of the gastrointestinal tract facilitate digestion and absorption and ensure that only useful digestive products are absorbed. Most absorption occurs in the small intestine, the absorptive area of which is enlarged by the presence of mucosal folds (**plicae**) and finger-like extensions of the lining (**villi**). Also, the cell membrane of absorptive columnar cells of the intestinal epithelium has special **membrane transport proteins** that enable these cells to absorb useful molecules, and the unabsorbed remainder becomes a residue to be voided. Selective absorption by these cells requires effective closing of the more direct paracellular route between the lateral borders of the numerous cells that comprise the epithelial lining. Continuous tight junctions accordingly seal off extracellular space from the gut lumen, and desmosomes minimize separation of the epithelial cells when luminal contents squeeze past them.

As a protection from gastric hydrochloric acid and the enzyme content of digestive juices, the epithelial lining of the gut produces copious **mucus**. A second function of this mucus is to reduce friction and ease the passage of bulky residue along the large intestine. Any kind of wet epithelial membrane that protects itself with mucus is known as a **mucous membrane** or **mucosa**. Also regarded as being part of the mucous membrane (mucosa) is the closely associated layer of loose connective tissue, the **lamina propria** (L. *proprius*, one's own). In addition, most mucous membranes have a basal layer of smooth muscle, the **muscularis mucosae** (L, for muscle of the mucosa). These three layers are represented schematically in Figure 13-9.

In addition to having a variety of mucosal cells producing hydrochloric acid, enzymes, and mucus, the gut mucosal epithelium contains cells that secrete hormones. The gut is therefore regarded as a diffuse kind of *endocrine organ*. Because the pancreas produces the hormones insulin and glucagon as well as digestive enzymes, it also is considered both endocrine and exocrine.

Another general feature of the gut mucosa is that considerable amounts of **lymphoid tissue** are present in the lamina propria under the lining epithelium. This layer contains large, permanent lym-

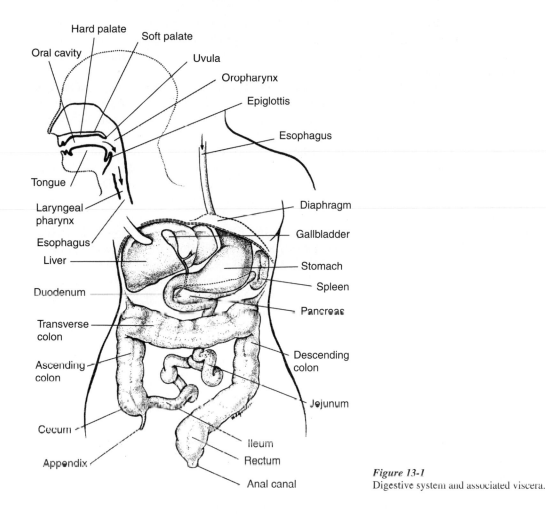

Figure 13-1
Digestive system and associated viscera.

phoid follicles strategically positioned along the digestive tract, primarily in the palatine and lingual tonsils, Peyer's patches, and appendix. Plasma cells derived from B cells of the numerous solitary lymphoid follicles present in this layer produce humoral antibodies to antigens gaining access through tiny breaches in the epithelial barrier. Moreover, some of the plasma cells produce immunoglobulins that belong to a class known as **secretory IgA**. The epithelial cells transport these antibodies into the gut lumen, where they protect the mucosa from invasion by pathogenic microorganisms.

ORAL CAVITY AND TONGUE

The epithelial lining of the oral cavity, subject to much wear and tear, is stratified squamous epithelium. On the underside of the tongue, floor of the mouth, and mucosal surfaces of the cheeks and lips, the epithelial lining remains nonkeratinized and relatively flexible. In contrast, the stratified squamous epithelium covering the gingivae (gums), hard palate (roof of the mouth), and most of the upper side of the tongue, is keratinized and firm. These surfaces need extra protection from abrasion during eating. Where the keratinized epithelium borders on nonkeratinized epithelium (and, to a certain extent, locally on the gingivae and hard palate), the epithelium may be parakeratinized (i.e., incompletely keratinized, in the sense that the stratum corneum remains indistinct), with the surface cells remaining nucleated even though they are close to forming keratin. Deep to the fibroelastic oral lamina propria lie numerous small **minor salivary glands** that are predominantly mucus secreting.

Representing a substantial mass of interlacing skeletal muscle fiber bundles and connective tissue, the **tongue** also contains mucous and serous glands and small pockets of adipose tissue. Because its muscle fibers are arranged in three different planes, the tongue can perform various complex movements. In contrast to the smooth nonkeratinized undersurface of the tongue, the **anterior (palatine) portion** of the mostly keratinized dorsal surface of the tongue is raised into small projections known as **lingual papillae**. The posterior third (**pharyngeal portion**) of the dorsal surface lacks papillae but is bumpy because of underlying aggregates of **lymphoid follicles**. Delineating the boundary between these two parts of the dorsal surface is a shallow groove called the **sulcus terminalis** (Fig. 13-2).

The lingual papillae consist of an epithelial covering and a core of lamina propria. The majority are known as **filiform papillae** (L. *filum*, thread) because of their long thread-like shape. **Fungiform papillae**, like button mushrooms, each have a globular tip. Slightly anterior to the sulcus terminalis is a V-shaped row of up to 12 large **vallate** (or **circumvallate**) **papillae**. Resembling large fungiform papillae, these projections are each surrounded by a moat-like trough. Underlying serous glands keep the troughs flushed out with watery secretion and also produce a lipase. **Foliate papillae**, which are small lateral folds of the mucosa, are only minimally represented in the human tongue. The filiform papillae impart a slight roughness to the dorsal surface and contain afferent nerve endings sensitive to touch. The vallate, foliate, and most of the fungiform papillae possess taste receptors situated in structures called **taste buds**. The taste receptors of a vallate papilla lie at its perimeter in the medial walls of the surrounding trough. The underlying serous glands provide enough fresh fluid to dissolve substances to be tasted and to clear away debris and lingering tastes.

Taste Buds

Bud-like or barrel-shaped **taste buds** (Fig. 13-3) are present on the vallate, foliate, and fungiform papillae, and are widely distributed in the oral and pharyngeal mucosa. Taste buds contain epithelially derived **taste receptor cells, sustentacular cells** (a general term for the *supporting cells* of sensory receptors), and **basal cells** from which both of these cell types are renewed. The taste receptor cells and sustentacular cells surround a small central cavity that opens onto the surface at a tiny taste pore (see Fig. 13-3B, *arrow*).

Chemoreceptive taste receptors are stimulated by direct contact with dissolved substances that enter through the taste pore. When these receptors are stimulated, they initiate impulses in the afferent nerve fibers with which they synapse. All flavors are perceived as various combinations of four basic tastes—sweet, sour, bitter, and salty. Also, olfactory stimuli received by the nasal **olfactory organ** while food is being eaten greatly enhance the taste of certain foods.

Lingual Tonsil

The lamina propria under the posterior third of the dorsal surface of the tongue is characterized by having prominent aggregates of lymphoid follicles. Arrangements in which multiple confluent lymphoid follicles lie in permanent close association with wet epithelial membranes are called **tonsils**, so this nodular region of the tongue is known as the **lingual tonsil** (see Fig. 13-2). The overlying stratified squamous nonkeratinizing epithelium extends down into the lymphoid tissue as deep pits called **crypts**, and lymphocytes are able to migrate through this epithelium into the oral cavity. Mucous glands secrete into the crypts and keep them free of debris.

m
tra
th
se
of
a
bo
th
me
str
tee
bo
the
an

co
aln
cro
2 f

De

Ap
con
we
pro
stri

mas
root
hen
stay
Der
tivi
den
also

Bloc
in pu

Odo
(sing

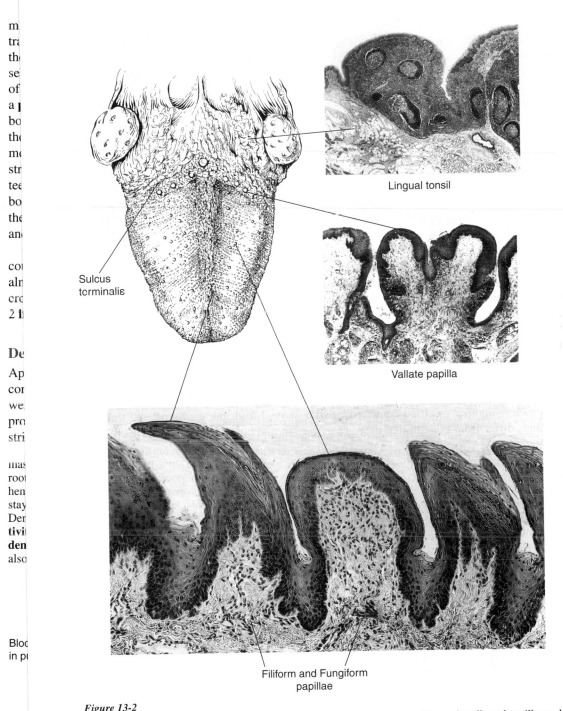

Sulcus terminalis

Lingual tonsil

Vallate papilla

Filiform and Fungiform papillae

Figure 13-2
Histological features of the dorsal surface of the tongue. The respective sites of the various lingual papillae and the lingual tonsil are indicated.

compound alveolar or tubuloalveolar glands of the **mixed** type. **Serous** secretory units generally predominate and most of the mucous secretory units are capped with **serous demilunes** (see Plate 4-4).
The serous secretion from the serous cells in the demilune enters the lumen of the mucous secretory
unit by way of small intercellular **secretory canaliculi** between the mucous cells. In common with
the parotids, the submandibular glands have a strong fibrous capsule and fairly conspicuous ducts.

Sublingual Glands

The **sublingual glands** lie bilaterally under the tongue, beneath the mucosal lining of the floor of the
oral cavity. Their multiple ducts open near the orifices of the submandibular ducts. The sublingual
glands are compound tubuloalveolar glands of the **mixed** type. They differ from the submandibular
glands in that commonly, the majority of secretory units are **mucus-secreting**. Some mucous secretory units in the sublingual glands possess serous demilunes. The capsule is not thick but the septa
are fairly substantial.

Salivary Ducts

Salivary glands have **intralobular ducts** of two different kinds. Leading from their secretory units are **intercalated ducts**. These small ducts are lined with a simple low cuboidal epithelium that is partly invested by
myoepithelial cells. The intercalated ducts (which are rather long in the parotids) continue on as **striated ducts**,
so called because after suitable staining, fine striations may be detected in the basal part of their columnar lining cells. These striations correspond to basal infoldings and interdigitations of the cell membrane with numerous more or less parallel associated mitochondria. The folds provide a large expanse of cell membrane for
active transport of substances into or out of the duct. A major role of the striated ducts (which are comparatively
long in the submandibular glands) is to modify ionic composition of the secretion. The striated ducts open into
interlobular ducts, known also as **terminal secretory (excretory) ducts**, lined with a tall columnar epithelium that becomes pseudostratified columnar, and then stratified columnar, as the luminal diameter increases.

Salivary Secretion

The mixed secretion of major and minor salivary glands, **saliva**, contains mucus and two digestive enzymes
(salivary α amylase and a lipase). Besides keeping the lips and oral mucosa moist and lubricated, saliva moistens
ingested food, enabling it to be tasted and then swallowed with ease. It also buffers the prevalent acidic conditions in the oral cavity. Furthermore, it contains IgA antibodies capable of reducing microbial attachment to the
gut mucosa. Salivary secretory activity is stimulated by autonomic efferent impulses. Parasympathetic impulses
elicit the production of copious watery secretion, whereas sympathetic impulses elicit the production of much
smaller volumes of thick viscid secretion, which often results in the feeling that the oral cavity has gone dry.

PALATE AND PHARYNX

Forming the upper part of the digestive tract, the palate and pharynx are characterized by the presence of protective devices and features that promote immunity to ingested microorganisms.

Hard and Soft Palates

The part of the oral mucosa that lines the roof of the mouth is a site where the lamina propria is
strongly bound to the periosteum of overlying maxillae and palatine bones. This part of the palate is
able to withstand forceful movements of the tongue in the process of eating and swallowing. The epithelium that lines the anterior two-thirds of the palate, which because of its bony roof is known as
the **hard palate**, is stratified squamous keratinizing epithelium with occasional areas of local para-
keratinization.

Posterior to the hard palate is the **soft palate**, the undersurface of which is lined with stratified squamous nonkeratinizing epithelium. The mucous membrane of the nasopharynx is separated from that of the oropharynx by a layer of skeletal muscle that contracts during swallowing. This action raises the soft palate so that it presses against the posterior wall of the pharynx, closing off the nasopharynx and stopping food from going down the wrong way during the process of swallowing.

Palatine Tonsils

The paired **palatine tonsils** are prominent ovoid masses of lymphoid tissue that contain large aggregates of confluent lymphoid follicles. They are situated bilaterally in the lamina propria of the pharyngeal mucosa between the glossopalatine and pharyngopalatine arches. The overlying stratified squamous nonkeratinizing epithelium invaginates as deep **crypts** (Fig. 13-8). The associated lymphoid tissue consists of a dense accumulation of separate and fused **lymphoid follicles**, many with large pale-staining germinal centers. Lymphocytes are able to pass through the crypt epithelium into the lumen of the pharynx and thereby gain access to the saliva. Associated with the palatine tonsils are underlying mucous glands with ducts that rarely open into the crypts. Debris therefore tends to collect in the crypts, predisposing the palatine tonsils to infection. If palatine tonsils become persistently inflamed due to unremitting infection, their surgical removal (**tonsillectomy**) may be considered expedient.

Pharynx

Besides guiding food from the oral cavity to the esophagus, the pharynx conducts air between the nasal cavities and the larynx. Hence it serves both as a digestive passageway and as a respiratory airway. The **nasopharynx** is the airway that lies above the soft palate. It is lined with pseudostratified ciliated columnar epithelium. In contrast, the **oropharynx** and **laryngeal pharynx** are lined with

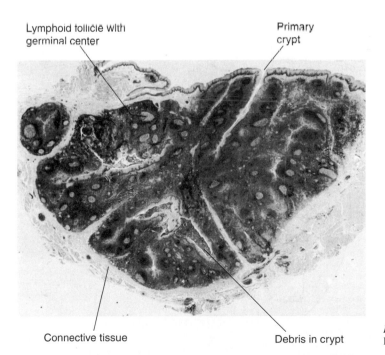

Lymphoid follicle with germinal center

Primary crypt

Connective tissue

Debris in crypt

Figure 13-8
Palatine tonsil (very low power).

stratified squamous nonkeratinizing epithelium. Lying in the midline of the posterior wall of the nasopharynx is a single **pharyngeal tonsil** (see Fig. 14-1) made up of multiple confluent lymphoid follicles in intimate association with overlying pseudostratified epithelium. If the pharyngeal tonsil becomes unduly enlarged it chronically obstructs nasal breathing, a condition known as **adenoidal lymphoid hyperplasia** or **adenoids**.

The various tonsils that we have described are distributed as an incomplete ring around the digestive and respiratory tracts at the level where the two tracts intersect. Lymphocytes of lymphoid follicles in tonsils may become repeatedly exposed to antigens from a multitude of potentially infective microorganisms that can enter either tract from the outside world. Immunoglobulins, especially IgAs, produced in response to such antigens provide substantial protection against infection by pathogenic microorganisms (as described under Gut-Associated Lymphoid Tissue in Chapter 7).

DIGESTIVE TRACT: WALL STRUCTURE

The remainder of the digestive tract has walls made up of four major layers called the **mucosa (mucous membrane), submucosa, muscularis externa,** and **serosa** or **adventitia** (Fig. 13-9), the general features of which are outlined in the following sections.

Mucosa (Mucous Membrane)

The mucosa of the digestive tract consists of 1) the lining **epithelium** with its glandular invaginations; 2) an underlying layer of loose connective tissue, termed the **lamina propria**, that supports

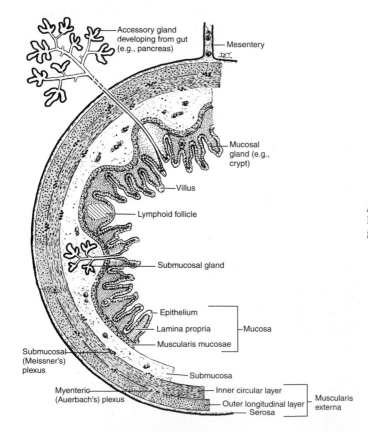

Accessory gland developing from gut (e.g., pancreas)

Mesentery

Mucosal gland (e.g., crypt)

Villus

Lymphoid follicle

Submucosal gland

Epithelium

Lamina propria

Muscularis mucosae

— Mucosa

Submucosal (Meissner's) plexus

Submucosa

Myenteric (Auerbach's) plexus

Inner circular layer

Outer longitudinal layer

Serosa

Muscularis externa

Figure 13-9
Basic wall organization in the gastrointestinal tract.

the epithelium and accommodates its associated **mucosal glands**; and 3) in many parts of the tract, a thin basal layer of smooth muscle called the **muscularis mucosae**.

Epithelium

The type of epithelium and the distinctive features of any mucosal or submucosal glands reflect the individual functions of each part of the tract.

The esophagus is efficiently protected from abrasion by being lined with stratified squamous nonkeratinizing epithelium. The stomach has a simple columnar epithelium entirely made up of cells that secrete protective mucus. The small and large intestines possess a simple columnar epithelium with columnar absorptive cells and mucus-secreting goblet cells. Copious quantities of mucus are required in the duodenum (the first part of the small intestine) to combat gastric acidity. Here, supplementary supplies come from **submucosal** mucous glands (shown at left in Fig. 13-9). The esophagus, too, has a few submucosal mucous glands.

Gastric pits are tiny recesses in the epithelial lining of the stomach. From these pits, simple tubular mucosal glands called **gastric glands** extend into the lamina propria. Simple tubular mucosal glands called **crypts** (of **Lieberkühn**) similarly extend into the lamina propria of the small and large intestines. In addition to mucosal and submucosal glands, the digestive tract possesses several **accessory glands** situated outside its walls (upper left in Fig. 13-9). The chief accessory glands are the liver, pancreas, and salivary glands.

Lamina Propria

Extensively provided with lymphatic capillaries as well as fenestrated blood capillaries, the lamina propria is the neighboring loose connective tissue layer that nourishes the mucosal epithelium and its associated mucosal glands. Various products of digestion pass into capillaries or lymphatics in the central cores (i.e., lamina propria) of finger-like **villi** of the small intestine (see Fig. 13-9). Unencapsulated lymphoid follicles and plasma cells are also commonly found in the mucosal connective tissue layer. Immunoglobulin secretion by plasma cells is an important part of the local defense strategy for discouraging mucosal invasion by pathogenic ingested microbes and gut parasites.

Muscularis Mucosae

The muscularis mucosae is typically a thin, double layer of smooth muscle. In the digestive tract, the muscle cells are arranged circularly or helically in the inner layer and longitudinally in the outer layer. Contractile activity of the muscularis mucosae results in an independent local moving and folding of the mucosa that facilitates digestion and absorption. Tonus of smooth muscle cells extending from the muscularis mucosae to tips of villi can regulate villous height in the small intestine.

Submucosa

Between the mucosa and muscularis externa lies the **submucosa**, a loose connective tissue layer with comparatively large blood vessels and also lymphatics. Each mucosal fold has a submucosal core (see Fig. 13-9, *top*). Near the border between the submucosa and the muscularis externa lies a plexus of autonomic ganglion cells and nerve fibers, the **submucosal (Meissner's) plexus** (see Fig. 13-9, *bottom left*). This nerve plexus is not easy to find in routine sections, however. Its postganglionic fibers supply the muscularis mucosae and mucosal glands. In the duodenum and esophagus, the submucosa also contains **mucus-secreting glands** (see Fig. 13-9, *left*).

Muscularis Externa

The most substantial layer of the wall is generally the **muscularis externa**, which typically consists of two layers of smooth muscle, the inner one circular and the outer one longitudinal. Actually, the muscle cells in both layers follow a slightly helical course, but in transverse sections of the tract, cells of the inner layer are cut more or less longitudinally and those of the outer layer are generally cut transversely. The muscularis externa is the muscle coat responsible for moving luminal contents along the tract. Rhythmic waves of contraction (**peristaltic waves**) that propel the contents along are coordinated by efferent impulses from another autonomic plexus called the **myenteric (Auerbach's) plexus**. This plexus of interneurons, motor neurons, and unmyelinated fibers lies between the circular and longitudinal layers of the muscularis externa (see Fig. 13-9, *bottom left*). It may be seen to advantage in sections of large intestine (see Plate 9-8). The luminal diameter of the intestine is regulated chiefly by the tonus in the circular layer of the muscularis externa.

The myenteric plexus and submucosal plexus are both integral parts of the **enteric nervous system**, a regional component of the nervous system that functions semi-independently of the CNS.

Serosa or Adventitia

In those regions of the gastrointestinal tract where the outermost loose connective tissue coat of the wall is covered by visceral peritoneum, this coat is referred to as a **serosa**. But in those regions where a mesothelial covering is lacking (e.g., retroperitoneal segments of the intestine attached to the posterior abdominal wall), the outermost connective tissue coat is called an **adventitia**. Many blood vessels, lymphatics, and nerves lie in this coat. Gut **mesenteries** (see Fig. 13-9, *top*) are serosal suspensory folds representing double sheets of peritoneal mesothelium with a thin layer of loose connective tissue sandwiched between them. This middle layer contains blood vessels, lymphatics, nerves, and variable numbers of fat cells.

ESOPHAGUS

The relatively muscular walls of the esophagus convey chewed food rapidly from the pharynx to the stomach. The lining layer of stratified squamous nonkeratinizing epithelium (Plate 13-2) withstands intermittent abrasion, and mucus from small numbers of submucosal **esophageal glands** can ease the passage of swallowed food. Also, some simple tubular mucous glands known as **cardiac glands** are present in the lamina propria, both at the upper end and at the lower end of the esophagus. The **muscularis mucosae** of the lower part of the esophagus is substantial. In the middle third, its smooth muscle is mostly longitudinal. The muscle constituting the **muscularis externa** of the top third is skeletal, whereas in the bottom third it is smooth. In the middle third, the muscularis externa contains both types of muscle. The outermost layer of most of the esophagus is an **adventitia** that binds it to adjacent structures.

STOMACH

Digestion and absorption begin in the stomach, an expandable muscular-walled reservoir that retains swallowed food by maintaining tonus in its outlet muscle, the **pyloric sphincter** (Gk. *pylōrus*, gate guard). **Gastric juice** secreted by gastric mucosal glands contains **hydrochloric acid, mucus,** the proteolytic enzyme **pepsin** (secreted as its precursor, **pepsinogen**), and **lipase**, which breaks down fats. **Intrinsic factor**, an absolute requirement for vitamin B_{12} absorption, comes from the cells that produce gastric hydrochloric acid. The surface epithelial cells lining the stomach produce a thick coating of mucus that protects the gastric mucosa from acid and enzymes in the lumen, but even so the surface mucous cells need to be replaced after 4 to 6 days of contact with the stomach contents. The churning action of gastric contractions reduces semisolid chewed food to semifluid **chyme**. Absorption of drugs, alcohol, salts, and water begins when food is still undergoing digestion in the stomach.

Anatomically, the stomach is made up of a superior region called the **fundus**, a main region known as the **body**, and a distal part consisting of the **pyloric antrum, pyloric canal,** and **pylorus** (Fig. 13-10). Histologically, only three regions are readily distinguishable: 1) the **cardiac region** surrounding the cardiac orifice; 2) the **body of the stomach** or **fundic region**, which includes both the fundus and the body; and 3) the **pyloric region**, which includes the pyloric antrum, pyloric canal, and pylorus. A characteristic feature seen in the gastric mucosa of the empty stomach is that it is raised into longitudinal branching folds termed **rugae** (L. for wrinkles; see Fig. 13-10). These folds and their submucosal cores (Plate 13-3A) become flattened out if a substantial meal is ingested. Another characteristic of the gastric mucosa is its dense distribution of simple tubular mucosal glands. Supplemental submucosal glands are not present, except near the pyloric-duodenal junction. The gastric **muscularis externa** varies from the usual plan in that it has *three layers* instead of two, the innermost one being oblique, the middle one circular, and the outermost one, longitudinal. A serosa covers the external surface of the stomach.

Gastric Epithelium, Pits, and Glands

The epithelial lining layer of the stomach consists entirely of **mucous columnar cells**, not the mixture of columnar absorptive cells and goblet cells that characterizes the intestine. In H&E-stained sections, the columnar gastric epithelial lining cells are pale staining owing to their content of mucus-filled secretory granules (see Plate 13-3B).

Fundic Region

Opening into each **gastric pit (foveola)**, the term for tiny epithelial recesses in the gastric lining, are several **gastric glands** (Fig. 13-11). Mucous columnar cells resembling those of the gastric lining epithelium also line the pits. A variety of cell types is found in gastric glands, depending on the region of the stomach in which they lie. The mucosal glands of the cardiac region (**cardiac glands**) are small and predominantly mucus secreting. Those of the fundic region (**fundic glands**) are larger and secrete almost all the hydrochloric acid and enzymes produced by the stomach, together with some of the mucus. Also known as **zymogenic glands**, fundic glands are long and fairly straight, and some of them branch toward their base (see Fig. 13-11), which explains the many oblique and transverse sections of gland **bases** that are also seen (see Plate 13-3B). The middle part of the gastric

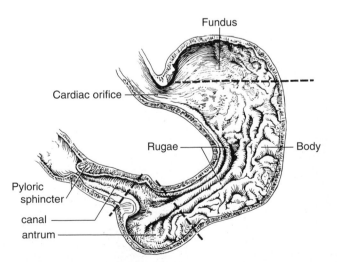

Cardiac orifice

Fundus

Rugae

Body

Pyloric sphincter

canal

antrum

Figure 13-10
Regions and internal features of the stomach (showing internal aspect of posterior wall).

gland is called its **neck** region, and the upper part opening into a gastric pit is called its **isthmus** (see Fig. 13-11). The isthmus and neck regions contain dividing cells, immature cells, and maturing surface epithelial cells, and they constitute the germinal zone from which surface and glandular epithelial cells of the fundic mucosa are renewed. The neck region contains mucus-secreting **mucous neck cells**. Interspersed with these mucus-producing cells are acidophilic **parietal (oxyntic) cells** that commonly appear large, rounded, and pale-staining, with a central spherical nucleus (see Plate 13-3 and Figs. 13-11 and 13-12). Parietal cells produce gastric **hydrochloric acid** and the secretory glycoprotein **intrinsic factor**, without which adequate amounts of vitamin B_{12} cannot be absorbed from the small intestine. If intrinsic factor is underproduced, erythropoietic activity of myeloid tissue is impaired (**pernicious anemia**). Distributed chiefly in the neck region of the gland, parietal cells are also scattered through the isthmus and base.

Parietal cells are characterized by having intracellular channels (**canaliculi**) that produce hydrochloric acid and deliver it to the gland lumen. Many mitochondria border on these canaliculi and numerous long microvilli project from the canalicular surface (Fig. 13-12). The canalicular membrane actively transports hydrogen ions and chloride ions into the canaliculi. Bicarbonate ions produced along with the hydrogen ions diffuse from the cell into the interstitial spaces, and subsequently enter the bloodstream. The local interstitial concentration of bicarbonate ions protects the mucosa from hydrogen ions leaking from the gastric lumen through the mucosal epithelium. The substantial coating of mucus above the gastric lining acts as an important diffusion barrier between the mucosal bicarbonate and the luminal hydrogen ions.

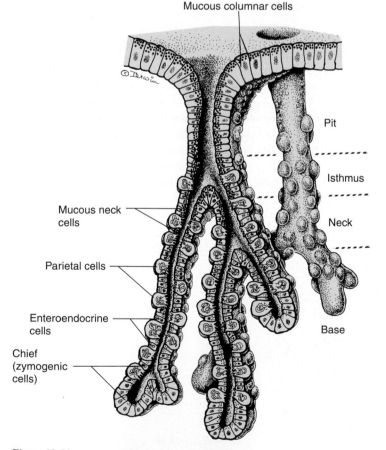

Figure 13-11
Gastric pit and associated gastric glands in the gastric fundic region.

cretory unit such as that found in other glands. Corresponding roughly to an ovoid mass of liver parenchyma, it incorporates contiguous parts of two adjacent classic lobules (Fig. 13-22). To understand the basic concept of the liver acinus, it is necessary to appreciate which components constitute its axial vasculature. The dual blood supply to hepatic sinusoids is delivered by tiny terminal branches of arterial and portal venous vessels following the portal area distribution (see Fig. 13-20A). These terminal branches are fed by side branches that emerge from the vessels in the portal areas as shown in the middle of Figure 13-22. Each side branch of the hepatic artery is accompanied by a side branch of the portal vein, and the two vessels constitute the vascular backbone and morphological axis of the liver acinus. The peripheral landmarks of the acinus are two neighboring **central veins** (known also as **terminal hepatic venules**) and a **portal area.**

Once the liver is viewed as being made up essentially of acini, it becomes evident that whereas the nearest hepatocytes to the vascular backbone of the acinus border on blood that is rich in nutrients and oxygen, those situated farther away from the axial vessels are to some extent deprived. Also, these more distant cells are exposed to higher concentrations of the liver's metabolic byproducts. The preferential positioning of hepatocytes constitutes the basis for **zonation** within the acinus. Thus, **zone 1** represents a relatively privileged part of the acinus where hepatocytes are able to synthesize glycogen and plasma proteins actively. **Zone 2** is a nondescript intermediate region that receives second-rate blood as far as nutrients and oxygen are concerned. **Zone 3** extends as far as the central veins, now more often referred to as terminal hepatic venules. Its hepatocytes have to depend on blood that is relatively low in nutrients and oxygen (see Fig. 13-22). Zone 3 represents the major site of alcohol and drug detoxification, and its cells are much more susceptible than those of zone 1 to hypoxia and toxic damage by reactive and toxic metabolites. Because zone 3 borders on central veins, histological evidence of cell death is sometimes seen in the vicinity of the central veins.

Hepatic Sinusoids

Hepatocyte surfaces bordering on liver sinusoids are covered with microvilli (see Figs. 13-20B and 13-23). These projections expand the surface area for glucose absorption from the blood. They occupy a **perisinusoidal space (space of Disse)** that lies between hepatocytes and the endothelial lining of their associated sinusoids. Because the endothelial layer excludes blood cells and platelets from the perisinusoidal space, the projecting microvilli are bathed only by plasma, facilitating two-way exchanges across the cell membrane. In addition to plasma, the perisinusoidal space contains

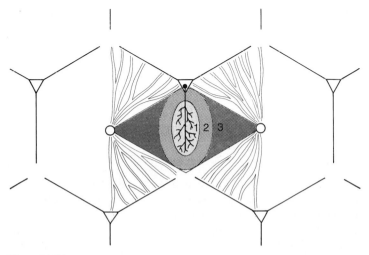

Figure 13-22
Schematic diagram showing the three zones of a liver acinus. Two classic lobules are outlined for orientation. The three possible directions followed by vascular backbones of acini are indicated by the straight lines extending from each triangular portal area.

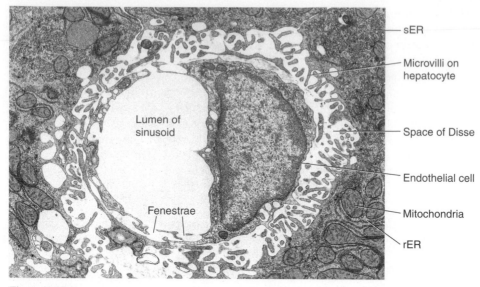

Figure 13-23
Electron micrograph of a hepatic sinusoid (rat liver, ×14,300).

reticular fibers and small amounts of discontinuous, nonobstructing basement membrane. Plasma has free access to this space, entering through large open fenestrae and sieve-like areas furnished with smaller pores that traverse the endothelial cell cytoplasm.

The liver contains a resident permanent population of sinusoid-associated macrophages known as **Kupffer cells** (see Fig. 13-20*A*). Many of these monocyte-derived macrophages are incorporated into the lining of sinusoids; others are stretched across the lumen (Fig. 13-24). These actively phagocytic stellate cells engulf senescent erythrocytes, potentially obstructive debris, and particulate matter. They also capture any bacteria that may arrive in the portal blood. Also present in the perisinusoidal space are **lipocytes (hepatic stellate cells, Ito cells)**, which are fat-storing cells that store vitamin A and provide support. In response to liver damage, these fat-containing perisinusoidal cells can proliferate, become contractile, and produce collagen fibers. They play a major role in the extensive bridging fibrosis with progressive parenchymal disruption that characterizes the potentially fatal liver disease, **cirrhosis** (Gk. *kirrhos*, orange-brown; *ōsis*, condition).

Hepatocytes

Hepatocytes are densely packed with all kinds of organelles and inclusions. Energy-providing mitochondria are particularly abundant (see Fig. 13-23). The extensive rER synthesizes plasma proteins and constituent proteins of lipoproteins. The lipids incorporated into these molecules are synthesized by the cell's profuse sER. The large Golgi complex packages plasma proteins and lipoproteins into secretory vesicles ready for their release into hepatic sinusoids. The extensive sER is the major site of transformation and conjugation reactions that can convert or detoxify potentially damaging endogenous and exogenous compounds, such as ammonia, steroids, alcohol, drugs, and a variety of absorbed toxic chemicals. Prolonged exposure of hepatocytes to some of these compounds can lead to supplementary formation of more sER, providing additional supplies of the necessary sER-associated enzymes. Also metabolized by the sER of hepatocytes is stored glycogen, which is present in these cells as sER-associated particles (see Fig. 3-17). The peroxisomes of hepatocytes assist to a more minor extent in metabolizing alcohol (see Chapter 3 under Peroxisomes).

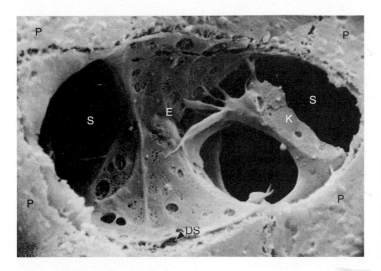

Figure 13-24
Scanning electron micrograph showing a Kupffer cell (K) situated at a bifurcation between sinusoids (S) of the liver ($\times$ 6,000). The space of Disse (DS) between fenestrated sinusoidal endothelial cells and the parenchymal hepatocytes (P) is just discernible.

Bile

The exocrine secretion of hepatocytes, **bile**, contains bilirubin, bile salts, IgA, cholesterol, and steroids. The **bile salts** facilitate fat digestion and absorption. **Bilirubin** is an iron-depleted degradation product of heme produced during the disposal of worn-out erythrocytes by splenic macrophages and Kupffer cells. This pigmented breakdown product passes into the plasma, from which it is absorbed by hepatocytes. Glucuronyl transferases associated with their sER conjugate bilirubin with glucuronic acid and render it water soluble. The conjugated bilirubin then becomes secreted into bile canaliculi as soluble **bilirubin glucuronides**.

CLINICAL IMPLICATIONS: JAUNDICE

If the bilirubin clearance capacity of hepatocytes becomes inadequate, this waste pigment gradually accumulates in the blood (**hyperbilirubinemia**) and also in several body tissues. Enough of it may collect in the skin and sclerae (whites of the eyes) for these to acquire a distinctly yellow color. Known as **jaundice** (Fr. *jaune*, yellow), this condition may reflect excessive destruction of erythrocytes, some incapacity for uptake or processing of bilirubin by hepatocytes, or inadequate drainage of bile due to some obstruction of the duct system. If the jaundice results from only limited numbers of damaged hepatocytes, gradual recovery of normal liver function may be expected as this organ has a remarkable potential for regenerating new hepatocytes.

Bile Ducts

Intrahepatic bile ducts are situated in portal areas. The narrowest ducts, called **bile ductules**, have a low cuboidal lining. They drain by way of small ducts into larger ducts lined with simple columnar epithelium. Emerging from the porta hepatis are the **right** and **left hepatic ducts**, which unite as the **common hepatic duct**. The tall columnar epithelium of these extrahepatic ducts is surrounded by smooth muscle cells and strong connective tissue.

Bile reaches bile ductules by the following route. Anastomosing **bile canaliculi** channel it toward a portal area, near which it drains into short **canals of Hering** that are bordered partly by hepatocytes and partly by duct cells. These small tributaries open directly, as well as indirectly, by way of tiny bypass ducts lined entirely by duct cells (**preductules** or **cholangioles**) into a **bile ductule** in the portal area.

Gallbladder

The gallbladder is a thin-walled, elongated sac that stores and concentrates bile. If undistended, its mucosa is highly folded and has an unusual and distinctive appearance in sections (Fig. 13-25). In

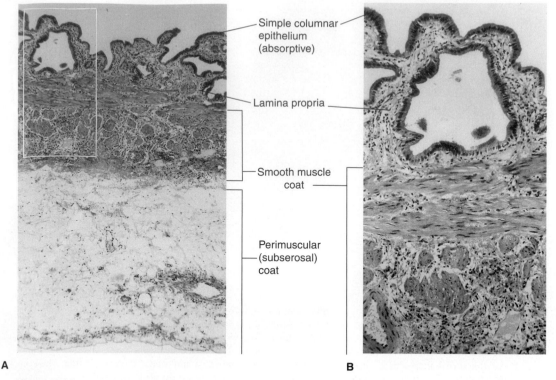

A   B

Figure 13-25
Gallbladder. (*A*) Low power view. (*B*) Same area seen under higher magnification.

contrast to other parts of the digestive tract, most regions of the mucosa lack mucosal glands. The tall columnar absorptive cells that constitute the epithelial lining (see Fig. 13-25*B*) possess apical microvilli. Below the **lamina propria** that supports the folded surface epithelium lies a skimpy **muscle coat** made up of circular, longitudinal, and oblique smooth muscle (see Fig. 13-25*A*). The muscular coat is equivalent in position to the **muscularis externa**; the muscularis mucosae is not represented. The outermost layer, known as the **perimuscular (subserosal) coat**, consists of loose connective tissue. A mucosal **spiral fold** extends from the cystic duct into the neck of the gallbladder. Its role seems to be that of keeping the lumen open and facilitating the passage of bile in either direction.

The **cystic duct** (leading from the gallbladder) and the **common hepatic duct** (leading from the liver) unite as the **bile duct**, the outlet of which is guarded by the **choledochal sphincter**. In the duodenal wall, the **bile duct** generally unites with the **main pancreatic duct**, forming a mutual lumen that opens into the duodenum at the **major duodenal papilla**. By remaining closed between meals, the choledochal sphincter stops bile from passing continuously into the duodenum. Closure of the sphincter causes bile to back up through the cystic duct and collect in the gallbladder, where a substantial proportion of its water is resorbed while it is being stored. Gallbladder contraction and emptying after meals are induced by CCK, a hormone that is released by enteroendocrine cells when significant concentrations of free fatty acids, peptides, or amino acids enter the small intestine. Fatty foods are known to be particularly effective in triggering gallbladder emptying.

Summary

The main features of the digestive system are shown in summary form in Table 13-3.

TABLE 13-3

DIGESTIVE SYSTEM: SUMMARY OF FEATURES OF MAJOR COMPONENTS

Part	Main Functions	Distinctive Features	General Features
Esophagus	Conveys food rapidly to the stomach	Stratified squamous nonkeratinizing epithelium; muscularis externa with skeletal muscle in top third, smooth muscle in bottom third, and mixture in middle third	
Stomach	Retains food and thoroughly mixes it with gastric juice	Simple columnar mucus-secreting epithelium (mucous columnar cells, all alike) with gastric pits and glands; no villi or goblet cells	Rugae; muscularis externa has 3 layers
Gastric fundus (body)	Adds hydrochloric acid and enzymes that initiate digestion; begins absorption	Pits are shallow, glands long and fairly straight; several cell types in glands (parietal, chief or zymogenic, mucous, enteroendocrine, and immature); main enzyme- and acid-producing region	Produces acid, enzymes, gastrointestinal hormones, and mucus
Gastric pylorus and antrum	Pyloric sphincter regulates emptying of the stomach	Pits are deep, glands shorter and more branched; mostly mucous cells in glands; pyloric sphincter	Produces mucus and gastrointestinal hormones
Small intestine	Adds enzymes that continue digestion, e.g., brush border enzymes; absorbs nutrients; produces gastrointestinal hormones	Villi; Paneth, crypt base columnar, goblet, absorptive, and enteroendocrine cells in crypts	Plicae, villi, and microvilli; absorptive cells and goblet cells; produces mucus; crypts also produce enzymes and hormones; lymphoid follicles; renewal from crypt base columnar cells
Duodenum		Mucus-secreting submucosal (Brunner's) glands; high broad villi	
Jejunum		Lacks large submucosal glands and lacks large confluent lymphoid follicles	
Ileum		Large confluent lymphoid follicles (Peyer's patches); low narrower villi	
Large intestine		Villi are absent; crypts generally lack Paneth cells; goblet cells abundant	Absorptive columnar cells and goblet cells; crypts longer
Colon	Retrieves water and sodium; produces gastrointestinal hormones but not enzymes; completes digestion and absorption	Teniae coil	

(continued)

TABLE 13-3

DIGESTIVE SYSTEM: SUMMARY OF FEATURES OF MAJOR COMPONENTS *(CONTINUED)*			
Part	Main Functions	Distinctive Features	General Features
Appendix	Promotes immune responses, particularly IgA-mediated responses, to ingested antigens	Prominent aggregates of lymphoid follicles; small lumen	
Accessory Structures			
Tongue	Facilitates eating, tasting, and swallowing	Lingual papillae and taste buds on palatine portion; lingual tonsil on pharyngeal portion	Skeletal muscle fibers with multiple orientation
Teeth	Prepare food for tasting, swallowing, and digestion	Hard dentin covered by even harder enamel; central pulp cavity; cementum; periodontal ligament	20 primary and 32 secondary teeth; 3 mineralized tissues; enamel not regenerated
Tonsils	Promote immune responses, particularly IgA-mediated responses, to ingested antigens	Large aggregates of lymphoid follicles; all except pharyngeal tonsil are covered by stratified squamous nonkeratinizing epithelium; underlying mucous glands and clear crypts (lingual) or accumulated debris in crypts (palatine)	Lingual (multiple), palatine (paired), and pharyngeal (single)
Salivary glands	Secrete saliva	Parotid is serous, submandibular mostly serous, and sublingual mostly mucous; intralobular ducts prominent; centro-acinar cells are absent	Compound exocrine glands; paired
Pancreas		Loose connective tissue sheath and septa are very thin	Compound exocrine and endocrine gland; single
Exocrine	Produces alkaline pancreatic juice containing a wide range of digestive enzymes	Brightly staining acinar cells; intralobular ducts are few and inconspicuous; centro-acinar cells are present	
Endocrine	Produces hormones; insulin and glucagon regulate carbohydrate metabolism	Pale-staining islets; no ducts	
Liver	Converts glucose into stored glycogen; secretes plasma proteins, lipoproteins, bilirubin, bile salts, and IgA; metabolizes alcohol, drugs, and toxins	Portal areas and central veins (terminal hepatic venules); indistinct lobular organization; acinar parenchymal organization; hepatocytes with bile canaliculi; Kupffer cells	Portal and systemic circulations; sinusoids; perisinusoidal space (= space of Disse) for hepatocyte-plasma exchanges; gallbladder for bile storage and concentration

Bibliography

Teeth

Eisenmann DR. Enamel structure. In: Ten Cate AR. Oral Histology: Development, Structure, and Function, ed 3. St. Louis, CV Mosby, 1989.

Pashley DH. Dentin, a dynamic substrate: a review. Scanning Microsc 3:161, 1989.

Sigal MJ, Aubin JE, Ten Cate AR, Pitaru S. The odontoblast process extends to the dentinoenamel junction: an immunocytochemical study of rat dentine. J Histochem Cytochem 32:872, 1984.

Ten Cate AR. Oral Histology: Development, Structure, and Function, ed 3. St. Louis, CV Mosby, 1989.

Oral Cavity, Pharynx, and Esophagus

Beidler LN, Smallman RLS. Renewal of cells within taste buds. J Cell Biol 27:263, 1965.

Brandtzaeg P. Immune functions of human nasal mucosa and tonsils in health and disease. In: Bienenstock J, ed. Immunology of the Lung and Upper Respiratory Tract. New York, McGraw-Hill, 1984, p 28.

Dale AC. Salivary glands. In: Ten Cate AR. Oral Histology: Development, Structure, and Function, ed 3. St. Louis, CV Mosby, 1989.

Murray RG. The ultrastructure of taste buds. In Friedmann J, ed. The Ultrastructure of Sensory Organs. Amsterdam, North Holland Publishing, 1973, p 1.

Riva A, Lantini MS, Testa Riva F. Normal human salivary glands. In: Riva A, Motta PM, eds. Ultrastructure of the Extraparietal Glands of the Digestive Tract. Boston, Kluwer Academic Publishers, 1990, p 53.

Riva A, Tandler B, Testa Riva F. Ultrastructural observations on human sublingual gland. Am J Anat 181:385, 1988.

Young JA, Van Lennep DW. The Morphology of Salivary Glands. New York, Academic Press, 1978.

Stomach and Intestine

Abbas B, Hayes TL, Wilson DJ, Carr KE. Internal structure of the intestinal villus: morphological and morphometric observations at different levels of the mouse villus. J Anat 162:263, 1989.

Cheng H, Leblond CP. Origin, differentiation and renewal of the four main epithelial cell types in the mouse small intestine: I. Columnar cells. Am J Anat 141:461, 1974.

Delvalle J, Yamada T. The gut as an endocrine organ. Annu Rev Med 41:447, 1990.

Doe WF. The intestinal immune system. Gut 30:1679, 1989.

Ferguson A. Mucosal immunology. Immunol Today 11:1, 1990.

Ito S, Lacy ER. Morphology of gastric mucosal damage, defenses and restitution in the presence of luminal ethanol. Gastroenterology 88:250, 1985.

Jarry A, Robaszkiewicz M, Brousse N, Potet F. Immune cells associated with M cells in the follicle-associated epithelium of Peyer's patches in the rat. An electron- and immuno-electron-microscopic study. Cell Tissue Res 255:293, 1989.

Komuro T, Hashimoto Y. Three-dimensional structure of the rat intestinal wall (mucosa and submucosa). Arch Histol Cytol 53:1, 1990.

Lee ER, Trasler J, Dwivedi S, Leblond CP. Division of the mouse gastric mucosa into zymogenic and mucous regions on the basis of gland features. Am J Anat 164:187, 1982.

Magney JE, Erlandsen SL, Bjerknes ML, Cheng H. Scanning electron microscopy of isolated epithelium of the murine gastrointestinal tract: Morphology of the basal surface and evidence for paracrinelike cells. Am J Anat 177:43, 1986.

Ouellette AJ, Selsted ME. Paneth cell defensins: endogenous peptide components of intestinal host defence. FASEB J 10:1280, 1996.

Owen D. Normal histology of the stomach. Am J Surg Pathol 10:48, 1986.

Silen W, Ito S. Mechanisms for rapid epithelialization of the gastric mucosal surface. Annu Rev Physiol 47:217, 1985.

Takagi T, Takebayashi S, Tokuyasu K, Tsuji K. Scanning electron microscopy on the human gastric mucosa: fetal, normal, and various pathological conditions. Acta Pathol Jpn 24:233, 1974.

Wolfe MM, Soll AH. The physiology of gastric acid secretion. N Engl J Med 319:1707, 1988.

Exocrine Pancreas and Liver

Erlinger S. Bile secretion. Br Med Bull 48:860, 1992.

Frizzell RA, Heintze K. Transport functions of the gallbladder. In: Javitt NB, ed. International Review of Physiology: Liver and Biliary Tract Physiology I, vol 21. Baltimore, University Park Press, 1980, p 221.

Gumucio JJ. Hepatocyte heterogeneity: the coming of age from the description of a biological curiosity to a partial understanding of its physiological meaning and regulation. Hepatology 9:154, 1989.

Hall JG, Andrew E. Biliglobulin: a new look at IgA. Immunol Today 1(5):100, 1980.

Horn T, Junge J, Nielsen O, Christoffersen P. Light microscopical demonstration and zonal distribution of parasinusoidal cells (Ito cells) in normal human liver. Virchows Arch [A] 413:147, 1988.

Howat HT, Sarles H, eds. The Exocrine Pancreas. Philadelphia, WB Saunders, 1979.

Jones AL, Schmucker DL. Current concepts of liver structure as related to function. Gastroenterology 73:833, 1977.

Kardon R, Kessel RG. Three-dimensional organization of the hepatic microcirculation in the rodent as observed by scanning electron microscopy of corrosion casts. Gastroenterology 97: 72, 1980.

McCuskey RS, McCuskey PA. Fine structure and function of Kupffer cells. J Electron Microsc Tech 14:237, 1990.

Miyai K. Structure-function relationship of the liver in health and disease. In: Gitnick G, Hollander D, Kaplowitz N, Samloff IM, Schoenfield LJ, eds. Principles and Practice of Gastroenterology and Hepatology. New York, Elsevier, 1988, p 1051.

Motta PM. Three-dimensional architecture of the mammalian liver. A scanning electron microscopic review. In: Allen DJ, Motta PM, DiDio JA, eds. Three Dimensional Microanatomy of Cells and Tissue Surfaces. New York, Elsevier/North Holland Biomedical Press, 1981.

Motta P, Muto M, Fujita T. The Liver. An Atlas of Scanning Electron Microscopy. Tokyo, Igaku-Shoin, 1978.

Rappaport AM. Physioanatomical basis of toxic liver injury. In: Farber E, Fisher MM, eds. Toxic Injury of the Liver, pt A. New York, Marcel Dekker, 1979, p 1.

Rappaport AM, Macphee PJ, Fisher MM, Phillips MJ. The scarring of the liver acini (cirrhosis): tridimensional and microcirculatory considerations. Virchows Arch [A] 402:107, 1983.

Reichen J, Paumgartner G. Excretory function of the liver. In: Javitt NB, ed. International Review of Physiology: Liver and Biliary Tract Physiology I, vol 21. Baltimore, University Park Press, 1980, p 103.

Sarles H. The exocrine pancreas. Int Rev Physiol 12:173, 1977.

Schmid R. Bilirubin metabolism in man. N Engl J Med 287:703, 1972.

Tanikawa K. Ultrastructural Aspects of the Liver and Its Disorders, ed 2. Tokyo, Igaku-Shoin, 1979.

Wake K, Decker K, Kirn A, et al. Cell biology and kinetics of Kupffer cells in the liver. Int Rev Cytol 118:173, 1989.

CHAPTER 14

Respiratory System

OBJECTIVES

On completing this chapter, you should be able to the following:

- List and describe in some detail the succession of airways and air conducting passages
- Recognize bronchi and bronchioles in lung sections and explain why their microscopic structure is not identical
- Outline the importance of elastin in the respiratory system
- Draw a labeled diagram showing the histological organization of an interalveolar wall and the alveolar–capillary barrier
- Explain the functional significance of secretory epithelial cells of interalveolar walls
- Outline two mechanisms that keep the lungs free of obstructing particulate matter

The main parts of the respiratory system are the lungs, which provide an expansive interface for gas exchange between air and blood, and a branching system of airways for conducting air to and from the lungs as a result of respiratory movements of the thoracic walls and diaphragm. Acting in conjunction with the cardiovascular system, it supplies the necessary oxygen for oxidative metabolism and discards the metabolic byproduct, carbon dioxide. Blood returning from the systemic circulation to the right heart is rich in carbon dioxide but depleted of oxygen. Gaseous exchange in the lungs replenishes the oxygen and dissipates the carbon dioxide. Blood pumped through the systemic circulation by the left side of the heart has thus become reoxygenated (see Fig. 11-1). Components of the respiratory system that we describe in this chapter are listed in Table 14-1.

The **lungs** develop in gland-like manner from foregut endoderm. They lie protected by the **thoracic cage**, an expandable cage-like structure having the ribs, costal cartilages, and sternum as its walls and the diaphragm as its floor (Fig. 14-1). Each lung is invaginated into its own **pleural cavity**, which is accordingly reduced to a narrow potential space (Fig. 14-1). This cavity is lined with simple squamous serosal mesothelium, which together with a subserosal layer of dense fibroelastic connective tissue constitutes a lining layer known as the **pleura**. At the **hilum** of the lung, the site at which major blood vessels, air passages, lymphatics, and nerves enter or emerge, the **parietal pleura** lining the walls of the pleural cavity is continuous with the **visceral pleura** investing the lung. Friction between these apposed serosal membranes during respiratory movements is

TABLE 14-1

RESPIRATORY SYSTEM: PRINCIPAL COMPONENTS

Conducting Portion

Nasal cavities
   Nasal conchae
   Olfactory areas

Nasopharynx
   Pharyngeal tonsil

Larynx
   Epiglottis

Trachea

Bronchi
   Extrapulmonary (primary)
   Intrapulmonary (secondary and tertiary)

Bronchioles

Respiratory Portion

Respiratory bronchioles

Alveolar ducts

Alveolar sacs

Alveoli

External Pulmonary Investing Layer

Visceral pleura

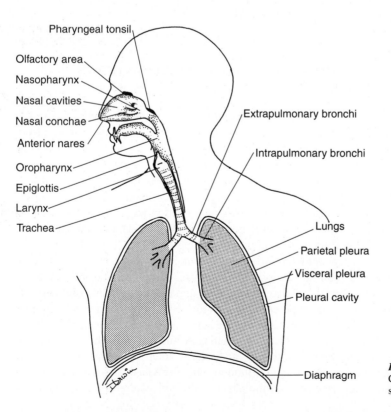

Figure 14-1
Conducting portion of the respiratory system.

counteracted by a thin film of tissue fluid in the pleural cavity. During **inspiration**, contraction of the diaphragm and outward movement of the ribs expand the thoracic cage, drawing air into the lungs. This action increases elastic tension in the visceral pleura, stretches the entire tracheo-bronchial tree, and expands the finer components of lung tissue, all containing abundant elastin. *Passive recoil* of stretched elastin is the chief factor that expels air when the thoracic cage assumes its former dimensions on **expiration**.

The parts of the respiratory system responsible for supplying the lungs with air are collectively referred to as its **conducting portion**, as distinct from the **respiratory portion** responsible for gas exchange.

CONDUCTING PORTION

The main conducting airways in the upper part of the respiratory tract have walls that are reinforced with bone or cartilage to keep them open, and their mucosal lining is adapted for cleaning and conditioning air on its way to the lungs. The incoming air passes through a succession of cavities and passageways, namely the **nasal cavities, nasopharynx, larynx**, and **trachea**, and next enters several generations of progressively smaller **bronchi**, followed by a larger number of different orders of **bronchioles**. It then reaches the **alveolar ducts, alveolar sacs**, and **alveoli**, the sites where gas exchange occurs. We begin by considering the airways that constitute the conducting portion of the system.

Nasal Cavities and Olfactory Areas

The bilateral **nasal cavities** open anteriorly at the nostrils (**anterior nares**) and posteriorly into the **nasopharynx** at the **choanae**. Their roof, floor, and walls are strong because they are supported by bone and cartilage. Epidermis bearing coarse filtering hairs lines the anterior region of each cavity. Posterior to a transitional zone lined by stratified squamous nonkeratinizing epithelium, the lining membrane becomes pseudostratified ciliated columnar epithelium with goblet cells. The nasal mucus picks up coarse dust particles and is carried posteriorly to the oropharynx by ciliary action. The underlying lamina propria, supplied with serous and mucous glands that also contribute mucus, is firmly bound to periosteum of nasal bones or perichondrium of nasal cartilages. It is profusely vascular and serves to warm (or cool) the incoming air.

Three curved shelves, supported by cancellous bone and covered by nasal mucous membrane, project medially from the lateral wall of each nasal cavity. Because of their shell-like appearance, they are known as the **superior, middle**, and **inferior conchae** (L. *concha*, shell) or **turbinates**. The lamina propria of the middle and inferior conchae is particularly vascular, possessing many thin-walled veins. Under certain conditions these vessels, which most of the time are almost collapsed, become congested with blood. The two lower pairs of conchae may thus become sufficiently swollen to impede free passage of air, which explains why persons may experience a stuffed-up nose in an overheated environment or as a result of infections such as the common cold.

Each nasal cavity has in its roof an **olfactory area** representing half of the **olfactory organ**, one of the so-called organs of special sense. These distinctive sensory areas of the nasal mucosa extend laterally over the superior conchae and medially along the superior border of the nasal septum. Their extra-thick pseudostratified epithelium is made up of **olfactory receptor cells**, supporting (**sustentacular**) cells, and **basal cells**, but lacks goblet cells. In this case, the **receptor cells** are modified **bipolar neurons** with a dendrite reaching the free surface of the olfactory area and an axon that extends into the lamina propria (Fig. 14-2). The bulbous tip of the dendrite bears long **olfactory cilia** that are almost immotile. Lying flat along the exposed surface, above the microvilli on the sustentacular cells, these entangled long cilia are bathed in the serous secretion of associated glands

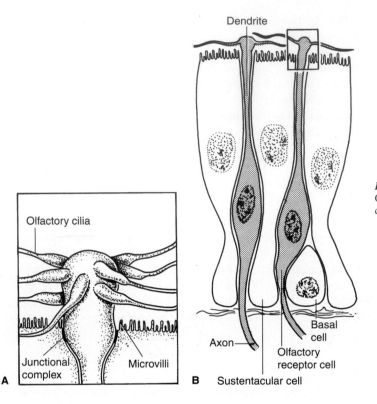

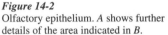

Figure 14-2
Olfactory epithelium. *A* shows further
details of the area indicated in *B*.

situated in the lamina propria of the olfactory areas. The unmyelinated axon of each receptor cell extends into the lamina propria and, along with others, traverses the cribriform plate of the ethmoid bone. Olfactory nerve fibers then enter the **olfactory bulbs,** which represent anterior extensions of the olfactory cortex.

The tall **sustentacular cells** of the olfactory areas have many microvilli on their free surface and contain a pigment similar to lipofuscin that imparts a characteristic yellowish color to the olfactory areas. Also bordering on the basement membrane of the epithelium are scattered unspecialized **basal cells**.

Evidence suggests that the basal cells are incompletely differentiated and have the potential to produce new olfactory receptor cells. Such a capacity for renewal is warranted in view of the vulnerable situation occupied by these neurons at a body surface so susceptible to infection. However, this represents an exception to the general rule that damaged neurons are not routinely replaced in postnatal life.

When dissolved in the serous secretion that bathes the olfactory cilia, odoriferous substances directly stimulate the chemoreceptive olfactory receptor cells. The manner in which odors are perceived, however, remains unclear. Individual olfactory receptors can respond to many different odors, so odor discrimination may depend on recognition of spatial patterns of stimulated receptor cells.

Nasopharynx

Most of the **nasopharynx** is lined by pseudostratified ciliated columnar epithelium with goblet cells. The **pharyngeal tonsil,** an unpaired median mass of unencapsulated lymphoid tissue, lies in the lamina propria of the roof and posterior wall of this part of the pharynx (see Fig. 14-1). Its histological organization is similar to that of the palatine and lingual tonsils except that 1) it is more diffuse, and 2) it is covered, at least in part, by pseudostratified epithelium instead of stratified squamous onkeratinizing epithelium. Also, the covering epithelium extends into the lamina propria as folds rather than crypts. If the pharyngeal tonsil becomes overly enlarged owing to persistent infection, a condition known as **adenoidal lymphoid hyperplasia** or **adenoids**, the swelling may impede or obstruct free passage of air through the nasopharynx and become a cause of chronic mouth-breathing.

Larynx and Epiglottis

Situated between the laryngeal pharynx and the trachea is the **larynx**, the body's complex sound-producing organ (Fig. 14-3). The strong supporting framework of the laryngeal walls is made up of several cartilages interconnected by ligaments and voluntary muscles. Key functions of the larynx are 1) to stop inhaled objects, liquids, or food from entering the trachea, 2) to produce vocal sounds (**phonation**) through the voluntary regulation of airflow, and 3) to counteract obstruction or irritation through **coughing**. Bilateral **vestibular folds** of mucous membrane project medially into the lumen. Below these upper protective folds lie paired **vocal folds**, responsible for phonation. The cores of the vocal folds contain bundles of elastic fibers (**vocal ligaments**) and also skeletal muscle fibers. The tension and length of the vocal ligaments, and the clearance gap between them, determine the kinds of sounds that are uttered. The vocal cords are covered by protective stratified squamous nonkeratinizing epithelium, whereas most of the remainder of the larynx is lined by pseudostratified ciliated columnar epithelium with goblet cells and has mucous and serous glands in its lamina propria. Laryngeal cilia beat toward the pharynx.

The **epiglottis** is an upward flap-like extension of the anterior wall of the larynx. It is supported by a plate of **elastic cartilage** (Fig. 14-4), the fibrous perichondrium of which is bound to the lamina propria of the mucosal covering on its two surfaces. The anterior surface and the upper part of the posterior surface, both subject to minor abrasion during swallowing, are covered with stratified squamous nonkeratinizing epithelium. The lower, more protected part of the posterior surface has a pseudostratified ciliated columnar epithelium with goblet cells and associated underlying mucous glands containing some serous acini.

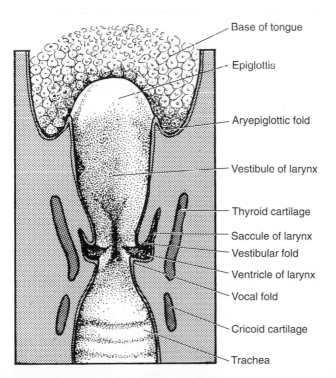

Base of tongue

Epiglottis

Aryepiglottic fold

Vestibule of larynx

Thyroid cartilage

Saccule of larynx

Vestibular fold

Ventricle of larynx

Vocal fold

Cricoid cartilage

Trachea

Figure 14-3
Schematic diagram of the anterior half of the larynx (posterior view without tracheal cartilages; coronal section).

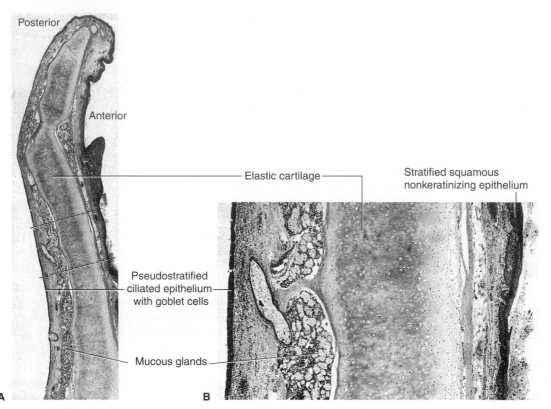

Figure 14-4
(*A*) Epiglottis (low power). (*B*) The area between the dotted lines seen under higher magnification.

Trachea

The **trachea** is a relatively wide, flexible air tube that extends from the larynx into the thorax, where it bifurcates into two extrapulmonary (primary) bronchi (see Fig. 14-1). Its lumen is kept open by a series of up to 20 **tracheal cartilages**. Basically horseshoe-shaped, the tracheal cartilages are strong rings of hyaline cartilage that remain incomplete posteriorly where the trachea lies against the esophagus (Plate 14-1). Some of the cartilages are partially subdivided into superior and inferior halves. The gap between the posterior ends of each incomplete ring is bridged by interlacing bundles of smooth muscle (shown in Fig. 14-6*A* and termed the **trachealis** muscle), together with fibroelastic connective tissue. The more flexible regions between the tracheal cartilages are supported by dense fibroelastic connective tissue continuous with the perichondrium, a strong arrangement that permits extension of the trachea if the head is tilted back as well as during respiratory elongation of the tracheobronchial tree.

The epithelium that lines the trachea and bronchi (**tracheobronchial epithelium**) is pseudostratified ciliated columnar epithelium with goblet cells, also known as **respiratory epithelium**. Hormone-producing **neuroendocrine cells (Kulchitsky cells)** that belong to the same large family as those present in the digestive tract are scattered throughout this epithelium. Some of the products that they release are calcitonin, somatostatin, serotonin, and a gastrin-releasing peptide called bombesin. Ciliary activity of surface cells transports a continuous blanket of sticky mucus up the trachea to the pharynx (Fig. 14-5). Any particles large enough to settle out of the inhaled air become trapped on this creeping coat of mucus, which represents a major protective device for keeping the

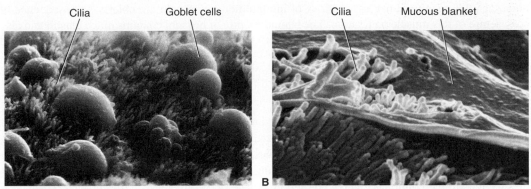

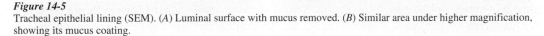

Figure 14-5
Tracheal epithelial lining (SEM). (*A*) Luminal surface with mucus removed. (*B*) Similar area under higher magnification, showing its mucus coating.

lungs clear of extraneous particulate matter and infecting bacteria. The lamina propria of the trachea contains abundant elastin that plays a major role in elastic recoil of this passageway, such as during expiration. This underlying connective tissue also contains scattered solitary lymphoid follicles. Much of the tracheal mucus comes from mucoserous (mixed) submucosal glands.

Bronchi

Each **main (primary) bronchus** extends from the lower end of the trachea to the hilum of a lung. Here, it is associated with the major blood vessels and lymphatics of the lung and invested with dense ordinary connective tissue. Extrapulmonary bronchi perform the same functions as the trachea and closely resemble them in histological structure.

The wall structure of the **intrapulmonary bronchi** also basically corresponds to that of the trachea. The supporting cartilage plates, however, are more irregular and do not all fully encircle the circumference of the lumen. In sections, they generally appear as separate *islands* of hyaline cartilage (Plate 14-2). Dense fibroelastic connective tissue, continuous with the perichondrium, supports the flexible regions between them. Crisscrossing bundles of smooth muscle are arranged helically around the lumen, between the mucosa and the cartilage plates (Fig. 14-6*B*). The longitudinal

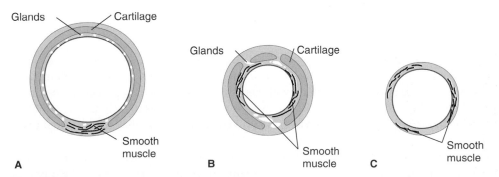

Figure 14-6
Comparative wall structure of (*A*) the trachea, (*B*) a bronchus, and (*C*) a bronchiole, showing their respective content and the position of hyaline cartilage, mucoserous glands, and smooth muscle.

mucosal folds seen in transverse sections of intrapulmonary bronchi are chiefly a consequence of contracture of this muscle on fixation. The lamina propria of bronchi contains much elastin and also solitary lymphoid follicles. Bronchi are lined with the respiratory epithelium described above and have mucoserous submucosal glands.

Bronchioles

With continuing dichotomous branching, the conducting passages become reduced to a diameter of 1 mm or less and acquire a simpler wall structure. Certain features are helpful in distinguishing these small airways, which are termed **bronchioles**, from bronchi. First, they are lined by a *simple epithelium* instead of a pseudostratified epithelium, without associated glands. The larger bronchioles have a simple columnar ciliated epithelium (Plate 14-3), whereas smaller bronchioles have a simple cuboidal epithelium without cilia. Serous secretory cells called **Clara cells** are present in the lining epithelium. More numerous in the smaller bronchioles, these cells are believed to be protective. They secrete glycoproteins, and the cytochrome P-450 complement of their sER has considerable potential for detoxifying noxious inhaled particulate matter. Goblet cells disappear from the lining epithelium just above the level where ciliated cells begin to give way to nonciliated cells. Small bronchioles are either incompletely ciliated or else lack cilia, and they have no goblet cells. Another distinguishing feature of bronchioles is that generally they *lack glands* in their walls. A third difference is that bronchioles also *lack cartilages*. Because they are soft-walled and surrounded on all sides by a respiratory spongework that becomes stretched during inspiration, bronchioles are pulled open by expansion of the tissue attached to their perimeter. External to the thin elastic lamina propria of bronchioles lies a helical crisscrossing arrangement of **smooth muscle** bundles (see Fig. 14-6C). The tonus in the smooth muscle cells regulates the luminal diameter of these narrow passageways.

CLINICAL IMPLICATIONS

Asthma

The absence of cartilages from the walls of bronchioles poses a potential hazard since it allows these air passages to constrict to the point of almost closing down when the tonus in their smooth muscle cells becomes excessive. Bronchoconstriction can become acute in **asthma**, a respiratory condition generally of allergic origin that is commonly exacerbated by nonspecific lung irritants. Patients with asthma often experience more difficulty with expiration than with inspiration. This is because bronchioles drawn open during inspiration are also required to remain open during expiration to permit the rapid outflow of air caused by elastic recoil of lung tissues. Thus, in an asthmatic attack, more wheezing noises and breathing difficulty may be associated with air expulsion than with inhalation.

Two orders or so of distal conducting passages called **terminal bronchioles** have a moderate content of smooth muscle cells in their walls. Their lining layer ranges from simple columnar ciliated epithelium to simple cuboidal epithelium with nonciliated as well as ciliated cells, but without goblet cells. The slightly larger bronchioles bringing air to lung **lobules**, which are the structural units discernible through the visceral pleura as small polygonal areas, are called **preterminal bronchioles**.

The final three orders or so of bronchioles have a scattering of thin-walled air pouches (alveoli) extending from their walls. Known as **respiratory bronchioles**, they are the sites where gas exchange begins, so they represent the beginning of the **respiratory portion** of the lung. Each first-order respiratory bronchiole supplies air to a small unit of lung structure called a lung **acinus**.

RESPIRATORY PORTION

The individual components in the respiratory portion of the lung are harder to discern than conducting passages. This is partly because the lungs, stretched in the living state, collapse when the pleural cavities are opened for lung removal. Furthermore, in contrast to the conducting passages described above, not even major components of the respiratory portion such as alveolar ducts have much of a wall structure. So instead of dealing with air tubes that have walls of their own, we are now considering *air spaces* of particular shapes and sizes, with walls that are *shared* with other air spaces. The three orders of air spaces described below are present in the sponge-like arrangement of pulmonary capillaries, supporting fibers, and flimsy intervening walls. The gas mixture inside them, renewed 12 to 15 times per minute at rest, lies as close as 0.2 μm to blood streaming through pulmonary capillaries. Because gases readily diffuse over this distance, a highly efficient arrangement exists for oxygen uptake and dissipation of carbon dioxide.

Alveolar Ducts and Sacs

Distally in the bronchial tree, respiratory bronchioles (the only kind with alveoli in their walls) open into two to nine orders of less discernible tubular passages known as **alveolar ducts** (Fig. 14-7). Alveolar ducts may be thought of as long corridors flanked by many rooms. So many rooms flank the corridor, however, that its walls are difficult to recognize. They are generally represented only by small, isolated clusters of nonciliated cuboidal epithelium, associated with minimal amounts of loose connective tissue and occasional smooth muscle cells. Instead of bordering directly on the corridor, many rooms are arranged as small groups opening into the same lobby, so that access to them is gained by passing through the lobby. The rooms represent **alveoli**, and the lobby around which they are grouped represents a composite air space called an **alveolar sac** (several of which, marked with asterisks, are discernible in Fig. 14-6*B*).

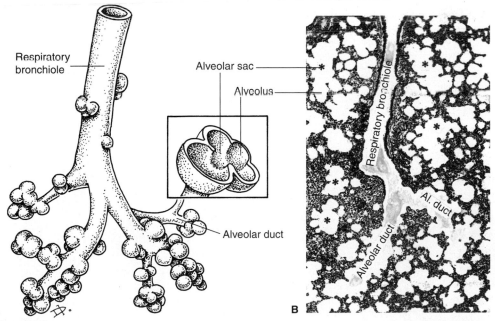

Figure 14-7
Schematic diagram (*A*) and low power view (*B*) of a respiratory bronchiole leading to alveolar ducts (child's lung). Asterisks in *B* indicate alveolar sacs.

Alveoli

The basic structural and functional gas exchange unit is the pulmonary **alveolus**. Since this term denotes an *air space* (L. *alveolus*, small hollow space), the flimsy partitions between alveoli are strictly regarded as **interalveolar walls (septa)**. An alveolus may open into an alveolar sac, alveolar duct, or respiratory bronchiole. Its interior may also communicate directly with that of a neighboring alveolus by way of a perforation through the intervening partition known as an **alveolar pore** (Fig. 14-8). The alveolar pores provide parallel alternative routes for passage of air under conditions of significant resistance to airflow.

New alveoli continue to develop in infancy. When children reach the age of about 8 years, the total adult complement of approximately 300 million alveoli is attained, representing roughly an 8-fold increase over the number that was present at birth.

The delicate **interalveolar walls** are supplied with abundant **capillaries** but *lack* lymphatics. They are supported by **elastic fibers** and a network of **reticular fibers**, as well as by **basement membranes** (Figs. 14-9 and 14-10). The covering epithelium on the free surface of their walls is composed chiefly of extremely flat squamous epithelial cells called **type I pneumocytes** (see Figs. 14-10 and 14-11), interconnected by continuous tight junctions. The short diffusion path over which gas exchange occurs between alveolar air and capillary blood is made up of the attenuated cytoplasm and underlying base-

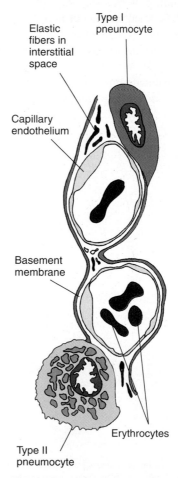

Figure 14-9
Structural basis of the interalveolar wall.

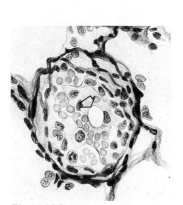

Figure 14-8
Alveolar pore (*arrow*) seen in a thick section of lung.

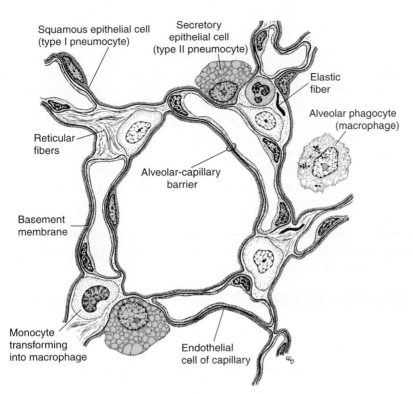

Figure 14-10
Key histological components of the interalveolar wall.

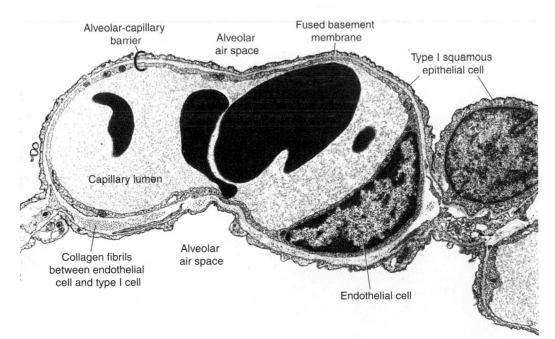

Figure 14-11
Electron micrograph showing an interalveolar capillary, a type I pneumocyte, and other components of the interalveolar wall. The three layers of the alveolar–capillary barrier are discernible. A narrow interstitial space with collagen fibrils may be seen along the lower margin of the capillary.

ment membrane of these type I cells, along with the thin layer of cytoplasm and surrounding basement membrane of capillary **endothelial cells** (see Fig. 14-10). At sites where these two basement membranes lie in intimate apposition they fuse, hence most of the **alveolar–capillary barrier** appears to have three layers rather than four. The total thickness of this barrier varies from 0.2 to 2.5 μm.

Scattered between the type I pneumocytes are rounded secretory epithelial cells called **type II pneumocytes** (see Fig. 14-9). These cells also belong to the covering epithelium of the interalveolar walls and are joined to the other constituent cells by continuous tight junctions (Fig. 14-12). Type II pneumocytes may be distinguished from type I pneumocytes by their more rounded shape, relatively large nucleus, and foamy-looking cytoplasm (see Fig. 14-10). Their somewhat vacuolated appearance is due to their content of highly distinctive granules containing an electron-dense lamellar material rich in phospholipids. These membrane-bounded granules are known as **lamellar bodies** because of their characteristic layered appearance in electron micrographs (see Fig. 14-12). Although conventionally regarded as secretory granules, lamellar bodies may be more complex in origin. When their phospholipid secretory product is released, it spreads over the thin film of tissue fluid that covers the exposed surface of interalveolar walls. Its role is to reduce surface tension forces at the air–water interface and thus to facilitate expansion of alveoli.

CLINICAL IMPLICATIONS

Pulmonary Surfactant

Lung alveoli have an inherently unstable configuration, behaving as incomplete bubbles with a marked tendency to collapse during expiration as a result of surface tension forces. However, this tendency is minimized by the presence of a surface layer of the phospholipid secretory product of type II pneumocytes, the molecular structure of which gives it detergent-like surfactant activity. Pulmonary surfactant decreases alveolar surface tension forces to minimal levels. Its presence in alveoli is essential for newborns, whose lungs were filled with fluid (primarily amniotic fluid) during gestation, to obtain their first breath of air. Immaturity of type II cells at the time of delivery, a common complication if birth is premature and one that can affect full-term infants as well, can result in a critical deficiency of pulmonary surfactant at birth. This deficit may be severe enough to cause potentially fatal respiratory difficulty in the newborn (**respiratory distress syndrome**).

Pulmonary surfactant is a complex mixture containing phospholipids (chiefly **dipalmitoyl phosphatidylcholine**), proteins, and carbohydrates. The phospholipids become part of a lipoprotein complex.

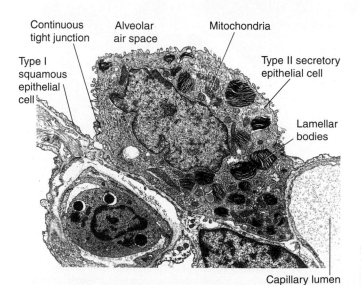

Figure 14-12
Electron micrograph showing a type II pneumocyte in an interalveolar wall (dog lung).

TABLE 14-2

SUMMARIZED MAJOR FEATURES OF THE RESPIRATORY SYSTEM

Part	Main Functions	Distinctive Features	General Features
Nasal cavities and nasal conchae	Filter, humidify, and warm or cool inhaled air	Bone or cartilage support in walls; mucosal glands	Nasal cavities lined mostly by pseudostratified ciliated columnar epithelium with goblet cells (= respiratory epithelium)
Olfactory areas	Chemoreceptors responsive to smells	Olfactory receptor cells (bipolar neurons with modified cilia); pigmented sustentacular cells; receptor cell replacement from basal cells; associated serous mucosal glands	Closely associated with olfactory bulbs of the brain
Pharyngeal tonsil	Site of immune responses to inhaled antigens	Diffuse lymphoid follicles covered by pseudostratified epithelium; causes adenoids if it enlarges	A component of the tonsillar ring in the nasopharynx and oropharynx
Larynx	Phonation; permits entry and exit of gases only	Framework made of cartilages and ligaments; skeletal muscles; protective vestibular folds; vocal folds with elastic vocal ligaments; stratified squamous epithelium on vocal folds and on anterior surface of epiglottis; elastic cartilage in epiglottis	Except for vocal folds and anterior surface of epiglottis, lining is mostly respiratory epithelium
Trachea	Conducts air into thorax; withstands stretch	Cartilages are horseshoe-shaped, incomplete posteriorly; trachealis muscle (smooth); fibroelastic tissue; submucosal mucoserous glands	Expiratory elastic recoil; respiratory epithelium contains neuroendocrine cells, transports mucus blanket
Bronchi	Conduct air into lungs	Extrapulmonary bronchial cartilages as in trachea; intrapulmonary bronchial cartilages are irregular in shape; fibroelastic tissue; helical smooth muscle; submucosal mucoserous glands	Same as for trachea
Bronchioles	Conduct air into respiratory tissue; gas exchange begins	Simple columnar or cuboidal epithelium; lack glands and cartilages; helical smooth muscle; discontinuation of goblet cells and then cilia with decreasing luminal diameter; respiratory bronchioles have some alveoli	Bronchiolar constriction impedes airflow, e.g., during expiration in asthmatics
Alveolar ducts	Conduct air to alveolar sacs and alveoli	Isolated groups of cuboidal epithelial cells; minimal wall structure	Recognizable only in favorable planes of section

(continued)

TABLE 14-2

SUMMARIZED MAJOR FEATURES OF THE RESPIRATORY SYSTEM *(CONTINUED)*

Part	Main Functions	Distinctive Features	General Features
Alveoli	Chief sites of gas exchange; surfactant production	Interalveolar walls contain pulmonary capillaries, elastic and reticular fibers, and basement membranes, but lack lymphatics; attenuated type I cells adapted for gas exchanges; rounded type II cells with lamellar bodies secrete surfactant; alveolar macrophages	Alveolar sacs have associated alveoli; alveoli have alveolar pores; continuing postnatal formation of alveoli
Pleura	Lining of pleural cavity; visceral pleura glides over parietal pleura	Simple squamous serosa with fibroelastic subserosa	Expiratory elastic recoil of subserosal elastic fibers of visceral pleura

In addition to **type I** and **type II pneumocytes** and **endothelial cells** of alveolar capillaries, it is possible to find occasional interstitial **fibroblasts** and even to spot **monocytes** transforming into **macrophages** in interalveolar walls (see Fig. 14-10). Large, rounded **alveolar macrophages (phagocytes)** with engulfed particles are sometimes seen bulging from interalveolar walls or seemingly lying free in alveolar air spaces. Alveolar macrophages can arise either directly or indirectly from monocytes escaping from alveolar capillaries because alveolar macrophages themselves can divide. Actively phagocytic macrophages carry engulfed particles through successive conducting passages to a mucus blanket that the tracheobronchial cilia sweep toward the pharynx (i.e., the **mucociliary escalator**). Macrophage clearance represents a second important mechanism for keeping the lungs clear of particulate matter. If a person inhales coal dust or soot or smokes too many cigarettes, however, daily overloading of the phagocytic clearance mechanism may lead to blackening of the lungs. Lymphatics in the visceral pleura commonly also appear blackened. Instead of being eliminated, many of the particles picked up from the inhaled contaminated air become more or less permanently included in interalveolar walls. This is because macrophages that scavenge them fail to reach the mucus blanket and hence fail to make an exit. The situation is worsened by any accompanying ciliary damage in the airways.

Summary

Essential features of the main parts of the respiratory system are shown in summary form in Table 14-2.

Bibliography

Conducting Airways

Bienenstock J. Bronchus-associated lymphoid tissue. In: Bienenstock J, ed. Immunology of the Lung and Upper Respiratory Tract. New York, McGraw-Hill, 1984, p 96.

Brandtzaeg P. Immune functions of human nasal mucosa and tonsils in health and disease. In: Bienenstock J, ed. Immunology of the Lung and Upper Respiratory Tract. New York, McGraw-Hill, 1984, p 28.

Breeze RG, Wheeldon EB. The cells of the pulmonary airways. Am Rev Respir Dis 116:705, 1977.

Davis AE, Smallman LA. An ultrastructural study of the mucosal surface of the human inferior concha: I. Normal appearances. J Anat 161:61, 1988.

Fink BR. The Human Larynx: A Functional Study. New York, Raven Press, 1975.

Graziadei PPC, Monti Graziadei GA. Continuous nerve cell renewal in the olfactory system. In: Jacobson M, ed. Handbook of Sensory Physiology, vol 9. Development of Sensory Systems. New York, Springer-Verlag, 1978, p 55.

Harding J, Graziadei PPC, Monti Graziadei GA, Margolis FL. Denervation in the primary olfactory pathway of mice: IV. Biochemical and morphological evidence for neuronal replacement following nerve section. Brain Res 132:11, 1977.

Plopper CG, Heidsiek JG, Weir AJ, St George JA, Hyde DM. Tracheobronchial epithelium in the adult rhesus monkey: a quantitative histochemical and ultrastructural study. Am J Anat 184:31, 1989.

Polyzonis BM, Kafandaris PM, Gigis PI, Demetriou T. An electron microscopic study of human olfactory mucosa. J Anat 128:77, 1979.

Rodger IW. Airway smooth muscle. Br Med Bull 48:97, 1992.

Weibel ER. Design and structure of the human lung. In: Fishman AP, ed. Pulmonary Diseases and Disorders. New York, McGraw-Hill, 1979.

Weibel ER. Looking into the lung: what can it tell us? AJR 133:1021, 1979.

Weibel ER. Lung cell biology. In: Fishman AP, ed. Handbook of Physiology, sect 3: The Respiratory System, vol 1. Circulation and Nonrespiratory Functions, Bethesda, MD, American Physiological Society, 1985, p 47.

Alveoli and Ancillary Pulmonary Functions

Bartels H. The air–blood barrier in the human lung: a freeze-fracture study. Cell Tissue Res 198:269, 1979.

Dobbs LG. Pulmonary surfactant. Annu Rev Med 40:431, 1989.

Heinemann HO, Fishman AP. Nonrespiratory functions of mammalian lung. Physiol Rev 49:1, 1969.

Kalina M, Socher R. Internalization of pulmonary surfactant into lamellar bodies of cultured rat pulmonary type II cells. J Histochem Cytochem 38:483, 1990.

Stern L, ed. Hyaline Membrane Disease: Pathogenesis and Pathophysiology. Orlando, Grune & Stratton, 1984.

Stratton JC. The ultrastructure of multilamellar bodies and surfactant in the human lung. Cell Tissue Res 193:219, 1978.

Takaro T, Price HP, Parra SC. Ultrastructural studies of apertures in the interalveolar septum of the adult human lung. Am Rev Respir Dis 119:425, 1979.

Van Furth R. Cellular biology of pulmonary macrophages. Int Arch Allergy Appl Immunol 1(Suppl 76):21, 1985.

Weibel ER, Gil J. Structure-function relationships at the alveolar level. In: West JB, ed. Bioengineering Aspects of the Lung. New York, Marcel Dekker, 1977, p 1.

CHAPTER 15

Urinary System

OBJECTIVES

The information in this chapter should enable you to do the following:

- Summarize with a labeled diagram the structural organization of a renal corpuscle
- Specify the glomerular components that produce the urinary filtrate, outlining the role of each component
- Name five major segments of the nephron and summarize the chief functions of each segment
- Recognize proximal and distal convoluted tubules and thin-walled segments of loops of Henle in sections
- State where juxtaglomerular cells are situated and discuss their functional importance
- Specify the lining epithelium and arrangement of smooth muscle in the urinary passages and bladder

The urinary system produces, stores, and voids the excretory product **urine**. This system is made up of the parts listed in Table 15-1. Representing large compound tubular glands, the **kidneys** eliminate the body's waste products, notably the toxic nitrogenous end-products of protein catabolism that come from the liver. In addition, the kidneys regulate the body's ion balance and water content and play a key role in stabilizing blood pressure. Finally, they maintain adequate oxygen-carrying capacity of the blood by secreting **erythropoietin**, the glycoprotein hormonal regulator of erythrocyte production in myeloid tissue. It is not clear, however, which kidney cells produce this hormone. In short, the essential role of the kidneys is to maintain the body's unique internal environment and to minimize unbalancing effects of processes that are inclined to alter its composition.

Urine draining toward the medial recess (**hilum**) of the kidney enters the **renal pelvis**, which is the funnel-shaped proximal end of the associated renal excretory duct or **ureter** (Fig. 15-1). Peristaltic contractions of the muscular walls of the ureters transport urine to the **urinary bladder**, the muscular-walled reservoir in which it is temporarily stored. Urine is voided through the **urethra**, an unpaired tubular excretory passage that opens to the exterior. In males, but not females, the urethra is considered a mutual component of both the urinary and the reproductive systems.

An essential structural and functional unit of the kidney is the **kidney (renal) tubule**. It is an epithelial blind-ending tubule with a compact mass of looped fenestrated capillaries called a

TABLE 15-1

URINARY SYSTEM: PRINCIPAL COMPONENTS
Kidneys
Cortex
Medulla
Renal pelvis (hilum)
Ureters
Urinary bladder
Urethra

glomerulus (L., small ball) invaginated into its closed proximal end (see Fig. 15-4). A special arrangement filters vast volumes of plasma, producing a filtrate that enters the kidney tubules. This initial **glomerular filtrate** contains nitrogenous waste products such as urea and uric acid, but minimal amounts of protein except some of low molecular weight. To avoid "throwing away the baby with the dirty bathwater", the kidney tubules then *resorb* those substances that are still useful to the body, including escaped plasma protein, amino acids, glucose, many different ions (notably sodium, chloride, calcium, and phosphate), and, above all, water. After the useful constituents have been extracted, only toxic substances and those not worth recycling remain in the filtrate, and these are voided in the urine. The cells that line the proximal segment of the kidney tubules are also able to *excrete* a few substances into the filtrate. Compounds eliminated in this manner include certain metabolites and the antibiotic penicillin.

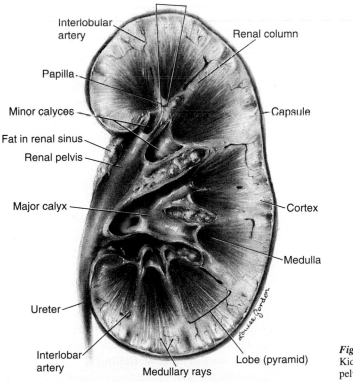

Figure 15-1
Kidney cut longitudinally to show the renal pelvis.

We shall first outline the general histological organization of the kidneys and then consider the various design features that enable the kidneys to eliminate end-products of metabolism without losing much of potential value.

KIDNEYS

Bilaterally attached to the posterior abdominal wall, the kidneys lie retroperitoneally on each side of the vertebral column. Each kidney is shaped like a lima bean. The associated ureter, renal artery, renal vein, major lymphatic vessels, and surrounding nerve plexus (renal plexus) emerge through adipose tissue at the **hilum** (see Fig. 15-1). Besides having a tough fibrous **capsule** made of irregular dense ordinary connective tissue, the kidneys are protected by large quantities of associated perirenal fat tissue. Their outer region, the **renal cortex**, has a granular appearance when cut, mainly because of its ovoid filtration units (Plate 15-1). The inner region, known as the **renal medulla**, has a more striated appearance (see Fig. 15-1). The human kidney is **multilobar**, meaning that it develops from a number of **lobes** (up to 18), each a conical mass (**pyramid**) of medullary tissue capped with cortex. Individual lobes (pyramids) are discernible where their lateral margins are delineated by **renal columns (of Bertin)**, which represent partitions of interlobar cortical tissue that penetrate deep into the medulla. The rounded-off apex of each medullary pyramid, termed its **papilla**, projects into the renal pelvis. Facilitating urine collection from the many papillae, the expanded proximal end of the associated ureter is subdivided into **major** and then **minor calyces**, small funnel-like structures that cap the renal papillae. The simple columnar epithelial covering of each papilla is continuous with the transitional epithelial lining of its associated calyx. Each lobe of the kidney is made up of several **lobules** that are less distinct than lobes. To explain what kidney lobules are, we need to describe the parts of a kidney tubule and discuss where they lie in the kidney.

Pathway of Nephron In Kidney Lobule

The unit of kidney structure responsible for filtration, excretion, and resorption is called the **nephron**. This term includes both the kidney tubule and its glomerulus. It does not, however, include the collecting tubule into which the nephron drains (Fig. 15-2). Each kidney is made up of more than a million nephrons, together with the branched system of collecting ducts into which they drain. The proximal end of each nephron is expanded into an ovoid to spherical filtration unit termed a **renal corpuscle** (Plate 15-2 and Figs. 15-3 and 15-4). This expanded proximal end opens into a proximal convoluted segment, a long loop of Henle, and then a distal convoluted segment, each with its own functional characteristics.

The **renal corpuscle** and **proximal convoluted tubule** both lie in the **renal cortex** (see Fig. 15-2). At the end of its tortuous course through the cortex in the vicinity of the renal corpuscle, the proximal tubule extends down into the **renal medulla** as the straight **descending portion of the loop of Henle**. Proximally, this looped segment is thick walled like the proximal convoluted tubule, but deeper in the medulla the loop is thin-walled (see Fig. 15-3). The thin-walled part of the loop descends farther into the medulla before making a U-turn and ascending to the cortex as the **ascending portion of the loop of Henle**. The ascending portion is thin-walled deep in the medulla but becomes thick-walled before it re-enters the cortex and continues on as the tortuous **distal convoluted tubule** (see Figs. 15-2 and 15-3). The beginning of the distal convoluted tubule lies in intimate association with the renal corpuscle of the same nephron (see Fig. 15-2), constituting an elaborate arrangement known as the **juxtaglomerular complex** (see later). The distal convoluted tubule then winds through the cortex, usually following along beside the proximal convoluted tubule, and joins a small tributary of a **main collecting duct (papillary duct** or **duct of Bellini)** that passes down through the medulla and opens onto a papilla. The reason for not considering collecting tubules to

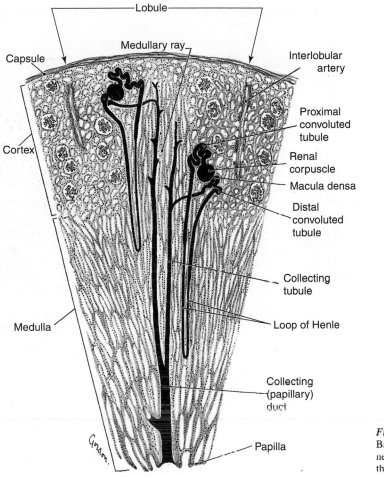

Capsule

Lobule

Medullary ray

Interlobular
artery

Cortex

Proximal
convoluted
tubule

Renal
corpuscle

Macula densa

Distal
convoluted
tubule

Collecting
tubule

Medulla

Loop of Henle

Collecting
(papillary)
duct

Papilla

Figure 15-2
Basic arrangement of the component
nephrons and collecting tubules of
the kidney lobule.

be integral parts of nephrons is that they develop independently as branching outgrowths of the ureteric bud and then connect with the nephrons they drain.

Thus, the granular appearance of the renal cortex reflects its content of renal corpuscles and convoluted tubules, and the striated appearance of the renal medulla reflects its content of loops of Henle and collecting tubules, which pursue a more or less straight course through this region. However, much as interlobar extensions of the renal cortex project down into the medulla as **renal columns**, minor extensions of the renal medulla project up into the cortex as ray-like groups called **medullary rays**. In Figure 15-2, it may be seen that 1) many nephrons drain into a main collecting duct and 2) the loops of Henle of these nephrons, along with the collecting tubules through which they drain toward the duct, lie in the same general region. The part of this region that extends into the cortex is a medullary ray.

In the case of the kidney, the term **lobule** means a group of nephrons that open into branches of the same main collecting duct, as in other compound glands with secretory units that open into branches of the same intralobular duct. Kidney lobules are not easy to discern, but their lateral margins are sometimes recognizable by the presence of arteries or veins that course between the lobules (e.g., **interlobular arteries**; see Fig. 15-2). These lobules may also be recognized by the fact that their central cores are medullary rays.

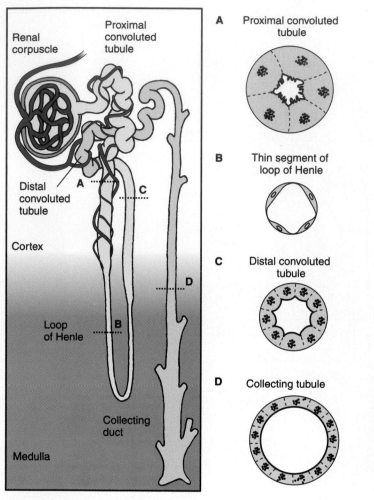

A Proximal convoluted tubule

B Thin segment of loop of Henle

C Distal convoluted tubule

D Collecting tubule

Figure 15-3
(*Left*) Relative positions of the parts of the nephron and a collecting tubule. (*Right*) Schematic diagrams showing the cross-sectional appearance of the parts of a nephron and a collecting tubule at the levels indicated at left.

Renal Corpuscle

The structure of the renal corpuscle is essentially determined by the manner in which it develops. When a tuft of glomerular capillaries grows into the blind end of a nephron, it becomes invested by a **visceral layer** of epithelium that invaginates along with it (see Fig. 15-4). The resulting proximal bulb-like expansion of the nephron, known as a **Bowman's capsule**, also retains a **parietal layer** of

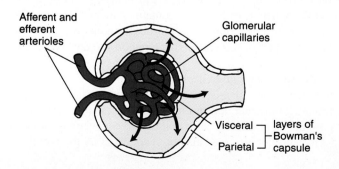

Figure 15-4
Essential organization of the renal corpuscle.

epithelium that remains continuous with the visceral layer. The glomerular filtrate produced by the glomerular capillaries passes through the visceral layer of epithelium into the **capsular (Bowman's) space**, as indicated by arrows in Figure 15-4. Whereas the **parietal** or **capsular epithelium** of Bowman's capsule (Fig. 15-5) is a simple squamous epithelium, the **visceral** or **glomerular epithelium** is made up of special cells called podocytes that are unique to the kidney (see later). A thick **glomerular basement membrane** lies between the podocytes and the capillary endothelial cells. Because of its glycoprotein content, this functionally important part of the glomerulus may be seen to advantage in kidney sections stained with PAS (see Plate 5-2).

Production of vast volumes of glomerular filtrate is facilitated by a structural arrangement that produces substantial hydrostatic pressure along the entire length of glomerular capillaries. Instead of draining into venules as in the other parts of the body, glomerular capillaries open into an **efferent arteriole** of similar construction to the **afferent arteriole** that supplies them (see Fig. 15-4). Both arterioles have smooth muscle cells in their media, and the contractile differential between these two vessels maintains a relatively high pressure along the full length of the glomerular

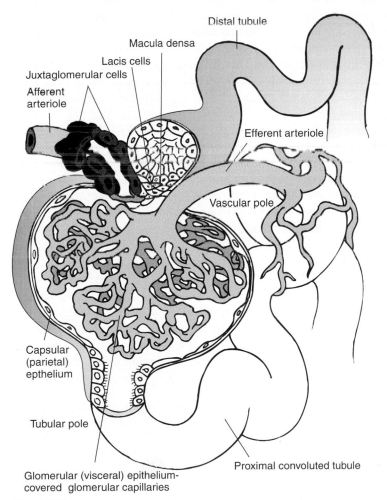

Figure 15-5
Anatomical relations of the parts of the juxtaglomerular complex to the associated parts of the nephron.

capillaries. A second factor facilitating filtration is that the capillary endothelial cells have numerous **open fenestrae** through which the blood plasma can freely pass.

The glomerular capillary loops are supported on delicate axial stalks made up of inconspicuous **mesangial cells** and an interstitial **mesangial matrix** that these cells produce. Besides having a supporting function and producing growth factors, mesangial cells are phagocytic and responsible for day-to-day upkeep of the glomerular basement membrane surrounding each capillary loop. They are able to remove macromolecular deposits that might otherwise interfere with the filtering action of this principal component of the glomerular filtration barrier.

Glomerular Filtration Barrier

The cells that constitute the **glomerular epithelium** (the **visceral layer** of Bowman's capsule) have a uniquely adapted, octopus-like structure that greatly facilitates the formation of glomerular filtrate. The unusual shape of these cells earned them the name **podocytes** (Fig. 15-6). Their cell bodies protrude into the capsular space (the lumen of Bowman's capsule) and their terminal branched extensions adhere to the basement membrane of glomerular capillaries. The several arm-like **primary processes** radiating from the cell body bear numerous **secondary processes** with side branches called **podocyte feet** (Gk. *podos*, foot) or **pedicels** that extend to the outer surface of the glomerular basement membrane. The tightly spaced foot processes of each podocyte interdigitate with those of other podocytes, leaving only narrow **filtration slits** 20 to 30 nm wide between the two arrays. Thus, the outer surface of glomerular capillaries is covered by closely approximated interdigitating foot processes with filtration slits between them.

Every molecule that enters the capsular space from a glomerular capillary has to pass through three layers. First, it must traverse the **fenestrated endothelium** that lines the capillary. This layer is provided with large open fenestrae, however, so it does not restrict passage of plasma and it behaves only as a pre-filter that excludes blood cells and platelets. The next layer, the **glomerular basement membrane**, is considered the main filtration barrier of the kidney. It is thicker than other basement membranes because essentially it is a fused basement membrane representing both an epithelial and an endothelial basement membrane. It has a three-layered appearance in the EM. The electron-lucent layer bordering on the endothelium is termed the **lamina lucida** (or **rara**) **interna** (see Fig. 15-6A). The comparatively electron dense middle layer is the **lamina densa**. The electron-lucent layer adjacent to the glomerular epithelium is the **lamina lucida** (or **rara**) **externa**. Because the epithelial and endothelial basement membranes are fused, a lamina fibroreticularis is lacking. Podocytes continuously produce additional basement membrane material in amounts that compensate for the phagocytic removal of damaged or deteriorating basement membrane by mesangial cells. The third component of the filtration barrier is the **glomerular epithelium** itself. Extending along each **filtration slit** between adjacent podocyte feet is a thin shelf-like **filtration slit diaphragm** with an axial supporting rib and somewhat zipper-like appearance (see Fig. 15-6B). Glomerular filtrate has to pass through this diaphragm to enter the capsular space.

The glomerular basement membrane behaves as a **molecular sieve** capable of sorting out molecules on the basis of molecular size and charge. This layer is impermeable to molecules with a molecular weight of more than 69,000 or a high negative charge. Although substances of low molecular weight are able to pass across the filtration barrier, useful ones are retrieved chiefly by the proximal tubule instead of being voided in the urine. Molecules of plasma albumin, with a molecular weight of 69,000 daltons, appear to be just small enough to pass the glomerular basement membrane, but they do not pass to any great extent because of their net negative charge. The glomerular basement membrane constituent that seems most responsible for excluding negatively charged macromolecules is heparan sulfate proteoglycan, which itself carries a substantial negative charge. The role of the filtration slit diaphragm, formerly thought to be an ancillary molecular sieve, remains unclear.

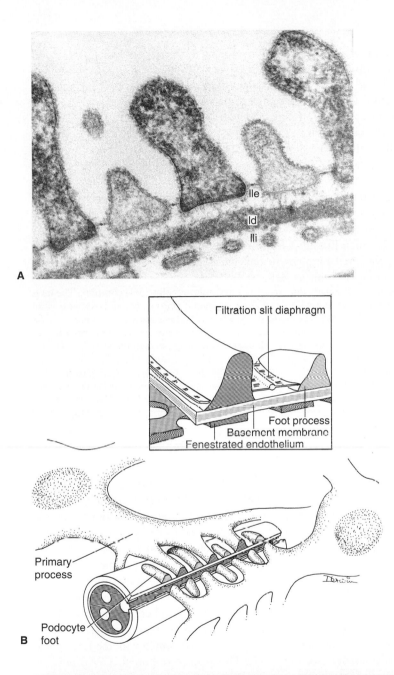

A

B

Figure 15-6
Glomerular filtration barrier. (*A*)
Electron micrograph (lle, lamina
lucida externa; ld, lamina densa; lli,
lamina lucida interna). (*B*)
Explanatory diagram.

CLINICAL IMPLICATIONS

Depletion of Plasma Protein Resulting From Glomerular Damage
The glomerular basement membrane loses its highly selective permeability properties when it deteriorates or becomes damaged. Certain kinds of antigen–antibody complexes formed when humoral antibodies combine with antigen are notorious for causing this kind of glomerular damage. Such complexes can become lodged in the glomerular basement membrane, whereupon they may elicit an acute inflammatory response. In severe cases, damage to the glomerular basement membrane may lead to massive and potentially fatal loss of plasma proteins into the urine (a complication in the **nephrotic syndrome**).

Juxtaglomerular Complex

The site where the afferent and efferent arterioles both converge on the renal corpuscle is termed its **vascular pole**, as distinct from the **tubular pole**, which is the site of origin of the proximal convoluted tubule (see Plate 15-2). From the renal cortex, the kidney tubule extends into the renal medulla as the loop of Henle and then returns to the vascular pole of the same renal corpuscle, where it fits into the notch lying between the afferent and efferent arterioles. Here, the side of the tubular wall that is nearest to the glomerulus is characterized by a densely nucleated spot called the **macula densa**, where the lining epithelial cells of the tubule are narrower and as a result their nuclei lie closer together (see Fig. 15-5 and Plate 15-2). This heavily nucleated region is generally regarded as indicating the site where the distal convoluted tubule begins. Interposed between the macula densa and the glomerulus lies a small group of cells with pale-staining nuclei. Known as **lacis cells**, these appear to be similar to mesangial cells. The most significant specialization at the vascular pole, however, is found in the wall of the afferent arteriole. Here, smooth muscle cells of the media are highly modified as special secretory cells called **juxtaglomerular (JG) cells**. These cells have large PAS-positive **secretory granules** that contain the proteolytic enzyme **renin** (see later). Small numbers of JG cells may be present in the efferent arteriole as well.

   The **JG cells** and **macula densa** are functionally integrated as a **juxtaglomerular (JG) complex**. The **lacis cells** are interconnected both with one another and with the JG cells by gap junctions, which is suggestive of some functional link with these cells. The JG complex monitors systemic blood pressure by responding to the **degree of stretch** in the wall of the afferent arteriole. At the same time, it monitors the **concentration of sodium and chloride ions** in the filtrate passing by the macula densa on its way through the nephron. The information gained helps to determine how much renin should be released to keep systemic blood pressure within normal limits and also to keep glomerular filtration rate virtually constant. Renin is also released in response to sympathetic nerve impulses. The role of **renin** in maintaining blood pressure is summarized in Table 15-2. **Angiotensinogen**, the substrate on which renin acts, is a plasma globulin produced in the liver. Chronic renal **ischemia** (impaired blood flow) can elevate renin levels, which in turn can be a contributing factor to high blood pressure (**hypertension**).

Proximal Convoluted Tubule

The longest part of the nephron is the **proximal convoluted tubule**. Leading from the tubular pole of the renal corpuscle, this segment winds through the renal cortex and then enters a medullary ray. Here, it becomes the thick descending portion of the loop of Henle, similar in histological appearance but not convoluted. These two upper parts of the nephron are therefore often referred to as the *convoluted part* and *straight part* of the proximal tubule, respectively. Several microscopic features permit proximal convoluted tubules to be differentiated from the distal convoluted tubules also seen in the cortex. Because of the longer length of the proximal tubule, sections of it usually outnumber those of the distal tubule. Also, its cells are larger and generally are better-stained (see Plate 15-2 and Figs. 15-3*A* and 15-7). Each cell appears wide and triangular, with a spherical nucleus and lateral cell margins that seem indistinct owing to interdigitation. The resorptive luminal surface of the proximal convoluted tubule cells bears numerous microvilli (Fig. 15-8), which with the LM appear as a fairly evident **striated (brush) border** (see Fig. 15-7). This resorptive border is PAS-positive owing to much glycoprotein in its cell coat. Numerous mitochondria provide the extra energy needed for pumping ions across the cell membrane (see Fig. 15-8). They are particularly abundant near the base of the cells, where they lie close to infoldings of lateral and basal regions of the cell membrane that increase the surface area available for ion transport.

   Cells of the proximal convoluted tubule actively resorb many constituents from the glomerular filtrate, including water, sodium, chloride, other ions, glucose, and amino acids. They are also able to retrieve escaped plasma proteins, break them down into amino acids, and release these into the interstitial spaces. In addition, they actively excrete certain metabolites, drugs, and dyes into the filtrate.

TABLE 15-2

ROLE OF RENIN IN BLOOD PRESSURE REGULATION

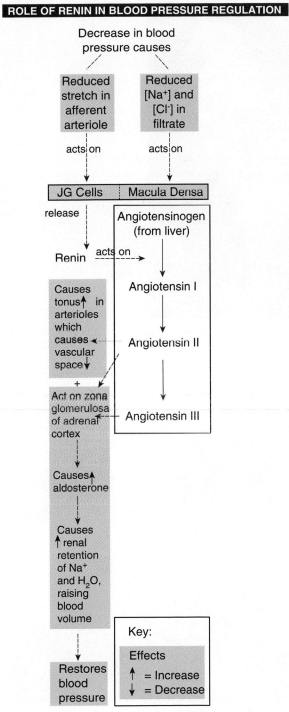

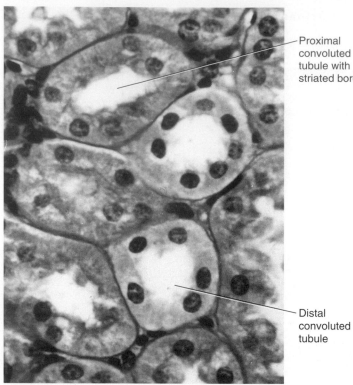

Figure 15-7
Proximal and distal convoluted tubules compared at the LM level (PAS and hematoxylin).

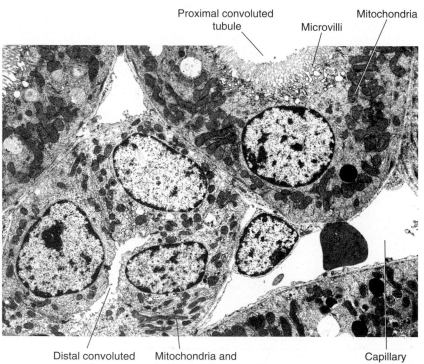

Figure 15-8
Proximal and distal convoluted tubules compared at the EM level.

Loop of Henle

The **loop of Henle** is made up of 1) an initial **thick descending portion**, representing a continuation of the proximal tubule and known also as the **pars recta** (straight part) of the proximal tubule, 2) a **thin descending portion**, 3) a **thin ascending portion**, and 4) a **thick ascending portion**, which represents the beginning of the distal tubule and resembles it in histological appearance and is accordingly known also as its **pars recta**. The ascending portion of the loop lies beside the descending portion, which extends for a variable distance into the renal medulla. A nephron with a glomerulus that lies near the corticomedullary border (a **juxtamedullary nephron**) has a relatively long loop of Henle that extends deep into the medulla. In contrast, most of the loop of Henle of a superficial nephron is generally situated in a medullary ray (see Fig. 15-2). The thin segment of the loop has a narrow lumen and a thin wall made up of squamous epithelial cells (see Figs. 15-3B and 15-9). Except for the absence of blood cells from its lumen, however, there is little to distinguish this part of the nephron from the numerous straight blood capillaries (**vasa recta**) that surround it.

Distal Convoluted Tubule

The final segment of the nephron, the **distal convoluted tubule**, lies in the renal cortex. From the heavily nucleated macula densa region apposed to the vascular pole of the renal corpuscle, the distal convoluted tubule pursues a winding course and then joins a collecting tubule. It is somewhat shorter than the proximal convoluted tubule and therefore less frequently represented in sections. Its cuboidal cells are also less well stained and somewhat smaller, giving this segment of the tubule a larger number of spherical nuclei in its walls and generally a wider-looking lumen (see Figs. 15-3C and 15-7 and Plate 15-2). The luminal surface of the distal convoluted tubule does not bear enough microvilli for this part of the nephron to have a distinct striated border (see Figs. 15-7 and 15-8). The lateral cell margins may be less indistinct than those of the proximal tubule. As in the proximal tubule, deep basal infoldings and interdigitations of the cell membrane are closely associated with numerous mitochondria. Sodium resorption by this last part of the tubule, and, to an even greater extent, by the cortical collecting ducts, is promoted by **aldosterone**, a steroid hormone produced by cells of the zona glomerulosa of the adrenal cortex.

Collecting Tubules

Small tributaries of the main collecting ducts, called **collecting tubules**, lie mostly in the medullary rays and medulla. They may be distinguished from the other kinds of tubules by the fact that they

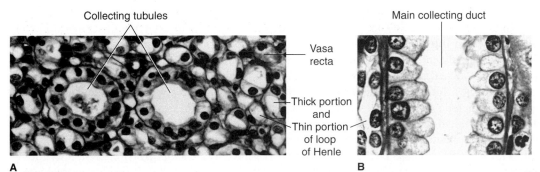

A   **B**

Figure 15-9
Renal medullary collecting tubules. (*A*) Representative collecting tubules (transverse section). (*B*) Main collecting duct (papillary duct, longitudinal section).

are composed of cuboidal to columnar cells with lateral margins that are *distinct* owing to lack of extensive interdigitation (see Figs. 15-3*D* and 15-9). Collecting tubules make up a branched system of drainage ducts that conveys urine to the renal pelvis. The main collecting ducts (**papillary ducts** or **ducts of Bellini**) that open onto renal papillae are easy to recognize because of their wide lumen and pale-staining columnar cells (see Fig. 15-9). Key activities of the renal collecting tubules are 1) to **resorb water** in response to vasopressin, as explained in the following section, and 2) to resorb sodium in response to aldosterone.

Filtrate Concentrating Mechanism

The various parts of the nephron and collecting tubule adjust the glomerular filtrate in such a way that by the time it reaches the renal pelvis, it is concentrated urine. The following briefly summarizes the main features of the **countercurrent mechanism** through which this is achieved.

Each region of the kidney tubule has distinctive permeability characteristics for water, ions, and urea. The thick ascending portion of the loop of Henle actively extracts chloride and sodium ions from the filtrate and transfers them to the interstitial spaces between the tubules. These ions can also pass passively into interstitial spaces from the thin ascending portion of the loop of Henle. As a result, chloride and sodium, and also urea, accumulate in the interstitial space and build up as an **interstitial concentration gradient** that increases with depth in the medulla and becomes maximal at the renal papilla (represented as shading in Fig. 15-3). This concentration gradient constitutes an increasingly **hypertonic environment** through which the filtrate must pass, within a collecting tubule, before draining from the papilla. The thin-walled capillaries of the medulla (**vasa recta**) have freely permeable walls that passively sustain the concentration gradient.

In the presence of the antidiuretic hormone **vasopressin** (ADH), released from the posterior lobe of the pituitary, a large proportion of the water is withdrawn osmotically from the urinary filtrate when it passes through medullary collecting tubules. The action of ADH is to increase the permeability of the medullary collecting tubules to water. If there is a deficiency of this hormone, the urine remains voluminous and hypotonic (dilute). Excessive production of dilute, pale-colored urine as a result of a **deficiency of ADH** is an indication of the condition **diabetes insipidus**.

Renal Blood Supply

The kidneys contain little connective tissue other than their thin fibrous capsule and the loose connective tissue associated with their blood vessels. Only small traces of loose connective tissue are found between their component nephrons. From renal corpuscle to papillary duct, each kidney tubule is nevertheless invested by a supporting basement membrane. Minimal amounts of loose connective tissue containing a few fibroblasts are also present between the medullary collecting tubules.

In the hilar region of the kidney, the **renal artery** branches into a number of **segmental arteries** from which **interlobar arteries** extend, between lobes, to the corticomedullary border (Fig. 15-10*A*). Here, the interlobar arteries give rise to **arcuate arteries**, so called because they arch over (L. *arcuatus*, arched), radiating from the tip of an interlobar artery like ribs of an umbrella. From the arcuate arteries, **interlobular arteries** ascend between lobules and give off lateral **intralobular arteries**, which lie within lobules and give rise to **afferent arterioles** supplying glomeruli (see Fig. 15-10*B*). Terminal branches of the interlobular arteries supply capsular capillaries. Blood reaches the cortical capillaries from efferent arterioles of more superficially situated glomeruli (levels 1 and 2 in Fig. 15-10*B*), whereas medullary capillaries (vasa recta) are supplied by efferent arterioles of deeper and juxtamedullary glomeruli (levels 3 and 4 in the same diagram). Blood leaves the kidneys by way of a roughly comparable distribution of veins (shown at right in Fig. 15-10*B*) and enters the renal veins, which open into the inferior vena cava.

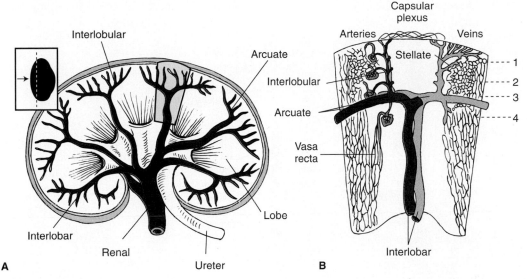

Figure 15-10
(*A*) Arterial blood supply of a kidney (cut as shown in the inset). (*B*) Blood vessels in the area indicated in *A*.

URETERS

Each **ureter** is essentially a long, straight, muscular-walled tube. Lying retroperitoneally, it extends from the renal pelvis (representing its funnel-shaped proximal end) to the urinary bladder. Major invaginated simple longitudinal folds of the mucosa give the lumen a characteristic *stellate* appearance (Fig. 15-11). The thick lining epithelium, **transitional epithelium,** is supported by a fibroelastic **lamina propria**. The deeply folded mucosa has a protective, accommodating function and usually allows any small kidney stones composed of insoluble substances (**urinary calculi**) to pass along the ureter along with the urine from which they formed. A ureter has no mucosal or submucosal glands and no submucosa. External to the mucosa lies a thick coat of smooth muscle. This **muscular coat** has two layers in the upper two-thirds of the ureter and three layers in the lower third. Surrounding the inner longitudinal layer is an outer circular layer (which is the *reverse* of the arrangement found in the gastrointestinal tract), and the additional third layer is again longitudinal. Peristaltic contractions of the muscular coat squeeze urine into the urinary bladder. The inferior end of each ureter takes an oblique course through the bladder wall, so its lumen closes down when the bladder becomes distended with urine. Folds of bladder mucosa covering the inferior orifices of the ureters act as flap valves and also help to protect against reflux of urine when the bladder is full. The outermost coat of the ureter, its **adventitia**, consists of fibroelastic connective tissue associated with blood vessels, lymphatics, and nerves.

URINARY BLADDER

The three layers of smooth muscle that make up the muscular coat of the urinary bladder are not readily discernible because the unvoided urine is stored in a sac-like structure and not a tube. In most other respects, however, the wall structure of the bladder resembles that of the ureters. The expansive lumen is lined with **transitional epithelium** (Plate 15-3). Substantial volume changes are accommodated through flattening of many mucosal folds, and the thick transitional lining epithelium is capable of stretching until it resembles stratified squamous epithelium. Although large bulging

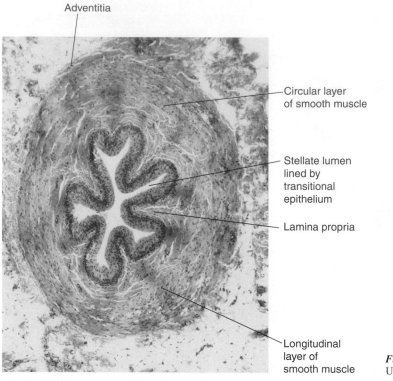

Adventitia

Circular layer
of smooth muscle

Stellate lumen
lined by
transitional
epithelium

Lamina propria

Longitudinal
layer of
smooth muscle

Figure 15-11
Ureter (low power).

polyploid cells on the luminal surface of the epithelium presumably facilitate stretching, a special structural adaptation in the luminal surface cells is required to accommodate the extreme changes in shape involved in bladder voiding and distention due to urinary accumulation. Rigid plate-like areas in the luminal domain of the cell membrane, with flexible interconnecting hinge-like regions, enable this region of the cell membrane to fold up like a concertina (though in a much less organized manner) when urine is voided and then stretch out flat when the bladder fills. The thicker, reinforced areas have attached membrane cytoskeletal filaments that presumably withstand and distribute much of the strain. In addition, desmosomes maintain strong intercellular adhesion, and continuous tight junctions minimize paracellular leakage between lateral margins of the superficial cells. This distinctive combination of cell junctions and plate-like thickenings of the luminal cell membrane maintains the osmotic barrier between urine and the interstitial space.

A fibroelastic lamina propria extends into the mucosal folds. The muscular coat of the bladder contains substantial bundles of smooth muscle arranged as indistinct inner and outer so-called longitudinal layers, with a thicker and predominantly circular middle layer between them (see Plate 15-3). In the neck region of the bladder, the smooth muscle coat forms the **internal sphincter** of the bladder, which is involuntary. The fibroelastic adventitia of the bladder is covered superiorly by peritoneum, forming a serosa.

URETHRA

The urethra is the unpaired excretory passage that conveys urine from the bladder to the exterior of the body. In males, the urethra is shared with the reproductive system (for a description, see Chap. 18). In females, the urethra is simpler and has the following characteristics. Although much shorter

TABLE 15-3

RENAL TUBULAR ORGANIZATION: KEY FEATURES

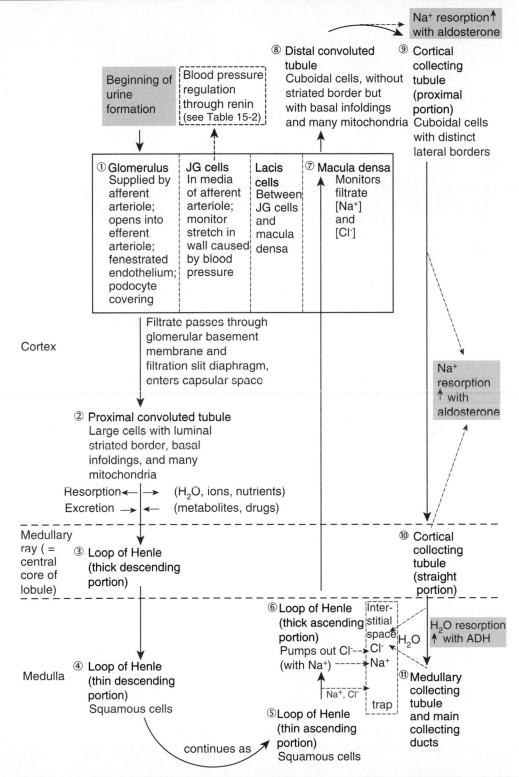

than the ureters, it, too, is a fairly straight muscular-walled tube. Its lumen, crescent shaped in transverse section, is kept closed unless urine is being passed. The female urethra is lined mostly by stratified (or pseudostratified) columnar epithelium, with associated small mucosal glands that secrete mucus. Near the bladder, however, the epithelium is transitional, and near the external urethral orifice, the lining membrane becomes stratified squamous nonkeratinizing epithelium. The thick fibroelastic lamina propria contains a plexus of thin-walled veins. The muscular coat consists of inner longitudinal and outer circular layers of smooth muscle, but these are not particularly distinct. Surrounding the external urethral orifice is a voluntary sphincter composed of skeletal muscle fibers, the **sphincter urethrae**. Posteroinferiorly, the urethra is tightly bound to the anterior wall of the vagina by an external layer of fibrous connective tissue.

Summary

All that should be necessary here is a review of the basic tubular organization of the kidney. A synopsis is given in Table 15-3.

Bibliography

General

Brenner BM, Rector FC, eds. The Kidney, vol 1, ed 4. Philadelphia, WB Saunders, 1992.

Bulger RE, Dobyan DC. Recent advances in renal morphology. Annu Rev Physiol 44:147, 1982.

Gosling JA, Dixon JS, Humpherson JR. Functional Anatomy of the Urinary Tract: An Integrated Text and Color Atlas. London, Gower Medical Publishing, 1983.

Maunsbach AB, Olsen TS, Christensen EI, eds. Functional Ultrastructure of the Kidney. New York, Academic Press, 1981.

Moffat DB. The Mammalian Kidney. London, Cambridge University Press, 1975.

Tisher CG. Functional anatomy of the kidney. Hosp Pract 13(5):53, 1978.

Nephron, Glomerular Filtration Barrier, and Mesangium

Ellis EN, Mauer SM, Sutherland DER, Steffes MW. Glomerular capillary morphology in normal humans. Lab Invest 60:231, 1989.

Farquhar MG. The glomerular basement membrane: a selective macromolecular filter. In: Hay ED, ed. Cell Biology of Extracellular Matrix. New York, Plenum, 1981, p 335.

Fujita T, Tokunaga J, Edanaga M. Scanning electron microscopy of the glomerular filtration membrane in the rat kidney. Cell Tissue Res 166:299, 1976.

Kanwar YS, Linker A, Farquhar MG. Increased permeability of the glomerular basement membrane to ferritin after removal of glycosaminoglycans (heparan sulfate) by enzyme digestion. J Cell Biol 86:688, 1980.

Karnovsky MJ, Ryan GB. Substructure of the glomerular slit diaphragm in freeze-fractured normal rat kidney. J Cell Biol 65:233, 1975.

Kriz W, Elger M, Lemley K, Sakai T. Structure of the glomerular mesangium: a biomechanical interpretation. Kidney Int 38(Suppl 30):S2, 1990.

Laurie GW, Leblond CP, Inoué S et al. Fine structure of the glomerular basement membrane and immunolocalization of five basement membrane components to the lamina densa (basal lamina) and its extensions in both glomeruli and tubules of the rat kidney. Am J Anat 169:463, 1984.

Lea PJ, Silverman M, Hegele R, Hollenberg MJ. Tridimensional ultrastructure of glomerular capillary endothelium revealed by high-resolution scanning electron microscopy. Microvasc Res 38:296, 1989.

Michielsen P, Creemers J. The structure and function of the glomerular mesangium. In: Dalton AJ, Haguenau F, eds. Ultrastructure of the Kidney. New York, Academic Press, 1967, p 57.

Ohno S, Baba T, Terada N, Fujii Y, Ueda H. Cell biology of kidney glomerulus. Int Rev Cytol 166:181, 1996.

Savage COS. The biology of the glomerulus: endothelial cells. Kidney Int 45:314, 1994.

Walker F. The origin, turnover, and removal of glomerular basement membrane. J Pathol 110:233, 1973.

Juxtaglomerular Complex

Barajas L. Anatomy of the juxtaglomerular apparatus. Am J Physiol 237:F333, 1979.

Briggs JP, Skott O, Schnermann J. Cellular mechanisms within the juxtaglomerular apparatus. Am J Hypertension 3:76, 1990.

Gibbons GH, Dzau VJ, Farhi ER, Barger AC. Interaction of signals influencing renin release. Annu Rev Physiol 46:291, 1984.

Komadinović D, Krstić R, Bucher O. Ultrastructural and morphometric aspects of the juxtaglomerular apparatus in the monkey kidney. Cell Tissue Res 192:503, 1978.

Schiller A, Taugner R. Are there specialized junctions in the pars maculata of the distal tubule? Cell Tissue Res 200:337, 1979.

Skott O, Jensen BL. Cellular and intrarenal control of renin secretion. Clin Sci 84:1, 1993.

Renal Connective Tissue and Blood Supply

Brenner BM, Beeuwkes R. The renal circulations. Hosp Pract 13(7):35, 1978.

Kriz W, Barrett JM, Peter S. The renal vasculature: anatomical-functional aspects. In: Thurau K, ed. International Review of Physiology, vol 11. Kidney and Urinary Tract Physiology II. Baltimore, University Park Press, 1976, p 1.

More RH, Duff GL. The renal arterial vasculature in man. Am J Pathol 27:95, 1950.

O'Morchoe CCC. Lymphatic drainage of the kidney. In: Johnston MG, ed. Experimental Biology of the Lymphatic Circulation. Amsterdam, Elsevier Biomedical Press, 1985, p 261.

Urinary Bladder

Hicks RM, Ketterer B. Isolation of the plasma membrane of the luminal surface of rat bladder epithelium, and the occurrence of a hexagonal lattice of subunits both in negatively stained whole mounts and in sectional membranes. J Cell Biol 45:542, 1970.

Staehelin A, Chlapowski FJ, Bonneville MA. Lumenal plasma membrane of the urinary bladder: 1. Three-dimensional reconstruction from freeze-etch images. J Cell Biol 53:73, 1972.

Newman J, Antonakopoulos GN. The fine structure of the human fetal urinary bladder: development and maturation: a light, transmission and scanning electron microscopic study. J Anat 166:135, 1989.

CHAPTER 16

Endocrine System

OBJECTIVES

When you have read this chapter, you should be able to do the following:
- Recognize chromophils in the pituitary and list the hormones they produce
- State two functional consequences of surgical damage to the connection between the hypothalamus and the pituitary
- Outline how thyroid hormone is produced by thyroid follicular epithelial cells
- Specify two histological signs of trophic stimulation of the thyroid
- Name two hormones that regulate osteoclast activity and summarize their action
- Draw a labeled diagram of an adrenal gland showing the sites of production of all the adrenal hormones
- Name three pancreatic hormones and state their chief functions

Many of the body's interdependent cellular processes are integrated and regulated through the secretory activity of cells of the **endocrine system**. This system is a body-wide communications network basically representing a long-acting, far-reaching extension of the nervous system. It provides numerous graded or absolute go-ahead or stop signals for a variety of important cellular activities. Such broad-based intercellular communication ensures that the body's important processes are all performed in a thoroughly coordinated manner that is appropriate to the needs of the body as a whole. In contrast to chemical neurotransmission (the fast, short-range neural signaling that occurs across synaptic clefts), **endocrine** signaling involves dissemination of signal molecules over relatively long distances by way of the blood circulation. Intermediate in speed between synaptic transmission and this slower means of communication is short-range lateral (**paracrine**) signaling, a localized kind of humoral communication. Such short-range diffusion of signal molecules is typical of some of the **enteroendocrine cells** of the gut, known alternatively as **paraneurons** because in common with neurosecretory cells they respond to certain stimuli by secreting peptides or monoamines. It is now recognized that many neural and endocrine mechanisms of coordination are interdependent, with much functional overlap, and they continue to be studied separately only as a matter of convenience. Thus, many functions conventionally considered to be endocrine are best thought of as endocrine activities of a highly integrated **neuroendocrine system**.

The various kinds of signal molecules produced by endocrine cells are termed **hormones**. Most hormones are liberated by exocytosis, but a few of them are able to diffuse through the cell membrane. They pass into interstitial spaces that border on wide fenestrated capillaries and enter the bloodstream, which transports them to **target cells** on which they exert their effects. Hormones have either **stimulatory** or **inhibitory** effects on target cells that recognize molecules of the hormone by means of a specific hormone receptor and respond accordingly. Hence, for each hormone it is useful to know the cellular source, target cells, and target cell responses. Some basic features of endocrine glands, such as absence of ducts and fundamental concepts of feedback regulation, were outlined under Endocrine Glands in Chapter 4.

INTRACELLULAR AND CELL SURFACE HORMONE RECEPTORS

Whereas **steroid** hormones are derived from cholesterol, the remainder, that is, **peptide, protein,** and **glycoprotein hormones** and modified amino acids such as **catecholamines**, are derived from amino acids. Because the various steroid hormones and thyroid hormone are lipid soluble, they are able to diffuse through the cell membrane and bind to **intracellular hormone receptor proteins** in their target cells. In contrast, except for thyroid hormone, the amino acid-derived hormones are water soluble and hence unable to diffuse through the cell membrane. These hormones bind to specific **hormone receptors** in the **cell membrane** of their target cells.

When a **steroid hormone** complexes with its intracellular receptor protein, the hormone-receptor complex binds to specific DNA sequences of the promoter region of specific genes, thus facilitating transcription of those genes. **Thyroid hormone** also facilitates gene transcription. In most cases, when an **amino acid-derived hormone** interacts with its receptor in the cell membrane, it mobilizes an intracellular second messenger such as **cyclic adenosine monophosphate (cAMP)** or cytosolic free **calcium ions**. The second messenger then mediates the action of the hormone.

Table 16-1 lists the primary sources of the body's hormones, some of which are regarded as having an ancillary role with respect to the endocrine system. Because the endocrine activities of ovaries

TABLE 16-1

MAJOR ENDOCRINE COMPONENTS OF THE BODY

Pituitary
    Associated regions of hypothalamus
    Anterior lobe
    Posterior lobe

Thyroid
    Follicular epithelial cells
    Parafollicular cells

Parathyroids

Adrenal cortex
    Zona glomerulosa
    Zona fasciculata
    Zona reticularis

Adrenal medulla

Pancreatic islets

Pineal

Sex glands
    Ovaries
    Testes

Others (selected)
    Thymus
    Gut enteroendocrine cells
    Tracheobronchial neuroendocrine cells
    Kidneys

and testes (organs that are common to both the endocrine system and the reproductive system) are central to reproductive biology, their description is deferred to Chapters 17 and 18. The thymic hormone requirement for T-cell differentiation, the epithelial hormone-producing cells of the gastrointestinal and respiratory tracts, and erythropoietin formation in the kidneys were described in previous chapters.

PITUITARY

Also known as the **hypophysis**, the **pituitary** is a small and rather complex endocrine organ that in many ways represents an endocrine extension of the hypothalamus. The **hypothalamus** is the part of the brain concerned with integration of autonomic responses, initiation of feeding and drinking, regulation of reproductive activities, adaptation to stress, and other so-called visceral functions of the body. Attached superiorly by its infundibular stalk to the median eminence of the tuber cinereum (the basal hypothalamic region that constitutes the floor of the third ventricle), the pituitary lies well protected within the sella turcica of the sphenoid bone. This small but important endocrine gland is made up of two different parts: 1) a glandular **anterior lobe** that develops from oral ectoderm by upgrowth of a diverticulum from the roof of the oral cavity, and 2) a neural **posterior lobe** that develops by downgrowth of the part of the diencephalon that forms the floor of the third ventricle (Figs. 16-1 and 16-2). When the ectodermal and neural components become closely apposed, epithelial continuity with the oral cavity is lost. Along the posterior border of the anterior lobe, where it adjoins the posterior lobe, a narrow region called the **pars intermedia** also develops, but its cells invade the anterior lobe and become diffusely distributed in it, with the result that the human pituitary has only an ill-defined pars intermedia. The glandular epithelial part of the pituitary, termed the **adenohypophysis**, is made up of 1) the **pars anterior** or **pars distalis**, which constitutes the principal part of the anterior lobe, 2) the **pars tuberalis**, a collar-like extension of the pars anterior that lies around the infundibular stalk, and 3) the **pars intermedia**, which is rudimentary and hard to discern in the human pituitary. In many cases, however, its position is roughly indicated by the presence of nearby colloid-filled vestigial cysts (see Figs. 16-1 and 16-3). The neural component of the pituitary, known as the **neurohypophysis** or **pars nervosa** because it is composed of nervous tissue, constitutes the **posterior lobe**. The entire pituitary is enclosed by a dura-derived fibrous capsule and covered superiorly by a thin fibrous shelf also derived from the dura.

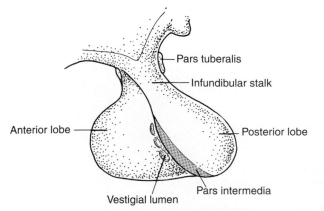

Figure 16-1
Principal parts of the pituitary.

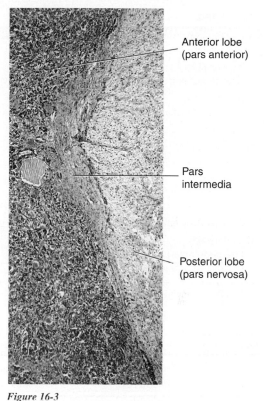

Anterior lobe
(pars anterior)

Pars
intermedia

Posterior lobe
(pars nervosa)

Figure 16-3
Principal parts of the pituitary (horizontal section, low
power). A colloid-filled follicle (*left of center*) indicates the
anterior boundary of the pars intermedia.

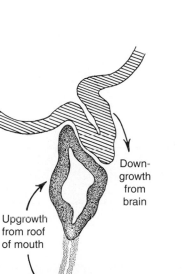

Down-
growth
from
brain

Upgrowth
from roof
of mouth

Figure 16-2
Pituitary development from its two primary sources.

Anterior Lobe

In marked contrast to the pale-staining posterior lobe of the pituitary, the anterior lobe stains brightly
with certain LM stains (**Plate 16-1**; see Fig. 16-3). It contains anastomosing cords of large secretory
epithelial cells that abut on wide fenestrated capillaries. Some of these cells, described as **chromophils**, stain very intensely due to abundant stored secretory granules. Other cells, with less hormone, appear smaller and do not stain brightly. Known as **chromophobes**, they are believed to represent the same cells in a quiescent, degranulated, or temporarily exhausted phase of secretion.
Depending on the affinity of their hormone-containing secretory granules for acid or basic stains, the
chromophils are broadly classified as pituitary **acidophils** or **basophils**. The difference between the
two, however, is not particularly striking in H&E-stained sections. It becomes obvious only if special staining methods are used. Three of the trophic hormones produced by basophils (thyroid-stimulating hormone [TSH], follicle-stimulating hormone [FSH], and luteinizing hormone [LH]; Tables
16-2 and 16-3) are glycoproteins, so the cells that produce them may be demonstrated (as a class) by
means of the PAS reaction. These three hormones, and also ACTH, are described as **trophic hormones** (Gk. *trophein*, to nourish) because they promote cellular growth and secretory activity in
other endocrine glands. To some extent, the different cell types in the anterior pituitary are distinguishable with the EM by the size and appearance of their stored granules (Fig. 16-4). Immunocytochemical staining, however, is necessary for their certain identification. In situations where the
cell's secretory activity has become suppressed by negative feedback, the content of the surplus secretory granules is subjected to lysosomal degradation.

TABLE 16-2

PRINCIPAL CELL TYPES AND HORMONES OF THE ANTERIOR PITUITARY

Acidophils

Somatotrophs
   Growth hormone (GH), alternatively known as somatotropin (STH)

Mammotrophs
   Prolactin (PRL), alternatively known as lactogenic hormone (LTH)

Basophils

Corticotrophs
   Adrenocorticotrophic hormone (ACTH), alternatively known as
   corticotropin
   Melanocyte-stimulating hormone (MSH)*

Thyrotrophs
   Thyroid-stimulating hormone (TSH), alternatively known as thyrotropin

Gonadotrophs
   Follicle-stimulating hormone (FSH)
   Luteinizing hormone (LH)

---

* ACTH has α-MSH activity; γ-MSH may also be released during ACTH formation and breakdown.

TABLE 16-3

ANTERIOR PITUITARY HORMONES

Hormone	Molecular Structure	Main Target Cells	Chief Actions
GH	Protein	Chondrocytes in epiphyseal plates + other body cells	In conjunction with insulin-like growth factors (somatomedins), promotes body growth and protein synthesis; also promotes carbohydrate and lipid utilization
PRL	Protein	Alveolar cells of breast	Brings about breast development during pregnancy and stimulates milk secretion
ACTH	Polypeptide	Corticosteroid secreting cells of adrenal cortex	Promotes growth and secretion of adrenal cortex
MSH*	Peptide	Melanocytes	Promotes melanin synthesis
TSH	Glycoprotein	Follicular epithelial cells of thyroid	Promotes growth and secretion of thyroid follicular epithelium
FSH	Glycoprotein	Follicular (granulosa) cells of ovaries	Promotes growth and maturation of ovarian follicles
		Sertoli cells of testes	Promotes androgen binding, which promotes spermatogenesis
LH	Glycoprotein	Thecal, preovulatory follicular (granulosa), and luteal cells of ovaries	Promotes ovulation and causes luteinization of ovarian follicles
		Interstitial (Leydig) cells of testes	Promotes androgen secretion, which promotes spermatogenesis

For names of the hormones abbreviated here, see Tables 16-2 and 16-4.
* Mostly α-MSH activity of ACTH.

Corticotroph

Non-secreting
(null) cell

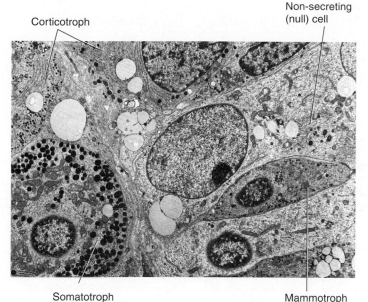

Figure 16-4
Electron micrograph showing four of
the epithelial cell types in the anterior
pituitary.

Somatotroph   Mammotroph

Table 16-2 lists the two principal types of acidophils and the three principal types of basophils, and specifies the chief sources of the six established anterior pituitary hormones, plus another (melanocyte-stimulating hormone [MSH]) that is a bit controversial. Besides these five main cell types, there are other chromophils that in common with gonadotrophs are able to produce more than one hormone. Thus, acidophils called **mammosomatotrophs** secrete growth hormone as well as prolactin, basophils called **corticothyrotrophs** secrete both ACTH and TSH, and basophils called **corticogonadotrophs** secrete ACTH, FSH, and LH. The main actions of the various anterior pituitary hormones are summarized in Table 16-3.

Hypothalamic–Anterior Pituitary Neuroendocrine Link

A special vascular arrangement expedites communication between 1) neural tissue of the infundibular stalk and adjacent region of hypothalamus (median eminence) and 2) secretory epithelial tissue of the anterior pituitary. Local plexuses of fenestrated capillaries are interconnected by **portal vessels** (portal venules and veins) extending down the pituitary stalk (Fig. 16-5). Venous blood from the neural capillary plexus (which lies outside the blood–brain barrier) passes down the portal vessels to the capillary plexus in the anterior lobe, an arrangement known as the **hypophysioportal circulation**. The significance of this essential vascular link is that it carries regulatory hormones produced by the hypothalamus to their target cells in the anterior pituitary.

The neurosecretory regions of the hypothalamus contain neurosecretory cells (secretory neurons) that release peptide hormones from their axon terminals. The peptide hormones that pass into the hypophysioportal circulation regulate the secretory activities of the various hormone-producing cells in the anterior pituitary. Vasopressin and oxytocin are somewhat different, since they pass into capillaries of the posterior lobe.

The hypothalamic hormones that regulate output of the anterior pituitary hormones are known as **hormone-releasing** and **hormone-inhibiting** hormones (Table 16-4). For two anterior pituitary hormones (growth hormone [GH] and prolactin [PRL]) there are inhibiting hormones as well as releasing hormones. The cell bodies of the neurosecretory cells that produce the releasing and inhibiting hormones are situated in several hypothalamic areas and nuclei (groups of nerve cell bodies) that constitute the **hypophysiotrophic area** of the

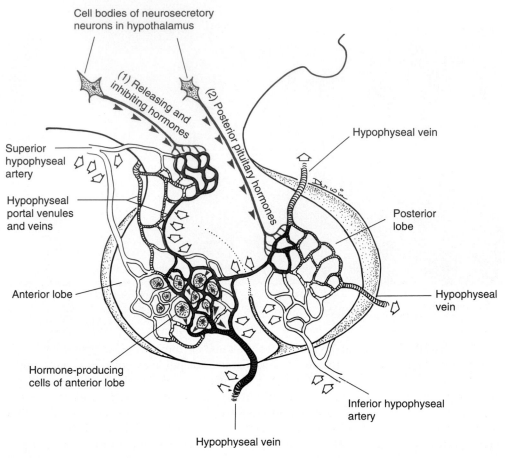

Cell bodies of neurosecretory
neurons in hypothalamus

(1) Releasing and
inhibiting hormones

(2) Posterior pituitary hormones

Hypophyseal vein

Superior
hypophyseal
artery

Hypophyseal
portal venules
and veins

Posterior
lobe

Anterior lobe

Hypophyseal
vein

Hormone-producing
cells of anterior lobe

Inferior hypophyseal
artery

Hypophyseal vein

Figure 16-5
Hypophysioportal circulation. Hypothalamic releasing and inhibiting hormones (1) reach anterior pituitary cells by way of this circulation (*left*). Posterior pituitary hormones (2) enter capillaries of the posterior pituitary (*right*). Open arrows indicate direction of blood flow; arrowheads indicate direction of hormone transport toward axon terminals.

hypothalamus. Most of their neurosecretory axon terminals are intimately associated with the fenestrated capillary plexus of the median eminence and infundibular stalk (see Fig. 16-5).

Posterior Lobe

The posterior lobe of the pituitary, alternatively known as the **pars nervosa** or **neurohypophysis**, is its pale-staining, neural part (see Fig. 16-3). It represents a posteroinferior extension of unmyelinated axons in the **hypothalamohypophyseal tracts**. Most of these axons belong to neurosecretory neurons with cell bodies that are situated in the **paraventricular nucleus** and **supraoptic nucleus** of the hypothalamus (Fig. 16-6). Neuronal cell bodies in these nuclei synthesize two peptide hormones that are released from axon terminals in the posterior lobe. The two peptides are produced by different cells. **Oxytocin** is synthesized chiefly by neuronal cell bodies in the paraventricular nucleus, whereas **vasopressin**, known also as **antidiuretic hormone (ADH)**, is synthesized chiefly by neuronal cell bodies in the supraoptic nucleus. Each hormone, complexed with its prohormone-derived carrier protein **(neurophysin)**, is transported in secretory granules to the axon terminals, where it is stored for release by exocytosis. Intracellular accumulations of these secretory granules may be

TABLE 16-4

HYPOTHALAMIC RELEASING AND RELEASE-INHIBITING HORMONES FOR ANTERIOR PITUITARY HORMONES

Growth hormone (GH)
   Releasing hormone (GHRH; somatocrinin)
   Inhibiting hormone (GIH or SRIH; somatostatin or SS)

Prolactin (PRL)
   Releasing hormone (PRH)
   Inhibiting hormone (PIH; dopamine or DA)

Adrenocorticotrophic hormone (ACTH; corticotropin)
   Corticotropin-releasing hormone (CRH)

Thyroid-stimulating hormone (TSH; thyrotropin)
   Thyrotropin-releasing hormone (TRH)*

Follicle-stimulating hormone (FSH) and luteinizing hormone (LH)
   Gonadotropin-releasing hormone (GnRH)**

---

* TRH also elicits prolactin secretion.
** Releases both FSH and LH.

discernible in appropriately stained LM sections as basophilic irregular masses called **Herring bodies**. The secreted hormone passes into fenestrated capillaries that border on the axon terminals. The posterior lobe also possesses its own population of small glial cells. Known as **pituicytes**, these inconspicuous cells are assumed to have a supporting function.

During labor, **oxytocin** (Gk. *oxys*, swift; *tokos*, birth) induces strong contractions of the myometrium (the uterine smooth muscle) that culminate in delivery of the newborn. Oxytocin also elicits the contraction of myoepithelial cells of mammary glands during nursing, causing milk ejection from the secretory alveoli (see Chapter 17). The antidiuretic action of **vasopressin**, namely that of augmenting the withdrawal of water from urinary filtrate passing along renal medullary collecting

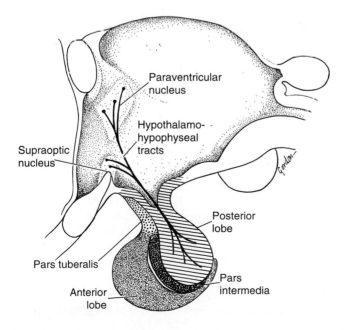

Figure 16-6
Hypothalamohypophyseal tracts extending from the paraventricular and supraoptic nuclei of the hypothalamus to the posterior lobe of the pituitary.

TABLE 16-5

PITUITARY DISORDERS: REPRESENTATIVE EXAMPLES			
Release Site and Hormone	Chief Target Tissues	Signs of Overproduction	Signs of Underproduction
Anterior Lobe			
Growth hormone (GH)	Skeletal tissues	**Gigantism**—long bones continue to grow after adolescence **Acromegaly**—some bones overgrow in response to late onset GH overproduction	**Dwarfism**—insufficient growth of long bones results in atypical short stature
Posterior Lobe			
Vasopressin (ADH)	Collecting tubules in kidney medulla	Excessive water retention leads to further complications	**Diabetes insipidus**—inadequate renal water resorption with voluminous watery urine requires excessive compensatory fluid ingestion

tubules, is described under filtrate Concentrating Mechanism in Chapter 15. Vasopressin also acts as a stimulus for ACTH secretion by corticotrophs.

CLINICAL IMPLICATIONS

Pituitary Disorders
The hypothalamus and its associated pituitary gland play key roles in adjusting the body's precise internal hormonal balance. Deficiencies or excesses of pituitary hormones, whether the result of substantially altered levels of hypothalamic stimulation, disease processes, or trauma affecting function of the pituitary itself, may profoundly affect metabolic processes. Many endocrine disorders are the result of exaggerated trophic responses to elevated levels of anterior pituitary hormones. Others are examples of inadequate trophic responses to diminished levels of these hormones. A few representative clinical disorders directly attributable to oversecretion or undersecretion of pituitary hormones are given in Table 16-5.

THYROID

The **thyroid gland** contains hormone-secreting cells of two distinct types. Endoderm-derived **thyroid follicular epithelial cells** produce **thyroid hormone**, which circulates predominantly as **thyroxine** (tetraiodothyronine, abbreviated to T_4) together with some **triiodothyronine** (T_3). Most of the circulating T_4 is converted into T_3, but both forms of the hormone can affect target cells. **Calcitonin**, the other hormone secreted by the thyroid, is made by **parafollicular cells** or **C cells** (C for *calcitonin*), which unlike the follicular epithelial cells are derived from neural crest.

The thyroid is a profusely vascular bilobed gland situated at the base of the larynx, largely inferior to it, with one lobe on each side of the trachea. This gland possesses an outer fascial sheath and an inner connective tissue capsule. Fine fibrous septa subdivide the parenchyma into poorly demarcated lobules essentially composed of spherical structural units called **thyroid follicles** (Plate

16-2). Simple cuboidal **thyroid follicular epithelial cells** constitute the epithelial lining of these extracellular storage compartments. Thyroid follicles are filled with the PAS-positive secretory glycoprotein, **thyroglobulin**. Known also as the **colloid** component of the gland, this stored glycoprotein undergoes **extracellular iodination** through combination of iodine with its tyrosyl residues. Thyroid peroxidase (**thyroperoxidase**), also produced by the follicular epithelial cells, promotes 1) oxidation of iodide, taken up from the circulation, to iodine and 2) binding of iodine to tyrosyl residues in the molecule. Stored extracellularly in its iodinated form, the thyroglobulin then remains continuously available for subsequent processing and production of thyroid hormone. Surrounding the follicle, and separated from it by the epithelial basement membrane, lies a minimal amount of delicate stromal connective tissue amply provided with fenestrated capillaries.

Thyroid Follicular Epithelial Cells

When stimulated to produce thyroid hormone, thyroid follicular epithelial cells show increased evidence of glycoprotein synthesis and secretion, including dilated rER, distended Golgi saccules, and abundant large secretory vesicles that deliver more thyroglobulin and thyroid peroxidase to the follicular lumen. The stimulated cells also bear more microvilli on their luminal surface, probably reflecting their increased resorptive activity. The supplementary peroxidase that they produce oxidizes the additional iodide that they take up from the circulation. Extracellular iodination takes place near the luminal surface of the cell membrane. Thyroglobulin secretion, intraluminal iodination, and formation of thyroid hormone through subsequent processing of the iodinated product proceed concurrently. To produce thyroid hormone, follicular epithelial cells submit globules of iodinated thyroglobulin that they have actively ingested to hydrolysis by lysosomal enzymes. Two products of this intracellular proteolysis are T_3 and T_4, which rapidly diffuse from the follicular cells and pass into the circulation by entering the adjacent fenestrated capillaries. T_3 and T_4, both regarded as constituents of thyroid hormone, play a key role in supporting the development, growth, and functional activities of most tissues and organ systems. Thyroid hormone is acknowledged as a virtually universal requirement for maintenance of normal levels of metabolic activity.

CLINICAL IMPLICATIONS

Level of Thyroid Activity
The functional activity of the thyroid is often indicated in part by the histological appearance of its follicles and their constituent follicular epithelial cells. Increased cell height (hypertrophy) and increased cell number in the follicular walls (hyperplasia) are indicative of *augmented* thyroid secretion. Increased thyroid secretion may be brought about by the trophic action of **TSH** from the anterior pituitary, but in many cases it is a trophic response to autoimmune antibodies (**thyroid-stimulating immunoglobulins, TSI**) to the TSH receptor. Other indications of TSH or TSI stimulation are 1) accelerated synthesis and iodination of colloid and 2) augmented endocytosis of colloid leading to increased production of thyroid hormone. The net result of such stimulation is depletion rather than expansion of the intraluminal colloid.

Dietary deficiency of iodide (which is broadly compensated for by the incorporation of iodide into table salt) does not permit normal levels of thyroid hormone production to be sustained. Diminished negative feedback on thyrotrophs by thyroid hormone leads to overproduction of TSH. The net result is marked hypertrophy and hyperplasia of thyroid follicular epithelial cells, with externally obvious enlargement of the thyroid (**goiter**). In contrast, elevation of the thyroid hormone level (**Graves' disease, hyperthyroidism**) is commonly associated with antibody-mediated inflammatory enlargement of the extrinsic eye muscles and intraorbital connective tissues, manifested by noticeable protrusion of the eyeballs (**exophthalmos**). Underproduction of thyroid hormone (**hypothyroidism**) in fetal life and infancy can lead to severe mental retardation and stunted body growth (**cretinism**), but consequences of hypothyroidism that is later in onset are less severe.

Parafollicular Cells (C Cells)

Widely dispersed throughout the thyroid are rounded, slightly larger pale-staining cells with a central spherical nucleus (see Plate 16-2). With the EM it may be seen that along with the follicular epithelial cells of a follicle, very small numbers of these larger cells lie internal to the follicular basement membrane. They are separated from thyroid colloid by attenuated interposed regions of follicular epithelial cells. Because of their position beside follicles, these larger cells are known as **parafollicular cells** (Gk. *para*, beside). Electron micrographs disclose that they have secretory granules containing the polypeptide hormone calcitonin, which accounts for their alternative name, **C cells**.

Calcitonin is a **calcium-lowering hormone** with antagonistic effects to parathyroid hormone (PTH). Whenever plasma calcium rises above its normal levels, parafollicular cells release their calcitonin by exocytosis. A primary target cell for calcitonin is the osteoclast. It will be recalled that the augmented bone resorption elicited by the antagonistic hormone, PTH, is the consequence of enlargement and increased resorptive activity of ruffled borders (the parts of osteoclasts specialized for matrix resorption). Calcitonin has an antagonistic effect, since it reduces the size and number of ruffled borders on stimulated osteoclasts and thus restricts the amount of calcium released through bone matrix resorption. Two other actions of calcitonin are that it reduces osteoclast numbers and augments renal calcium excretion. Because calcitonin overproduction or underproduction has no major consequences in humans, the physiological importance of calcitonin remains controversial.

PARATHYROIDS

Along the posterior border of the lobes of the thyroid, internal to its fascial sheath, lie four (occasionally two or six) **parathyroid glands**. These small, ovoid endoderm-derived glands are so named because of their anatomical position beside the thyroid. Each parathyroid possesses a thin capsule and delicate connective tissue septa that incompletely subdivide its parenchyma into lobules. Also present are capillaries, reticular fibers, and groups of fat cells that are seldom noticeable.

Chief Cells and Oxyphil Cells

The parenchymal cells of the thyroid, arranged as clumps and irregular wide cords, are of two distinct types, termed chief (principal) cells and oxyphil cells. The **chief cells** secrete PTH. They are small, round, and mostly pale-staining, with a central spherical nucleus (Plate 16-3). At first glance, they may seem to resemble a mass of small lymphocytes because of their small size and densely packed nuclei. Electron micrographs show that the chief cells contain a large Golgi complex, relatively few PTH secretory granules, and abundant glycogen, the presence of which accounts for their pale appearance in H&E-stained sections. Also present in the parathyroid glands is a smaller population of somewhat larger cells that are known as **oxyphil cells** because of their cytoplasmic acidophilia (one meaning of the Gk. *oxys* is acidic). These can often be recognized by their larger size and deeper pink color in H&E-stained sections (see Plate 16-3). Although larger than chief cells, the oxyphils generally have a smaller and slightly darker-staining nucleus. They are distributed as more or less isolated groups among the chief cells. Oxyphils appear in the parathyroids at around the age of puberty and are believed to represent chief cells that have reached a nonsecretory stage. In electron micrographs it may be seen that their cytoplasm is packed with large mitochondria, but the functional significance of this abundance is unclear.

Actions of Parathyroid Hormone

Parathyroid hormone (PTH) is a **calcium-raising hormone** antagonistic in action to calcitonin. Secreted by chief cells of the parathyroids whenever plasma calcium drops below normal, PTH stimulates osteoblasts to release several resorption-inducing factors. The osteoclast's response to these mediators is an increase of the combined area of its ruffled borders that leads to augmented resorptive activity. Following PTH administration, increased numbers of osteoclasts are present on resorbing bone surfaces. The possibility that PTH also regulates osteocyte functions is more controversial. Calcium ions liberated from bone matrix through increased bone resorption help to restore plasma calcium to normal levels. Other actions through which which PTH can compensate for a decrease in plasma calcium are by promoting 1) calcium resorption in the kidney tubules (while decreasing their phosphate resorption) and 2) the synthesis of **calcitriol**, a vitamin D_3 derivative that enhances gastrointestinal calcium absorption.

CLINICAL IMPLICATIONS

Tetany
Hormonally uncompensated trauma to the parathyroid glands during the course of neck surgery or unintentional removal of these glands (e.g., in thyroidectomy) is potentially fatal because the body depends on PTH secretion to maintain the normal plasma calcium level. If the plasma calcium concentration is allowed to drop, skeletal muscles in particular become hyperexcitable and overstimulated, undergoing uncontrolled contractile spasms (**tetany**). Severe laryngeal spasms may ultimately cut off the body's air supply and result in **asphyxia** (suffocation).

ADRENALS

The **adrenal (suprarenal) glands** secrete two classes of chemically unrelated adrenal hormones. The secretory epithelial cells in the outer region of the glands (the **adrenal cortex**, derived from mesoderm) secrete steroid hormones (**corticosteroids**) of three different subclasses. In contrast, the hormone-secreting cells in the central region (the **adrenal medulla**, derived from neural crest) secrete the catecholamine hormones **epinephrine** and **norepinephrine**. The distinctive association of two dissimilar kinds of hormone-producing cells with disparate developmental origins is due to the prenatal migration of neural crest derivatives from nearby developing sympathetic ganglia to the adrenal glands, in which they collect as a central diffuse mass. The adrenal medullary cells are therefore counterparts of **sympathetic ganglion cells** and in common with them produce **catecholamines**. The **fetal adrenal cortex** becomes active and then involutes. It is superseded by a **permanent adrenal cortex** that carries out the same activities postnatally. Appearing as a yellowish flattened mass, each adrenal gland is attached to the superomedial border of a kidney, internal to the surrounding fascia. Sections of an adrenal gland typically have a triangular outline (Fig. 16-7). The thick fibroelastic capsule, cortex, and medulla of the gland are readily distinguishable, especially under low magnification (see Fig. 16-7 and Plate 16-4). The cortical and medullary secretory cells abut on wide fenestrated capillaries into which the secreted hormones readily pass. The medulla receives both arterial blood and blood from the cortical capillaries, so cortical secretions can reach the medullary cells rapidly. The medullary venules empty into a large central medullary vein, the wide tributaries of which are often conspicuous in sections (see Plate 16-4*A*).

Adrenal Cortex

The unique organization of the adrenal cortex (see Fig. 16-7 and Plate 16-4) makes its histological recognition easy. From capsule to medulla, the cortex is made up of three zones, called the zona glomerulosa, zona fasciculata, and zona reticularis. Their names describe the arrangement of their respective hormone-secreting cells. The **zona glomerulosa** consists of more or less rounded groups of comparatively small secretory cells (L. *glomerulus*, little ball). The larger, more foamy-looking cells of the **zona fasciculata**, the thickest zone of the cortex, constitute slender radial columns, only one cell thick in some places, that border on long straight fenestrated capillaries. In the **zona reticularis**, comparable in thickness to the zona glomerulosa, the secretory cells are arranged as irregular anastomosing cords. Some of the nuclei in this zone have a pyknotic appearance. In all three zones, the secretory cells abut on fenestrated capillaries and synthesize steroid hormones, so they all contain abundant sER. In LM sections, it is common for zona fasciculata cells to appear foamy because of their substantial content of lipid droplets. Also present in these droplets are cholesteryl esters, required because all corticosteroids are derived from cholesterol.

CLINICAL IMPLICATIONS

Important Actions of Adrenocorticosteroids

The adrenocortical steroid hormones are of three major classes. **Mineralocorticoids** maintain the body's salt balance, **glucocorticoids** regulate carbohydrate and protein metabolism, and **sex hormones** affect reproductive function and promote development of secondary sexual characteristics. Adrenal mineralocorticoids and glucocorticoids play key roles in metabolic regulation and are absolutely essential to life. The main sources of the three classes of corticosteroids and the usual stimuli for their secretion are outlined in Figure 16-7. Only the zona glomerulosa cells have the enzymes necessary for synthesizing **aldosterone**. Representing the chief mineralocorticoid, aldosterone promotes sodium resorption from renal cortical collecting tubules and distal convoluted tubules. Aldosterone secretion is stimulated by angiotensins, which in turn are produced in response to renin released from renal JG cells (see Table 15-2). The steroid-secreting cells in the two inner zones (primarily those in the fasciculata, but also those in the reticularis) produce glucocorticoids, chiefly **cortisol (hydrocortisone)**. Important actions of cortisol are that it raises the blood sugar level by promoting production of glucose from proteins (notably, muscle proteins), and that it increases lipolysis in adipose tissue. Higher concentrations of cortisol can be used to alleviate inflammation and are immunosuppressive. Both the fasciculata and the reticularis also secrete **sex hormones**, which are chiefly weak androgens that if overproduced are potentially capable of 1) virilizing effects in women (**androgenital syndrome**) and 2) masculinizing effects on the external genitalia of female fetuses (**female pseudohermaphroditism**).

Actions of ACTH

The anterior pituitary hormone ACTH maintains the critical mass of the adrenal cortex by exerting a marked trophic effect on its steroid-producing cells. A plausible suggestion about the way ACTH maintains the secretory cell population and its corticosteroid secretory activity is through promotion of cell renewal and/or hypertrophy, especially in the zona glomerulosa, and functional maturation into cells of the fasciculata type. ACTH also maintains glomerulosa cell responsiveness to angiotensins, and stress-induced elevation of ACTH elicits a transient increase in their aldosterone output. A more long-lasting effect of ACTH, however, is that it augments the adrenal output of cortisol.

Adrenal Medulla

Simpler in organization than the adrenal cortex, the adrenal medulla contains anastomosing cords of rather pale-staining cells derived from neural crest. Grouped mainly around the medullary blood vessels, these large ovoid secretory cells border also on wide fenestrated capillaries (see Plate 16-4 and Figs. 16-7 and 16-8). Because their stored catecholamine has a strong affinity for chromium salts, the medullary secretory cells are known as **chromaffin cells**. With the EM, two types of chromaffin cells, one secreting **epinephrine** and the other, **norepinephrine**, are distinguishable on the

---

Figure 16-7
Cellular and functional organization of the three cortical zones and medulla of an adrenal gland.

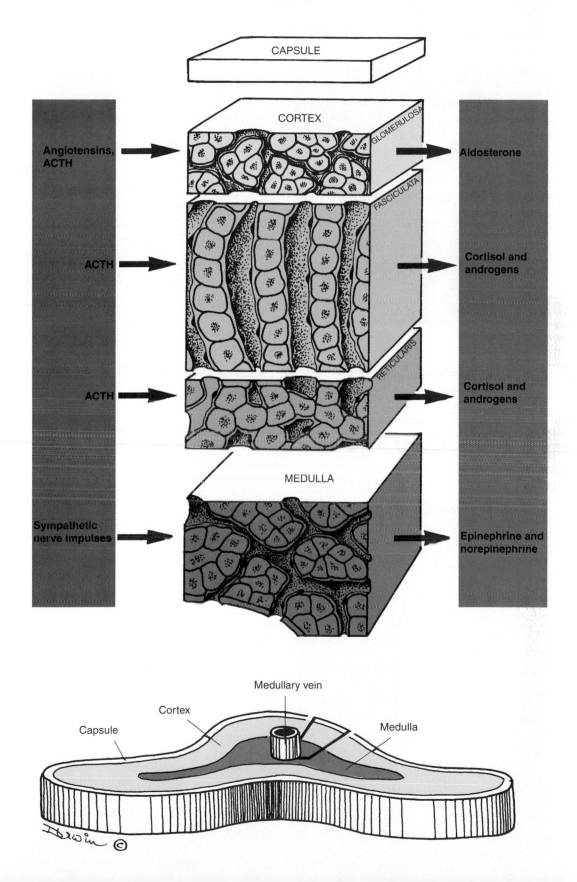

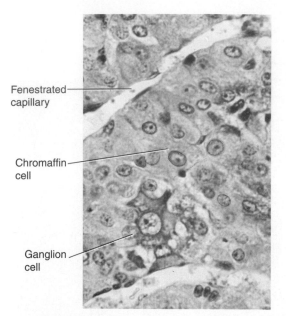

Fenestrated capillary

Chromaffin cell

Ganglion cell

Figure 16-8
Chromaffin cells and sympathetic ganglion cell of the adrenal medulla (high power).

basis of electron density and uniformity of shape of their storage granules (Fig. 16-9). Similar but much smaller aggregates of chromaffin cells present elsewhere in the body are known as **paraganglia**.

Adrenal medullary secretory cells are profusely innervated with **preganglionic sympathetic** fibers. Corresponding to **sympathetic ganglion cells**, they occupy the equivalent position in a sympathetic two-neuron chain. Sympathetic efferent impulses from preganglionic fibers are a stimulus

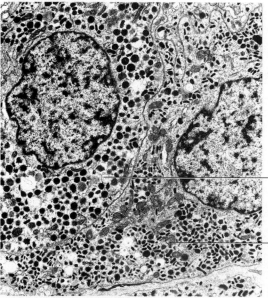

Epinephrine secreting chromaffin cell

Norepinephrine-secreting chromaffin cell

Figure 16-9
Electron micrograph showing the two secretory cell types in the adrenal medulla (baboon). Norepinephrine-containing secretory granules tend to be irregular or oval in appearance (a routine fixation artifact).

for exocytosis of their stored hormone (see Fig. 16-7). A small proportion of neural crest cells migrating to the adrenal medulla differentiate into multipolar sympathetic ganglion cells instead of chromaffin cells (see Fig. 16-8).

The chief adrenal medullary hormone is **epinephrine (adrenaline)**. Epinephrine and norepinephrine both exert profound effects on circulatory function. To different extents, they increase the force of cardiac contraction, accelerate heart rate, elevate blood pressure, and redirect blood to skeletal muscles and the liver. Among other effects, they also bring about the rapid conversion of glycogen to glucose and heighten the body's levels of awareness and responsiveness. These rapid, profound effects represent a major but relatively short-term response to emotional stress, physical stress, or physical exertion. Hence, the adrenal medullary hormones act as humoral extensions of the sympathetic nervous system that evoke rapid, bodywide responses in a variety of emergency situations.

PANCREATIC ISLETS

In addition to its acinar exocrine component, the pancreas possesses a diffuse endocrine component, also of endodermal origin, called the **pancreatic islets** or **islets of Langerhans**. Most numerous in the tail of the pancreas, these widely distributed groups of enteroendocrine cells produce the three amino acid-derived hormones **insulin, glucagon,** and **somatostatin**.

In H&E-stained sections, pancreatic islets appear as small, irregularly shaped light-staining areas sparsely scattered among the brightly stained acini (see Plate 13-8). Recognition of their specific secretory cell types requires immunofluorescent staining or other special staining. The Gomori method demonstrates large pink-staining **A (α) cells** distributed mostly in tiny groups around small blue-staining **B (β) cells** (Fig. 16-10). Other cell types, however, are also present but indistinguishable. Many fenestrated capillaries lie between the anastomosing cords of secretory cells, but they are

B (β) cells

A (α) cells

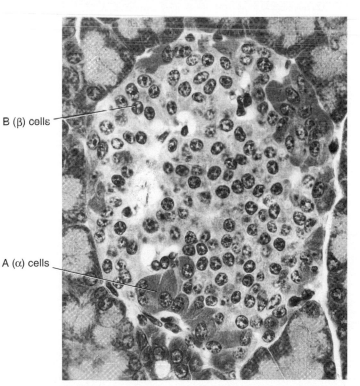

Figure 16-10
Pancreatic islet showing A and B cells (guinea pig pancreas, Gomori stain).

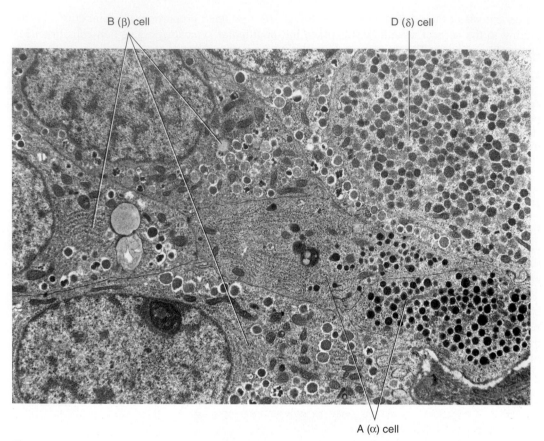

Figure 16-11
Electron micrograph showing three of the four secretory cell types in a pancreatic islet. Some B cell granules have irregularly-shaped crystalline contents.

inconspicuous in LM sections. From the surrounding sheath of loose connective tissue (which is so scant that it does not merit being called a capsule), reticular fibers extend into the islet and support its secretory cells and capillaries. Also, some of these cells are provided with autonomic efferent nerve endings. Parasympathetic stimulation of the pancreas, for example, augments secretion of insulin and glucagon by the islets.

TABLE 16-6

PANCREATIC ISLETS: SECRETORY CELL PRODUCTS

A (α) cells
  Glucagon

B (β) cells
  Insulin

D (δ) cells
  Somatostatin

F cells
  Pancreatic polypeptide

At the EM level, four different main secretory cell types are distinguishable in the islets, based on the size, electron density, and distribution of their granules (Fig. 16-11). For unequivocal identification by electron microscopy, however, specific immunocytochemical staining is essential for identification of their secretory product. The letters assigned to the pancreatic enteroendocrine cells, with the respective secretory product, are listed in Table 16-6. B (β) cells are the most common cells in the islets, whereas F cells are rare.

The main actions of the polypeptide hormone **insulin**, secreted in response to elevation of the blood sugar level, are to promote glucose transport into muscle cells and adipocytes, and to lower the blood sugar level still further by promoting glycogen synthesis in hepatocytes and muscle cells and also lipid synthesis in adipose tissue. The antagonistic polypeptide hormone **glucagon** raises the blood sugar level by promoting conversion of glycogen into glucose in the liver. In the metabolic disease **diabetes mellitus**, insulin deficiency or refractoriness to this hormone leads to an elevated blood sugar level (**hyperglycemia**), accompanied by glucose loss by way of the urine (**glycosuria**). The peptide hormone **somatostatin**, named from its first-discovered role as the hormone-inhibiting hormone for growth hormone, inhibits the release of many other hormones as well. Included among these are insulin, glucagon, and pancreatic polypeptide. Moreover, insulin inhibits glucagon secretion, and glucagon stimulates release of insulin and somatostatin. The intimate association of A, B, D, and F cells in the islets presumably facilitates paracrine regulation. **Pancreatic polypeptide**, secreted by F cells, exerts a suppressive action on pancreatic enzyme secretion, gallbladder emptying, and intestinal motility, thus reducing nutrient absorption. It also inhibits the somatostatin-releasing response triggered by intraluminal protein digestion.

PINEAL

Attached by a short stalk to the roof of the third ventricle is the **pineal body (epiphysis cerebri)**. Neuroectodermal in origin, this small median brain appendage is a tiny endocrine gland that produces the indoleamine **melatonin**. This hormone-like derivative of serotonin, or some related mediator, is believed to exert a suppressive effect on gonadotrophin secretion and thereby inhibit gonadal growth and function.

Extending into the pineal body from its thin, pia-derived connective tissue capsule are irregular trabeculae and septa that subdivide the interior of the gland into poorly demarcated lobules. Pineal secretory cells, termed **pinealocytes**, are large and pale-staining, with a large ovoid nucleus and cytoplasmic peripheral extensions that have club-shaped tips. To some extent, pinealocytes resemble neurons. Between these secretory cells lie numerous continuous capillaries and some neuroglia that resemble fibrous astrocytes. An additional feature of this gland is the presence of calcified concretions (**pineal sand** or **brain sand**) of unknown significance.

Pinealocytes synthesize and secrete **melatonin** primarily during periods when no light enters the eyes. Regulation of melatonin production is also dependent on sympathetic postganglionic efferent stimulation. The principal role of melatonin appears to be prevention of precocious gonadal function. Such a role is consistent with the fact that the pineal is relatively large during infancy but diminishes in size just before puberty. Melatonin, or some other mediator produced by the pineal, apparently exerts a suppressive effect on the release of gonadotrophin-releasing hormone, and it may also decrease the responsiveness of pituitary gonadotrophs to this releasing hormone.

Summary

The principal features of the endocrine organs described in this chapter are summarized in Table 16-7.

TABLE 16-7

ENDOCRINE ORGANS*: PRINCIPAL FEATURES

Endocrine Organ	Principal Secretory Cell Types	Hormone	Chief Direct or Indirect Target Cells	Principal Actions
Pituitary				
Anterior lobe (epithelial glandular tissue)	Somatotrophs (acidophil)	GH	Chondrocytes (in epiphyseal plates)	Promotes skeletal growth
	Mammotrophs (acidophil)	PRL	Mammary alveolar cells	Promotes milk secretion
	Corticotrophs (basophil)	ACTH	Adrenal cortical cells	Promotes growth and secretory activity of adrenal cortex
		MSH**	Melanocytes	Promotes melanization
	Thyrotrophs (basophil)	TSH	Thyroid follicular epithelial cells	Promotes growth and secretory activity of thyroid follicles
	Gonadotrophs	FSH	Ovarian follicular cells	Promotes ovarian follicular maturation
			Sertoli cells of testis	Promotes spermatogenesis through androgen binding
		LH	Ovarian thecal, follicular, and lutein cells	Promotes ovulation and luteinization
			Interstitial (Leydig) cells of testis	Promotes spermatogenesis by promoting androgen secretion
Posterior lobe (nervous tissue)	Secretory neurons in hypothalamic paraventricular nucleus	Oxytocin	Uterine smooth muscle cells; mammary myo-epithelial cells	Promotes parturition; promotes milk ejection when nursing
	Secretory neurons in hypothalamic supraoptic nucleus	Vasopressin (=ADH)	Renal medullary collecting tubules	Promotes water resorption by kidneys
Thyroid	Follicular epithelial cells	Thyroid hormone (T_4 and T_3)	Broad range	Maintains basal metabolic rate
	Parafollicular cells	Calcitonin	Osteoclasts; renal tubule epithelial cells	Decreases plasma calcium by inhibiting bone resorption and reducing renal calcium resorption
Parathyroid	Chief cells	PTH	Osteoclasts; renal tubule epithelial cells	Increases plasma calcium by promoting bone resorption and increasing renal calcium resorption
Adrenal cortex	Zona glomerulosa cells	Aldosterone	Renal cortical collecting tubules and distal convoluted tubules	Promotes sodium resorption
	Zona fasciculata and zona reticularis cells	Cortisol	Broad range, incuding hepatocytes and adipocytes	Promotes conversion of proteins to glucose + other effects on glucose availability
		Sex hormones (chiefly weak androgens)	Broad range	Masculinizing effects if overproduced

(continued)

TABLE 16-7

ENDOCRINE ORGANS*: PRINCIPAL FEATURES *(CONTINUED)*

Endocrine Organ	Principal Secretory Cell Types	Hormone	Chief Direct or Indirect Target Cells	Principal Actions
Adrenal medulla	Chromaffin cells	Epinephrine and norepinephrine	Broad range	Circulatory and other adjustments for dealing with emergency situations
Pancreatic islets	A (α) cells	Glucagon	Hepatocytes	Raises blood glucose
	B (β) cells	Insulin	Broad range	Lowers blood glucose
	D (δ) cells	Somatostatin	Broad range	Inhibits the release of insulin, glucagon, and several other hormones
Pineal	Pinealocytes	Melatonin	Hypothalamic neurons producing GnRH; gonadotrophs	Delays reproductive development until appropriate age (presumed role)

* Excluding ovaries (see Chap. 17) and testes (see Chap. 18).

** Activity largely attributable to ACTH.

Bibliography

General

Berridge MJ. The molecular basis of communication within the cell. Sci Am 253(4):142, 1985.

Fujita T, Iwanaga T, Kusumato Y, Yoshie S. Paraneurons and neurosecretion. In: Farner DS, Lederis K, eds. Neurosecretion: Molecules, Cells, Systems. New York, Plenum, 1982.

Ganong WF. Review of Medical Physiology, ed 17. Norwalk, CT, Appleton & Lange, 1995, pp 290–378.

Hadley ME. Endocrinology, ed 4. Upper Saddle River, NJ, Prentice-Hall, 1996.

Motta PM, ed. Ultrastructure of Endocrine Cells and Tissues. Boston, Martinus Nijhoff, 1984.

Snyder SH. The molecular basis of communication between cells. Sci Am 253(4):132, 1985.

Pituitary and Hypothalamus

Bergland RM, Page RB. Pituitary—brain vascular relations: a new paradigm. Science 204:18, 1979.

Bhatnagar AS, ed. The Anterior Pituitary Gland. New York, Raven Press, 1983.

Brownstein MJ, Russel JT, Gainer H. Synthesis, transport, and release of posterior pituitary hormones. Science 207:373, 1980.

Eipper BA, Mains RE. Structure and biosynthesis of pro-adrenocorticotropin/endorphin and related peptides. Endocr Rev 1:1, 1980.

Frawley LS, Boockfor FR. Mammosomatotropes: presence and functions in normal and neoplastic pituitary tissue. Endocr Rev 12:337, 1991.

Horvath E, Kovacs K. Pituitary gland. Pathol Res Pract 183:129, 1988.

McCann SM. Luteinizing-hormone-releasing hormone. N Engl J Med 296:797, 1977.

Page RB, Munger BL, Bergland RM. Scanning microscopy of pituitary vascular casts. Am J Anat 146:273, 1976.

Phillips LS, Vassilopoulou-Sellin R. Somatomedins. N Engl J Med 302:371, 1980.

Reichlin S. Somatostatin I. N Engl J Med 309:1495, 1983.

Reichlin S. Somatostatin II. N Engl J Med 309:1556, 1983.

Thyroid

Ekholm R. Biosynthesis of thyroid hormones. Int Rev Cytol 120:243, 1990.

Fujita H. Fine structure of the thyroid cell. Int Rev Cytol 40:197, 1975.

Fujita H. Functional morphology of the thyroid. Int Rev Cytol 113:145, 1988.

Oppenheimer JH. Thyroid hormone action at the cellular level. Science 203:971, 1979.

Parathyroids and Thyroid Parafollicular Cells

Austin LA, Heath H. Calcitonin: physiology and pathophysiology. N Engl J Med 304:269, 1981.

Bellows CG, Ishida H, Aubin JE, Heersche JNM. Parathyroid hormone reversibly suppresses the differentiation of osteoprogenitor cells into functional osteoblasts. Endocrinology 127:3111, 1990.

Bilezekian JP, Marcus R, Levine MA, eds. The Parathyroids: Basic and Clinical concepts. New York, Raven
Press, 1994.

Bonga SEW, Pang PKT. Control of calcium regulating hormones in the vertebrates: parathyroid hormone,
calcitonin, prolactin, and stanniocalcin. Int Rev Cytol 128:139, 1991.

Farley JR, Tarbaux NM, Hall SL, Linkhart TA, Baylink DJ. The anti-bone-resorptive agent calcitonin also
acts in vitro to directly increase bone formation and bone cell proliferation. Endocrinology 123:159, 1988.

King GJ, Holtrop ME, Raisz LG. The relation of ultrastructural changes in osteoclasts to resorption in bone
cultures stimulated with parathyroid hormone. Metab Bone Dis Rel Res 1:67, 1978.

Nunez EA, Gershon MD. Cytophysiology of thyroid parafollicular cells. Int Rev Cytol 52:1, 1978.

Talmage RV. The physiological significance of calcitonin. In: Peck WA ed. Bone and Mineral Research Annual, vol 1. Amsterdam, Excerpta Medica, 1983, p 74.

Adrenal Cortex

Blaschko H, Sayers G, Smith AD, eds. Adrenal Gland. In: Handbook of Physiology, sect 7. Endocrinology.
Washington, DC, American Physiological Society, 1975.

Idelman S. Ultrastructure of the mammalian adrenal cortex. Int Rev Cytol 27:181, 1970.

Long JA, Jones AL. Observations on the fine structure of the adrenal cortex of man. Lab Invest 17:355, 1967.

Neville AM, O'Hare MJ. The Human Adrenal Cortex. Berlin, Springer-Verlag, 1982.

Nussdorfer GC. Cytophysiology of the adrenal cortex. Int Rev Cytol 98:1, 1986.

Nussdorfer GC, Mazzocchi G, Meneghelli V. Cytophysiology of the adrenal zona fasciculata. Int Rev Cytol
55:291, 1978.

Adrenal Medulla

Brown WJ, Barajas L, Latta H. The ultrastructure of the human adrenal medulla: with comparative studies of
white rat. Anat Rec 169:173, 1971.

Carmichael SW. The Adrenal Medulla, vols 1–3. Annual Research Reviews. Montreal, Eden Press, 1979–
1984

Carmichael SW, Winkler H. The adrenal chromaffin cell. Sci Am 253(2):40, 1985.

Pancreatic Islets

Clemons DR, Cohick WS. The insulin-like growth factors. Annu Rev Physiol 55:131, 1993.

Cooperstein SJ, Watkins D, eds. The Islets of Langerhans: Biochemistry, Physiology, and Pathology. New
York, Academic Press, 1981.

Orci L, Perrelet A. The morphology of the A-cell. In: Unger RH, Orci L, eds. Glucagon: Physiology, Pathophysiology, and Morphology of the Pancreatic A-Cells. New York, Elsevier North-Holland, 1981, p 3.

Orci L, Vassalli J-D, Perrelet A. The insulin factory. Sci Am 256(9):85, 1988.

Steiner DF, James DE. Cellular and molecular biology of the beta cell. Diabetologia 35:S41, 1992.

Pineal

Brinkley S. The Pineal: Endocrine and Nonendocrine Function. Englewood Cliffs, NJ, Prentice Hall, 1988.

Hastings MH, Vance G, Maywood E. Some reflections on the phylogeny and function of the pineal. Experientia 45:903, 1989.

Reiter RJ. The pineal and its hormones in the control of reproduction in mammals. Endocr Rev 1:109, 1980.

Reiter RJ. Mechanisms of control of reproductive physiology by the pineal gland and its hormones. Adv Pineal Res 2:109, 1987.

Wurtman RJ, Axelrod J. The pineal as a neuroendocrine transducer. Hosp Pract 15(1):82, 1980.

CHAPTER 17

Female Reproductive System

OBJECTIVES

When you know the contents of this chapter, you should be able to do the following:

- Explain how haploid ova are derived from diploid oogonia
- Recognize four different maturation stages of ovarian follicles (including follicle-derived structures) present in the proliferative phase of the menstrual cycle
- Describe and discuss the significance of the distinctive blood vessels supplying the superficial part of the endometrium
- Recognize the endometrial histological changes associated with the proliferative and secretory phases of the menstrual cycle and state the hormones that characterize these phases
- Summarize how the body of the uterus differs from the cervix
- Name a peptide hormone released during labor and breast feeding and specify its target cells
- State the histological changes occurring in the breast during each half of pregnancy

Important functions of the female reproductive system are 1) to produce **ova** (female **germ cells**) through the process of **oogenesis**; 2) to facilitate meeting of female germ cells and spermatozoa and hence promote **fertilization**; 3) to maintain implanted conceptuses throughout their **gestation** period; and 4) to nurture infants postnatally through the process of **lactation**. The parts of the system that enable these various activities to be carried out are listed in Table 17-1. Ova are produced by the **ovaries**, which are bilateral almond-shaped organs lying in the pelvic cavity, attached to the uterus by the broad ligaments and ovarian ligaments. The relatively small central ovarian **medulla** is surrounded by a wide **cortex** that contains characteristic epithelial vesicular structures called **ovarian follicles**. Covering the peritoneal surface of the ovaries is a **simple cuboidal epithelium** that is continuous with peritoneal simple squamous mesothelium. When ovulation occurs, germ cells are therefore liberated into the peritoneal cavity. A fifth key function of the ovaries is that they produce the female sex hormones **estrogen** and **progesterone**.

Every 28 days or so, a ripening follicle becomes mature and releases a germ cell that has reached the **secondary oocyte** stage, which is the stage prior to formation of the ovum (see Fig. 17-1). No ovum is formed, however, unless fertilization ensues (see Table 17-3). Following oocyte release, which is known as **ovulation**, the residual follicular cells of the ruptured follicle transform into the

Table 17-1

FEMALE REPRODUCTIVE SYSTEM: COMPONENTS

Ovaries

Uterine tubes (fallopian tubes; oviducts)

Uterus
    Myometrium
    Endometrium
    Cervix

Placenta

Vagina

External genitalia

Mammary glands (breast)

---

predominant hormone-producing cell type of a **corpus luteum**. After functioning for 10 to 12 days, this generally short-lived endocrine gland involutes and becomes replaced by scar tissue (see Fig. 17-4). Gestation, however, requires the sustained secretory activity of an enlarged corpus luteum that remains active for 3 months or so before beginning to involute. At ovulation, the secondary oocyte liberated into the fluid-filled peritoneal cavity is swept into the associated **uterine tube** by ciliary action on finger-like **fimbriae** arranged as a fringe around the funnel-shaped proximal end or **infundibulum** (L., funnel) of the uterine tube. The ciliated, muscular-walled uterine tube undergoes

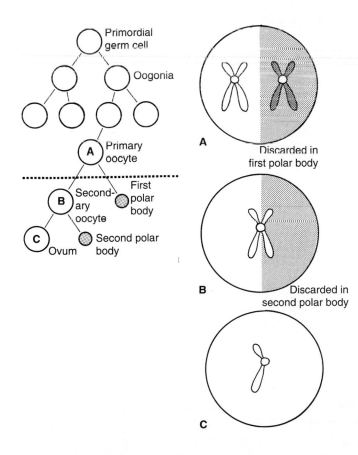

Figure 17-1
Schematic diagram of meiosis in females, showing a representative pair of homologous chromosomes in a primary oocyte (A) and their sequential segregation in the production of an ovum. Dotted line indicates the reduction division. (*A*) Primary oocyte (diploid); (*B*) secondary oocyte (haploid); (*C*) ovum (haploid).

peristaltic contractions that propel the oocyte toward the uterus. Fertilization generally occurs in the **ampulla**, a wide region of the uterine tube characterized by elaborate longitudinal folding of its lining (see Fig. 17-5 and Plate 17-4).

Lying medially in the pelvic cavity, the **uterus** has the shape of an inverted, slightly flattened hollow pear. The wide upper part is known as the **uterine body**, and the narrower inferior third is known as the **uterine cervix** (see Fig. 17-6). At the **uterine ostium** (the **external os** of the cervix) the **cervical canal** opens into the upper end of the **vagina** (see Fig. 17-6). The substantial smooth muscle coat that comprises the bulk of the uterine wall is called the **myometrium**. It is lined by the **endometrium** (Gk. *endon*, within), a mucous membrane with simple tubular exocrine glands. Phases of desquamation (sloughing) of most of the mucosa lead to subsequent phases of regeneration, glandular secretion, and regression (see Fig. 17-4). Every 28 days or so (L. *mensis*, month), a **menstrual cycle** begins when the endometrium begins to slough away. The menstrual cycle therefore starts on the first day of menstruation. Over the next 4 to 5 days, degenerating endometrial tissue, glandular secretions, and blood are lost as menstrual flow. This initial phase of the cycle is followed by the proliferative phase in which the endometrial cells divide, regenerating the endometrium. Approximately midway through the cycle, ovulation occurs and the endometrium enters the secretory phase (see Fig. 17-4). The endometrium is now appropriately prepared for supporting an implanted conceptus. If implantation occurs, cyclic loss and renewal of the endometrium is interrupted, and the next menstrual period does not occur when expected. Unless this happens, the ovarian hormone levels fall during the last day or two of the menstrual cycle. The sudden decline results in vascular disturbances that interfere with endometrial blood supply and bring about menstruation.

The **vagina** (L., sheath) is a muscular-walled, flattened tube. Its stratified squamous nonkeratinizing epithelial lining is raised into transverse folds (**rugae**). In addition to its role in sexual intercourse, it functions as the lower end of the birth canal. The **external genitalia (vulva)** include the mons pubis, labia majora and minora, and clitoris. The thin skin on the mons pubis and labia majora is supplied with hair follicles and supported by subcutaneous adipose tissue. The labia minora are delicate folds of thin skin that lack hair follicles. The clitoris, representing a rudimentary counterpart of the penis, contains erectile tissue and numerous sensory receptors, but does not enclose the urethra as is the case in males.

The early stages of **oogenesis** (**ovum** production) occur in prenatal life. Oogenesis and spermatogenesis nevertheless have certain features in common, so we shall begin with a description of the basis of germ cell formation.

OOGENESIS

Somatic cells typically contain 23 chromosome pairs. Each parent provides one chromosome of each pair. Because a somatic cell possesses two representations of each chromosome, the total complement of 46 chromosomes is designated the **diploid** (Gk. *diplous*, twofold) chromosome number. When a germ cell forms, it receives only one chromosome of each pair. Its complement of 23 chromosomes is therefore designated the **haploid** (Gk. *haplous*, single) chromosome number. The two-staged division process through which haploid germ cells are produced from their diploid precursor cells is known as **meiosis** (Gk., diminution). In females, the first meiotic division (**meiosis I**) is extremely prolonged (see Table 17-3). Meiosis I is the reduction division that results in the daughter cells receiving only the haploid number of chromosomes. The second meiotic division (**meiosis II**) is essentially a mitotic division that follows the first division without intervening replication of nuclear DNA. Only one ovum results from the two consecutive maturation divisions. The other daughter cells (**polar bodies**) are small and degenerate rapidly.

In females, **primordial germ cells** arising from yolk sac endoderm migrate to the developing ovaries and differentiate into **oogonia** (see top of Fig. 17-1 and also Table 17-3). In early fetal life, a series of consecutive mitotic divisions produces substantial numbers of oogonia, some of which survive and develop into larger cells called **primary oocytes**. Thus, primary oocytes are formed in prenatal life. These diploid cells then commence meiosis I. The first meiotic division is not completed until after puberty, however, and its completion occurs on an individual basis in follicles that are ready to rupture at the ovary surface (see Table 17-3).

First Meiotic Division

When a primary oocyte enters the long **prophase** of meiosis I, its 46 chromosomes become microscopically discernible as long, slender threads. This first stage of prophase I is therefore described as **leptotene** (Gk. *leptos*, slender; *tainia*, ribbon). Leptotene is followed by four further stages of prophase, making prophase I more complicated than a mitotic prophase (Table 17-2). In the next stage, called **zygotene** (Gk. *zygon*, yoked), the homologous chromosomes (and also the X and Y chromosomes if these are both present) pair with each other and become tightly apposed. Each pair of apposed homologues is termed a **bivalent**. In the third stage of prophase I, **pachytene** (Gk. *pachytes*, thickness), the homologues of each bivalent shorten and thicken owing to further chromatin condensation. By the fourth stage, **diplotene** (Gk. *diplous*, twofold), it is histologically evident that each homologue consists of two sister chromatids.

The bivalent now contains four chromatids. One homologue in the bivalent was originally entirely maternal. The other was entirely paternal. During diplotene, however, paired chromosomes can exchange gene-containing portions in the following way. Part of a chromatid (belonging to either homologue of the bivalent) may come to lie across a chromatid belonging to the other homologue, forming a **chiasma** (Gk., two crossing lines or X-shaped crossing). Configurations of this kind predispose chromatids to breakage at the sites where there is a crossover. When the broken ends reattach, the chromatid fragment may adhere to the remainder of the *homologous chromatid fragment* instead of reconstituting the original chromatid. The **crossing over** that occurs between homologous chromatids results in the exchange of some maternal and paternal genes, with resulting new gene combinations that are passed on to germ cells. After diplotene, both chromosomes of each bivalent may therefore bear genes from both parents.

Table 17-2

MEIOSIS STAGES
Meiosis I
Prophase
Leptotene
Zygotene
Pachytene
Diplotene
Diakinesis*
Metaphase
Anaphase
Telophase
Meiosis II
Prophase
Metaphase
Anaphase
Telophase

* In oogenesis, diakinesis is extended as **dictyotene**.

The last stage of prophase I is termed **diakinesis**. Prenatal development of the primary oocyte is completed by its entering a protracted resting stage known as **dictyotene** (see Table 17-2). The primary oocyte remains at this stage until sexual maturity has been attained. Throughout this long suspension of prophase, unique to oogenesis, the chromatin is partly extended (Gk. *diktyon*, net) and the nucleus, although still in prophase, appears as if it were in interphase. The primary oocyte stays in dictyotene from fetal life until just before the time of ovulation and release of the secondary oocyte (Table 17-3).

CLINICAL IMPLICATIONS

Down Syndrome

The length of dictyotene can be substantial because women are able to ovulate until they reach menopause, generally at the age of 45 to 55 years. This long delay is a predisposing factor for **Down syndrome (trisomy 21)**, the risk of which increases with maternal age at the time of the child's conception. In some cases of Down syndrome, the numerical chromosomal anomaly arises during anaphase I. Under normal circumstances, the two homologues of a bivalent would separate at this stage. Failure of two homologues to part company at anaphase is known as **nondisjunction**. If because of nondisjunction a secondary oocyte receives *two* number 21 chromosomes instead of one, and it then gives rise to a fertilized ovum, the infant has *three* number 21 chromosomes and has Down syndrome. In other cases, this syndrome results from inheritance of only an extra piece of a number 21 chromosome translocated onto another chromosome.

Completion of First Meiotic Division

In response to high LH levels, the process of meiosis resumes in the preovulatory primary oocyte that will give rise to the secondary oocyte. The nuclear envelope fragments, a spindle forms, and the primary oocyte enters metaphase I, at which stage its bivalents align in the equatorial plane. The centromeres of the two sister chromatids constituting each homologue of the bivalent, however, fail to dissociate from each other. As a result, when the primary oocyte reaches anaphase I, the two *homologues* of each bivalent separate from each other, but the two sister *chromatids* of each homologue do not. In other words, when the homologues segregate to the two daughter cells, each homologue remains represented by its paired sister chromatids. X and Y chromosomes, if present, also pair over a short distance, forming a partial bivalent, and then segregate to the two daughter cells. The fate of representative paired homologues is shown schematically in Figure 17-1. As a result of the **first maturation division** (conceptually represented by unshaded and shaded halves in Figure 17-1A), each daughter cell of the primary oocyte receives the dual chromosomes representing closely associated, paired sister chromatids. This unique chromosomal allocation results in each daughter cell receiving only 23 dual chromosomes (each representing paired sister chromatids) instead of 46 separate, single chromosomes as in a mitotic division. Thus, in contrast to the primary oocyte, which is *diploid* (see Fig. 17-1A), the secondary oocyte (derived from the left half of the primary oocyte as oriented in Fig. 17-1A, and shown again in Fig. 17-1B) is *haploid*. It should be appreciated that the terms *diploid* and *haploid* refer to the total number of chromosomes present in the cell, regardless of whether they are single (e.g., single, separate chromosomes characterizing G_1) or dual (e.g., paired sister chromatids in this case; pre-mitotically replicated chromosomes in G_2 cells). Individual chromosomes originating from either parent have an equal chance of segregating to either of the daughter cells. A further unusual feature of the first maturation division is that the two daughter cells are of unequal size. The larger cell has ovum-forming capability and is termed the **secondary oocyte**. The smaller cell, called the **first polar body**, is unable to produce an ovum.

Table 17-3

OOGENESIS STAGES

Primordial germ cells (2n)*
| Migrate from yolk sac to
| ovaries and differentiate
▼ into

Oogonia (2n)
| Proliferate by mitosis and
▼ differentiate into

Primary oocyte (2n)
| Enters prophase of 1st
| meiotic division, then
▼ passes into dictyotene

Oogenesis is suspended from
prenatal life until just before
ovulation, which is triggered
by the midcycle LH surge

| Completes 1st maturation
▼ (reduction) division

Secondary oocyte (n)* + 1st
polar body (n)

| Secondary oocyte released
| at ovulation
| Misses S phase
| Enters 2nd maturation
| division, but this stops
| in metaphase unless
| fertilization ensues
| Fertilization results in
| completion of 2nd
▼ maturation division

Ovum (n) + 2nd polar body (n)

* 2n denotes the diploid chromosome number, n denotes the haploid
number.

Second Meiotic Division

The only unusual feature of meiosis II (see Tables 17-2 and 17-3) is that the secondary oocyte undergoes its **second maturation division** without replicating nuclear DNA, that is, without first going through an S phase. At metaphase II, the 23 dual chromosomes (paired sister chromatids) present in the haploid secondary oocyte align in the equatorial plane. At anaphase II, the dual chromosomes split at their centromeres and their component sister chromatids separate as in an ordinary mitosis. The second maturation division is represented by the two halves of the secondary oocyte shown in Figure 17-1B. As a result of this division, each daughter cell receives one chromatid from each dual chromosome. Thus, the **ovum** (derived from the left half of the secondary oocyte as oriented in Fig. 17-1B, and shown again in Fig. 17-1C) is again *haploid*, receiving 23 single chromosomes. The other daughter cell, the **second polar body**, is much smaller and of no further use for reproduction.

At fertilization, a spermatozoon nucleus is introduced into the cytoplasm of the the ovum thus produced. The haploid nucleus of the ovum is called the **female pronucleus** and that of the spermatozoon, the **male pronucleus**. The pronuclei first pass through an S phase and then fuse, each contributing its 23 replicated (dual) chromosomes. A mitotic spindle forms, and the first two blastomeres each receive one of the chromatids of all 46 dual chromosomes and are therefore diploid.

OVARIES

Until menopause, postpubertal ovaries contain **ovarian follicles** showing various stages of maturation (Fig. 17-2). The connective tissue cortex in which they lie consists mainly of spindle-shaped, fibroblast-like stromal cells, interspersed with fine collagen fibers and arranged in a distinctive swirly pattern (Plate 17-1). Near the simple cuboidal surface epithelium of the ovaries, however, the stromal cells and fibers are arranged more or less parallel to the surface and constitute a whitish fibrous outer layer termed the **tunica albuginea** (L. *albus*, white; see Fig. 17-2). The ovarian medulla contains some relatively large blood vessels, notably coiled arteries and convoluted veins.

Follicular Maturation

The periphery of the ovarian cortex contains a number of follicles that have not yet responded to FSH. In the small **primordial follicles**, the primary oocyte, still at the dictyotene stage, is enclosed by a single layer of relatively flat **ovarian follicular epithelial cells**, also known as **granulosa cells** (see Fig. 17-2 and Plate 17-1). Beginning at puberty, a cyclic increase in the secretion of FSH by gonadotrophs of the anterior pituitary stimulates consecutive groups of follicles to enlarge and secrete

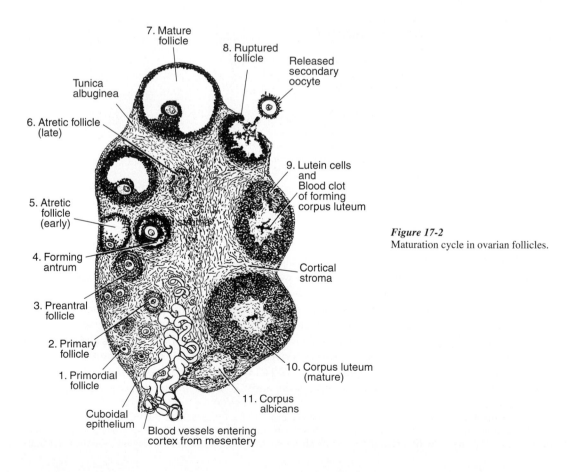

Figure 17-2
Maturation cycle in ovarian follicles.

estrogen in sufficient quantities to support full reproductive function. Twenty to 50 ovarian follicles respond to FSH each month. Before becoming stimulated by FSH, the follicular cells gain additional FSH receptors and become columnar in shape. The primary oocyte within them grows and acquires a refractile covering of extracellular glycoprotein, the **zona pellucida** (see Plate 17-1 and Fig. 17-3). This outer layer is traversed by tiny follicular cell processes and oocyte microvilli. A follicle that has begun to enlarge because of growth of its oocyte and follicular cells, and that has acquired at least two layers of these cells, is described as a **primary follicle** (see Plate 17-1 and Fig. 17-2). The next stage reflects a hypertrophic, hyperplastic response of the follicular cells to FSH. As a result of proliferation, the follicular walls become multilayered. The zona pellucida appears more distinct, and the stromal cells surrounding the follicle differentiate into a capsule-like **theca** (Gk. *theke*, box). Only one of the maturing follicles, however, completes the maturation process in each cycle; the remainder degenerate and become recognizable **atretic follicles**. Follicular maturation requires almost 3 months to reach completion and proceeds as follows. By the **secondary follicle** stage, tiny pools of **follicular fluid** begin to form among the follicular cells, which are more generally referred to as **granulosa cells** at this stage. The fluid-filled intercellular spaces gradually coalesce as an **antrum** containing follicular fluid (see Figs. 17-2 and 17-3). Supporting the oocyte in the midst of this nutritive fluid is a **cumulus oophorus** (Gk., egg-bearing heap) of granulosa cells.

Meanwhile, the surrounding theca gives rise to a cellular, well-vascularized **theca interna** that merges imperceptibly with a more fibrous **theca externa**. The vascular theca interna produces nutritive follicular fluid as an exudate. Its spindle-shaped **thecal cells** secrete **androgens** that pass inward to the granulosa cells, which

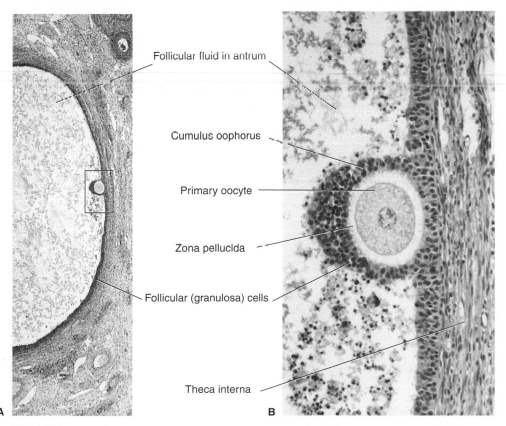

Follicular fluid in antrum

Cumulus oophorus

Primary oocyte

Zona pellucida

Follicular (granulosa) cells

Theca interna

A   B

Figure 17-3
Maturing ovarian follicle. (*A*) Very low power view. (*B*) Area outlined in *A* (medium power).

convert them into **estrogen**. Additional scattered groups of secretory stromal cells, collectively referred to as a diffuse ovarian **interstitial gland**, are believed to act as a subsidiary source of androgen substrate.

The dominant follicle of the cycle continues to grow until it approaches maturity and bulges from the ovarian surface as a **mature, tertiary,** or **graafian follicle** (see Fig. 17-2). **Ovulation** is triggered by a midcycle surge of LH (see Table 17-3), for which hormone the thecal cells and pre-ovulatory granulosa cells have the surface receptor. Oocyte release is preceded by follicular fluid accumulation, detachment of the oocyte and its investing granulosa cells from the cumulus oophorus, and completion of meiosis I (see Table 17-3). The secondary oocyte becomes extruded into the peritoneal cavity through rupture of the dominant follicle. Still enclosed by its **corona radiata** of attached granulosa cells, the secondary oocyte enters the associated uterine tube (see Fig. 17-5) and begins its second maturation division. Unless fertilization occurs, this maturation division proceeds only as far as metaphase II. Ovum formation is completed when fertilization occurs (see Table 17-3).

The second important action of LH is that of luteinizing ruptured follicles. Granulosa and theca interna cells remaining in the post-ovulatory follicle undergo LH-induced transformation and form a transitory endocrine organ known as a **corpus luteum**. Because of its content of pigmented **lutein cells** (L. *luteus*, yellow), the corpus luteum is yellow.

Corpus Luteum

Initially, minor bleeding caused by rupture of the mature follicle at ovulation results in the follicle filling with blood. Recognizable remains of the blood clot persist in the interior of the corpus luteum (see Fig. 17-2). In response to LH, the granulosa cells of the follicle hypertrophy and become transformed into **granulosa lutein cells**. The theca interna cells likewise become transformed into **theca lutein cells**, which look similar but are not as large (see Plate 17-2). The corpus luteum secretes both **progesterone** and **estrogen**, and again it is the granulosa cells (now **granulosa lutein cells**) that produce the estrogen and most of the progesterone necessary for preparing the endometrium for implantation. Subsidiary amounts of progesterone come from the theca lutein cells. Estrogen secretion is an FSH response; progesterone secretion is an LH response. Capillaries and other stromal elements extend in between the groups of lutein cells from the theca interna. The corpus luteum continues to enlarge through hypertrophy of the lutein cells, but involutes after approximately 14 days unless fertilization has occurred. The resulting decline in production of progesterone and estrogen (particularly the former) precipitates menstruation. Following involution, the corpus luteum becomes replaced by a small white fibrous scar called a **corpus albicans**.

Ovarian Hormone Secretion

Follicle-stimulating hormone from pituitary gonadotrophs stimulates follicular growth in the proliferative phase of the menstrual cycle (Fig. 17-4). Ripening of the follicles, however, raises the estrogen level. Below a certain concentration, estrogen suppresses further release of FSH (*negative* feedback). Follicular **inhibin**, a polypeptide produced by the ripening follicles, also inhibits FSH release.

Similarly, when LH from the pituitary elicits progesterone secretion in the secretory phase, the rising progesterone level suppresses further LH release. The brief midcycle surge of LH responsible for ovulation is elicited by the high estrogen level attained at this time. It is the result of a temporary *positive* feedback effect of the high estrogen level.

In the event that fertilization and implantation occur, the corpus luteum undergoes further growth instead of involuting (Plate 17-2). It continues to secrete progesterone and estrogen, in sufficient quantities to maintain the endometrium, until approximately the 9th or 10th week of gestation. At this time, the placenta takes over production of progesterone and, in collaboration with the fetal adrenal cortex and fetal liver, produces estrogen as well. The extended lifespan and prolonged

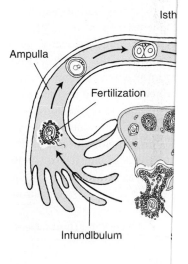

Ampulla

Fertilization

Isth...

Intundlbulum

Figure 17-5
Main parts of a uterine tube, showing

UTERUS

In the body of the uterus, the
myometrium. This muscle co
dometrium. The myometriur
tubes. Three indistinct layers o
and circularly arranged where
characterize the middle layer
pregnancy cause both hypertr
posterior pituitary peptide ho
ministered to induce labor an

Endometrium and Mens

The uterine mucosa (i.e., the
2) its associated simple tubu
substantial lamina propria, c
is considered to be made up
sloughs off during menstrua
generates a new functional l
functional layer change fror
menstrual cycle, convention
Each cycle begins with a **r**
phase is followed by a **pro**

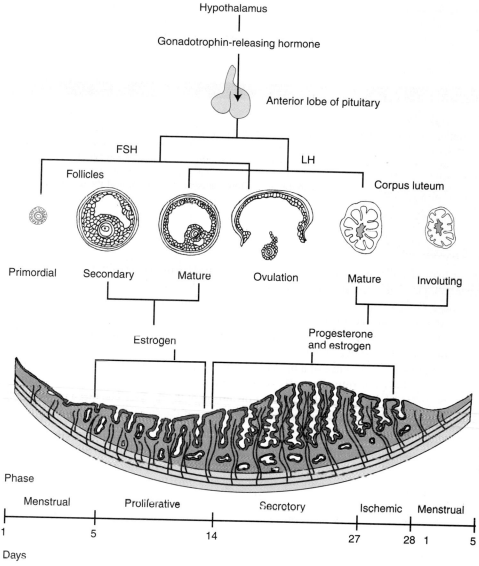

Figure 17-4
Regulation of ovarian hormone secretion and hormonal action on the endometrium over the course of the menstrual cycle.

secretory activity of the corpus luteum are due to the luteotrophic action of the glycoprotein hormone **human chorionic gonadotrophin (hCG)**, produced by trophoblast cells of the implanted conceptus (embryo and surrounding extraembryonic membranes). Production of hCG begins at approximately the 10th day of gestation. This hormone supersedes LH in maintaining the corpus luteum of pregnancy, and its detection in the maternal urine is the basis of pregnancy testing. In about the 3rd month of gestation, the corpus luteum of pregnancy involutes, becoming replaced by a large corpus albicans. The corpus luteum of pregnancy also produces relaxin, a hormone described under Uterine Cervix.

At **menopause**, ovarian f
mone production precludes fu
of discomfort (typically, vaso

Oral Contraceptives
Oral administration of progest
GnRH and LH. At the pharma
logues of progesterone and est
vent ovulation. Progesterone a
strual cycle, progesterone and

Follicular Atresia

In any given menstrual cycle
and liberates an oocyte. The
licular atresia, degeneration
ally resemble primary, secor
something going wrong with
later stages in which fibrobla
ognizing atretic follicles are
2) disorganized arrangement
tion of cell death), and 3) shr
of maturing follicles that bec
ovarian interstitial gland.

UTERINE TUBES

Each **uterine tube (fallop**
(fringed) **infundibulum**, 2)
4) an **intramural portion** th
the uterine lumen (Fig. 17-
age of the zygote (fertilizec
the blastocyst stage.

The ampullary lumen c
cosal folds (Plate 17-4). TI
mucosal folds. The simple
spersed with nonciliated, s
taining the liberated second
tle peristaltic contractions
The well-developed smoot
cular or spiral layer and ar
the isthmus and intramural
underlying loose connectiv

---

which the endometrium doubles or triples in thickness. This rapid regeneration is a result of cellular proliferation in response to **estrogen** primarily produced by ripening ovarian follicles. The term **interval phase** is sometimes applied to the latter part of the proliferative phase because although the endometrium has regenerated, its glands have not yet begun to secrete. At some time during the second or third week of the cycle, **ovulation** occurs. Conventionally, ovulation is assumed to occur on day 14 of the cycle (see Fig. 17-4). Following this is a **secretory (progestational, progravid) phase** of approximately 13 days duration when the endometrial glands start to secrete and the endometrium undergoes additional thickening. The secretory response is elicited by the **progesterone** that, together with estrogen, is produced by the corpus luteum. At the end of the cycle, as a consequence of the steep decline in ovarian hormone levels that results from involution of the corpus luteum, the endometrium enters an **ischemic phase**. In this last phase, a day or so in duration, the functional layer is subjected to sporadic interruption of its blood supply. The significant episodes of ischemic hypoxia result in necrosis and sloughing of the functional layer in the ensuing menstrual phase that marks the beginning of the next menstrual cycle.

At each phase of the menstrual cycle, the histological appearance of the endometrium reflects prevailing hormone production by the ovaries. During the proliferative phase, stromal and epithelial cells persisting in the basilar layer are acted on by estrogen alone, which causes them to proliferate. **Mitotic figures** can therefore be found in the stroma as well as in the epithelium. Epithelial cells that migrate from the tops of regenerating glands cover the raw surface left after menstruation. Throughout the proliferative phase, the endometrial glands remain fairly straight, narrow, and dark staining (Plate 17-5A) and the stroma between them appears rather cellular. In the second half of the cycle, progesterone is secreted (see Fig. 17-4). In combination with estrogen, it causes the endometrial glands to become sacculated and secretory. They widen and appear irregularly coiled or tortuous (see Plate 17-5B and C). If cut tangentially, their saccules may look almost ladder-like at low magnification. The hypertrophied secretory cells are pale staining because they store **glycogen**. When this accumulates they acquire a ragged appearance. Their copious viscid secretion is rich in glycogen and provides the appropriate nutritive environment for an implanted blastocyst. The secretory phase is further characterized by increasing vascularity of the stroma, lengthening of stromal blood vessels, stromal edema, and stromal cell enlargement.

The end of the secretory phase is characterized by intermittent **ischemia** (reduced blood flow) in the functional layer. This an endometrial response to declining levels of ovarian hormones, notably the fall in progesterone, is clearly related to the unusual vascular supply of this layer. Each small artery bringing blood from the uterine artery to the endometrium gives off a few straight branches that supply the basilar layer. It then continues on as a **spiral (coiled) artery** that supplies the functional layer (see bottom of Fig. 17-4). Thickening of the endometrium in the secretory phase results in substantial lengthening of the spiral arteries. When declining ovarian hormone levels lead to endometrial regression, the elongated spiral arteries buckle, kink, and undergo bouts of sustained vasoconstriction. The outcome is ischemic necrosis of the regions they supply. These and other vessels with walls damaged by hypoxia undergo sustained bleeding when the spiral arteries open up again. The vascular damage is manifested as stromal pools of extravasated blood and neutrophil invasion of the necrotic endometrial tissues. Sloughing of the necrotic tissues, accompanied by prolonged bleeding of damaged endometrial vessels onto the raw surface without the blood clotting, is manifested as **menstrual bleeding**. The basilar layer outlasts menstruation because of its uninterrupted, independent blood supply.

CLINICAL IMPLICATIONS

Endometrium in Atypical Cycles
About three or four times a year, **anovulatory cycles** may occur. Endometrial bleeding is experienced at the customary time for menstruation even in the absence of ovulation and formation of a corpus luteum. One cause of the anovulatory endometrial bleeding is the midcycle decline in estrogen level. In this case, menstruation represents a delayed response to the falling estrogen level that occurs after the dominant follicle has reached maturity. In other cases, endometrial bleeding is a consequence of prolonged estrogenic stimulation without the usual postovulatory rise and fall in progesterone level.

Uterine Cervix

The uterine cervix (L. for neck), which is the cylindrical inferior part of the uterus, opens by way of the **uterine ostium** into the upper end of the vagina (Fig. 17-6). Unlike the functional layer of endometrium in the uterine body, the cervical mucosa is not shed during menstruation because its lamina propria is not supplied by spiral arteries. The cervix is narrower than the uterine body and does not expand during pregnancy, so substantial dilatation is required during childbirth. Its strong fibrous walls are composed chiefly of irregular dense ordinary connective tissue with abundant collagen and contain relatively little smooth muscle. Toward the end of pregnancy, a softening-up process occurs in this dense connective tissue. The necessary change is brought about by **relaxin**, a polypeptide hormone produced by the corpus luteum of pregnancy and the decidual cells that underlie the implantation site. This hormone expedites delivery also by inducing slight slackening of the ligaments of the pubic symphysis.

Cervical Mucus

The flattened **cervical canal** is lined by a pale-staining simple columnar **mucus-secreting epithelium** that contains some ciliated cells. Tubular mucous glands lined with similar epithelium extend into the fibrous lamina propria, and elaborate mucosal folds account at least in part for the

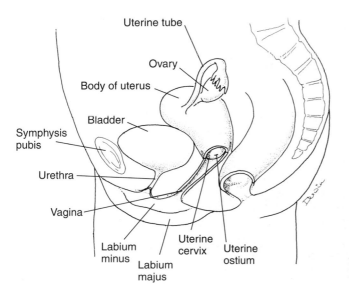

Figure 17-6
Principal parts of the female reproductive tract and associated viscera.

glandular appearance of the mucosa (Fig. 17-7). The secretory activity of this epithelium is sufficient to keep the cervical canal filled with mucus. Furthermore, the viscosity of cervical mucus
varies with ovarian hormone levels. Before ovulation the mucus has a relatively thin consistency,
making it comparatively easy for spermatozoa to negotiate, but following ovulation it becomes thick
and viscid and somewhat more difficult to penetrate. These changes reflect actions of estrogen and
progesterone, respectively.

CLINICAL IMPLICATIONS

Cervical Lesions and Cysts

Generally at a level slightly above the uterine ostium (external os of the cervix), the simple columnar epithelium that lines the cervical canal changes abruptly to the stratified squamous nonkeratinizing epithelium
that lines the vagina and covers the portion of cervix protruding posteroinferiorly into its upper end (see Fig.
17-6). This squamocolumnar junction (Plate 17-6) is clinically important because it is the site where **pre-
cancerous lesions** and **carcinomas of the cervix** are most likely to develop.

Over the course of a woman's lifetime, the level of the cervical squamocolumnar junction changes. In
her early reproductive years, it descends partway over the ectocervix. Then stratified squamous nonkeratinizing epithelium regrows over the ectocervix and extends up the cervical canal, usually to a level just
above the uterine ostium. In the course of replacing the downward extension of endocervical simple columnar epithelium, it is common for the regrowing stratified squamous epithelium to obstruct the lumen of
tubular mucous glands that have formed in the lamina propria in the vicinity of the ostium. This can lead to
the formation of mucus-filled cysts, lined with mucus-secreting epithelium, that are known as **nabothian
cysts (follicles)**.

When a pregnancy becomes established, the endometrial stromal cells in the body of the uterus
enlarge substantially, accumulating large amounts of glycogen and lipid in response to rising progesterone levels. This characteristic endometrial response is known as the **decidual reaction** (L. *de-
ciduus*, falling off) because the functional layer of endometrium is destined to be shed as the **decidua**
in the final stages of parturition.

Cervical glands

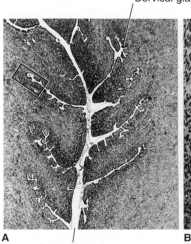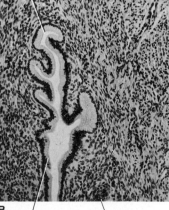

A   B

Figure 17-7
Uterine cervix. (*A*) Cervical
canal with its associated mucous
glands (very low power). (*B*)
Cervical mucous gland (medium
power).

Cervical canal   Simple columnar   Lamina propria
                      mucus-secreting
                      epithelium

PLACENTA

The placenta is a thickened disk-shaped structure growing to a diameter of about 20 cm. It is mostly fetal in origin but has a maternal component. The fetal portion is derived from the **chorion**, one of the surrounding extraembryonic membranes of the conceptus. The maternal portion is derived from the region of endometrium that underlies the implantation site (the **decidua basalis**). The placenta is the essential site of exchange of substances between maternal and fetal blood, including oxygen, nutrients, hormones, excretory products, humoral antibodies (IgG), and, unfortunately, any viruses or drugs that may be present in the maternal circulation. Also, the placenta is itself a major site of hormone production throughout pregnancy.

Placental Development

The late blastocyst consists of an **inner cell mass** that gives rise to the embryo and an outer, single layer of **trophoblast cells** (Gk. *trophein*, to nourish; *blastos*, germ) that encloses the blastocyst cavity. Generally, the blastocyst implants high up on the posterior wall of the uterus (see Fig. 17-5). Following implantation, the trophoblast cells become highly invasive and erode the endometrium. Their name reflects an essential role in deriving nourishment for the embryo. Intense invasive activity of these cells enables the blastocyst to implant in the secretory endometrium, where the embryo obtains nutrients from eroded vessels and glands.

The trophoblast gives rise to two layers, an inner pale-staining layer called the **cytotrophoblast** and an outer darker-staining layer called the **syncytiotrophoblast** (Fig. 17-8). The syncytiotrophoblast is a **syncytium** (Gk. *syn*, together), meaning that its component cells have fused together to form a continuous mass of multinucleated cytoplasm without any cell boundaries. In contrast, the cytotrophoblast remains made up of individual cells (see Fig. 17-8A). Irregular protrusions of the syncytiotrophoblast invade the endometrium and become surrounded by cavernous spaces (**lacunae**) filled with maternal blood. Finger-like extensions of the cytotrophoblast grow into these protrusions, and the resulting structures are called **primary placental villi**. Mesenchyme growing into the primary villi gives them a loose connective tissue core. Capillaries forming in this

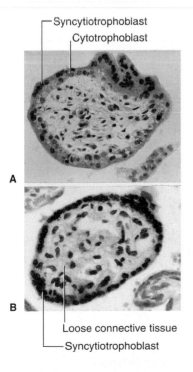

A

B

Figure 17-8
Chorionic villi. (*A*) From placenta in second trimester. (*B*) From full-term placenta.

tissue represent part of the embryonic circulation. Known at this stage as **chorionic villi** (because the trophoblast and its associated connective tissue, derived from extraembryonic somatic mesoderm, constitute the **chorion**), tufted extensions of the part of the chorion associated with the decidua basalis develop into large, elaborately branched outgrowths of the **villous chorion**. The disk-like area of chorion to which the irregularly shaped tufts are attached is known as the **chorionic plate** (Fig. 17-9). Many of the chorionic villi are anchored to the decidua. They are bathed with the maternal blood that circulates through the **intervillous space**, an extensive cavernous sinus forming from enlarging confluent lacunae. Maternal blood enters this space from eroded spiral arteries and returns through endometrial veins. By the fifth month of gestation, the cytotrophoblast cells have begun to disappear. By full term, almost all cytotrophoblast cells have fused with syncytiotrophoblast.

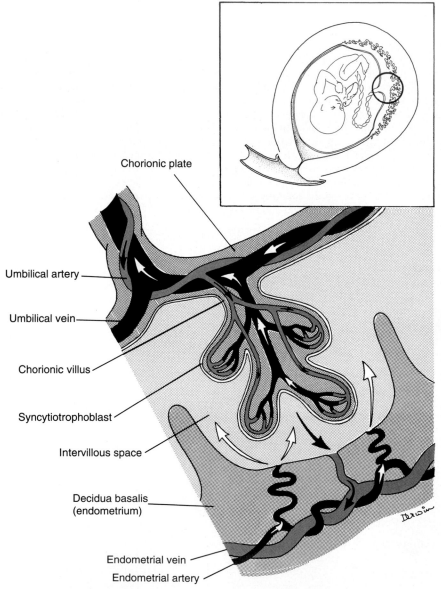

Figure 17-9
General organization of a placenta (showing area outlined in inset). Oxygenated blood is indicated in black.

Placental Barrier

In the first half of gestation, the six components of the **placental barrier** lying between the maternal and fetal circulations are as follows. First, the chorionic villi and chorionic plate are covered by 1) **syncytiotrophoblast** with its rather small, dark-staining nuclei, and 2) underlying **cytotrophoblast cells** with larger, lighter-staining nuclei (see Fig. 17-8A). Internal to these outermost layers of the fetal portion of the placenta are 3) the trophoblastic **basement membrane** and 4) fetal **loose connective tissue** constituting the core of each villus. The other components of the barrier are 5) the **endothelium** of the fetal capillaries and 6) its surrounding **basement membrane**. At full term, the cytotrophoblast is represented only as fragments; hence, the placental barrier comes to consist of five fetal components instead of six (see Fig. 17-8B).

Placental Hormones

The cytotrophoblast seems to be the initial chief placental source of **human chorionic gonadotrophin** (hCG), a glycoprotein hormone that mimics the luteotrophic effects of LH through the first few months of gestation, maintaining the corpus luteum of pregnancy. The syncytiotrophoblast is the chief source of **human chorionic somatomammotrophin** (hCS), a glycoprotein hormone with both lactogenic and growth-promoting activity. The steroid hormones **progesterone** and **estrogen** are made by both kinds of trophoblast, but estrogen formation requires the metabolic cooperation of the fetal adrenal cortex and fetal liver. Placental production of these glycoprotein and steroid hormones by the syncytiotrophoblast continues throughout gestation.

VAGINA

The sheath-like vagina is essentially a fibromuscular-walled canal, flattened anteroposteriorly, which leads from the exterior of the body (see Fig. 17-6). Lined by a fairly substantial stratified squamous nonkeratinizing epithelium, the vagina is without glands of its own but is kept moist by cervical mucus draining down through the cervical canal. The fibroelastic lamina propria contains a plexus of small veins and has a fairly vascular appearance (Plate 17-7). External to the lamina propria lies a smooth muscle coat. Some muscle bundles in the poorly demarcated inner region of this coat are circularly arranged, whereas those in the outer region are chiefly longitudinal. Surrounding the vaginal orifice are some skeletal muscle fibers. A fibrous adventitia binds the vagina to the urethra and other contiguous organs.

CLINICAL IMPLICATIONS

Vaginal and Exocervical Cytology
An established action of estrogen on the vaginal epithelium is augmented cell proliferation in the basal and parabasal layers, which results in epithelial thickening. Estrogen also elicits other cytological changes in this epithelium. The more superficial cells, still nucleated, become slightly more acidophilic as ovulation approaches. This change can be detected cytologically by special (Papanicolaou) staining of a **vaginal smear** consisting of exfoliated vaginal cells. The slight increase in acidophilia is considered a preliminary sign of keratinization, but under normal circumstances vaginal epithelial cells do not actually keratinize. The estrogen-stimulated cells also accumulate glycogen and lipid, giving them a characteristic pale, empty appearance in H&E-stained sections (see Plate 17-7). This glycogen undergoes bacterial fermentation to lactic acid, promoting acidic conditions that maintain a suitable intraluminal microflora.

Epithelial cells obtained for cytological evaluation from the lower region of the cervical canal or the vaginal surface of the exocervix and stained with the Papanicolaou stain may also show preliminary signs of becoming cancerous, indicating a need for more thorough examination.

MAMMARY GLANDS

Each **mammary gland (breast)** is essentially a group of up to 20 compound alveolar glands individually opening onto a surface elevation termed a **nipple**. Until pregnancy, mammary glands are represented solely by their branched duct systems opening onto the nipples. Stimulation of the female breasts by estrogen at puberty causes them to enlarge externally, but internally they still remain incompletely developed until the latter part of pregnancy, when they begin secreting in readiness for lactation. Characteristic enlargement and change of shape of the female breast at puberty are almost entirely due to accumulation of adipocytes in the stroma. Rising estrogen levels also cause enlargement of the nipples and further development of the duct system, but secretory alveoli do not develop at puberty. The elevated progesterone levels acquired during pregnancy, acting synergistically with estrogen, are necessary for mammary alveolar secretory units to form. Supplementary action of high prolactin levels brings about complete development and full secretory activity of the alveoli. Growth hormone, thyroid hormone, adrenal glucocorticoids, insulin, and hCS are also required for full mammary development and lactation.

At puberty, the mammary glands of boys generally remain flat. Small nodules of breast tissue, however, may develop at this time and regress after a year or so. If marked breast enlargement occurs in males, it is referred to as **gynecomastia** (Gk. *gynaikos*, woman; *mastos*, breast).

The nipples and their surrounding skin (areola) possess numerous sensory receptors and commonly are somewhat pigmented. Opening through separate orifices at the surface of each nipple are the **lactiferous ducts**, each representing the main duct of one of the many compound glands of the breast. The dense connective tissue supporting the nipple contains small bundles of smooth muscle, some arranged circumferentially and others lying parallel to the ducts. Each lactiferous duct is lined over most of its length by a double layer of columnar epithelium, and near the external orifice it widens into a **lactiferous sinus** large enough to store milk during milk ejection.

Resting Breast

The term **resting breast** denotes the breast that has not yet been stimulated to secrete. It is therefore still in an inactive state. In sections, the resting breast is represented only by its component duct systems and stroma (Fig. 17-10 and Plate 17-8). The parenchyma (i.e., ducts) and stroma are organized as follows. Each compound gland opens into a **lactiferous sinus** and constitutes a **lobe** made up of many **lobules**. As in other exocrine glands, it develops by downgrowth of the surface epithelium into the underlying connective tissue (see Fig. 4-8). Epidermis, taking with it the associated papillary layer of dermis, grows down through the reticular layer of dermis and forms the mammary duct system. The connective tissue that intimately invests the duct system is accordingly relatively cellular, resembling the papillary layer of dermis (see Fig. 17-10 and Plate 17-8). Regions of this relatively cellular **intralobular connective tissue** are widely separated by partitions of coarser and less cellular **interlobular connective tissue**, which is more comparable with the overlying reticular layer of dermis. The interlobular connective tissue also contains deposits of adipose tissue. The larger intralobular ducts are lined by a double layer of cuboidal to low columnar epithelial cells, but the smaller ducts have only a single layer of such cells. Finally, as an aid to recognition, resting breast is the only kind of gland that exhibits ducts without secretory units.

Lactating Breast

Further changes occur in the epithelial tissue of the breast during pregnancy. With the progressive rise in estrogen, progesterone, and maternal and placental lactogenic hormones, the profound *proliferative* response occurring in the epithelium during the first half of pregnancy gives way to a substantial *secretory* response. Development of the mammary glands is completed when **secretory**

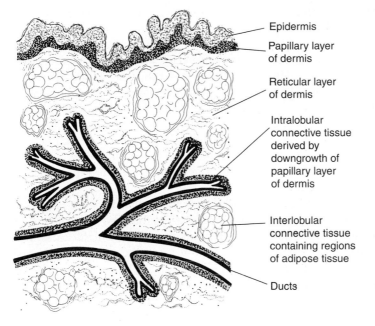

Epidermis

Papillary layer
of dermis

Reticular layer
of dermis

Intralobular
connective tissue
derived by
downgrowth of
papillary layer
of dermis

Interlobular
connective tissue
containing regions
of adipose tissue

Ducts

Figure 17-10
Tissue organization in resting breast.
Intralobular connective tissue arises
from the papillary layer of dermis
whereas interlobular connective
tissue arises from the reticular layer
of dermis.

alveoli bud from the intralobular ducts. By the second half of pregnancy, well-established lobules with secretory alveoli as well as ducts are evident. When the lobules enlarge, the interlobular connective tissue reduces to thin fibrous partitions. Mammary alveoli are made up of simple columnar secretory cells that secrete milk proteins and lipids (see Chapter 4 under Exocrine Glands), with investing myoepithelial cells. In the third trimester of pregnancy, the secretory cells begin producing a protein-containing serous fluid called **colostrum** and the breasts enlarge further. Milk is not secreted until a few days after parturition. Because of uneven rates of secretion, the alveoli and ducts become more distended in some lobules than in others.

In the **lactating breast** of nursing mothers, breast lobules appear even more rounded and distended because a greater number of alveoli is filled with secretion and only thin septa of interlobular connective tissue are seen (Plate 17-9). Again, although many alveoli are distended, some appear almost empty, a feature that aids recognition of actively secreting breast tissue.

Human breast milk, initially produced 1 to 3 days after parturition, has a substantial content of fat, proteins, lactose, and vitamins. It contains secretory IgA, affording temporary enteric passive immunity. Although milk is produced continuously (milk **secretion**), it is delivered only in response to suckling (milk **ejection** or milk **let-down**). Nursing sets up afferent impulses that are relayed to the hypothalamus, where they 1) stimulate oxytocin-producing neurons in the paraventricular nucleus to release oxytocin from their axon terminals lying in the posterior pituitary, and 2) suppress release of prolactin-inhibiting hormone (PIH; dopamine). The oxytocin then stimulates contraction of myoepithelial cells of the breast, causing milk to be expressed through the nipple (the **milk ejection reflex**). The suppressive effect of suckling on PIH release further augments prolactin secretion so that lactation continues.

Summary

Meiosis in females is summarized in Figure 17-1 and Table 17-3. Follicular maturation, the chief ovarian and endometrial interactions during the menstrual cycle, and developmental stages of the zygote leading to implantation are summarized in Figures 17-2, 17-4, and 17-5.

Surrounded by follicular cells, the primary oocyte remains suspended in prophase I. In response to FSH, its surrounding follicular cells enlarge, proliferate, and secrete estrogen. Mature follicles are characterized by a fluid-filled antrum. Theca interna cells synthesize androgen from which follicular (granulosa) cells produce estrogen. At ovulation, which is triggered by a midcycle surge of LH, the first maturation division occurs and the liberated haploid secondary oocyte enters a uterine tube. Also, the LH converts the residual granulosa cells and the theca interna cells into lutein cells. Granulosa lutein cells secrete both progesterone and estrogen. The corpus luteum produces these steroids for about 2 weeks but then involutes unless stimulated by hCG from trophoblast cells of an implanted conceptus, in which case it becomes a large corpus luteum of pregnancy. When a corpus luteum involutes, it is replaced by a corpus albicans. At any stage of maturation a follicle may become atretic. Fertilization leads to completion of the second maturation division. While the zygote is being transported along the uterine tube by peristalsis it cleaves. The blastocyst reaching the uterus implants in the endometrium.

The functional layer of endometrium, but not the basilar layer, is supplied by spiral arteries. It begins sloughing on day 1 of the menstrual cycle. The menstrual phase is followed by a phase of endometrial repair elicited by estrogen. Proliferation restores the endometrium to full thickness, with straight tubular glands. The secretory phase is a response to progesterone and estrogen from the corpus luteum. Tortuous, sacculated endometrial glands produce a glycogen-rich secretion suitable for nourishing an implanted conceptus. Unless implantation occurs, the corpus luteum regresses after 2 weeks or so. The resulting fall in progesterone, along with the decline in estrogen, affects the spiral arteries supplying the functional layer of endometrium. Intermittent vasospasm of these arteries causes regional hypoxia and necrosis during the short ischemic (premenstrual) phase, followed by menstruation.

If pregnancy ensues, the region of endometrium eroded by trophoblast cells becomes the maternal component of the placenta (the decidua basalis). The fetal component is essentially the chorionic plate with its tufted chorionic villi, which are bathed by the maternal blood present in the intervillous space. Covering the villi is the syncytiotrophoblast, with underlying cytotrophoblast during the first half of gestation. Some of the hormones secreted by the trophoblast are hCG, hCS, progesterone, and estrogen.

The secretory epithelium of the uterine cervix produces mucus. The cervical mucosa remains intact throughout menstruation. The fibrous cervical walls become stretched during childbirth because this part of the uterus does not dilate in pregnancy. This stretching is facilitated by relaxin. Properties of cervical mucus and cytological characteristics of vaginal epithelium are indicators of ovarian hormone levels.

Each breast contains up to 20 compound glands opening individually onto the nipples by way of lactiferous sinuses. Before pregnancy, mammary glands are represented solely by their duct systems. Augmented estrogen secretion at puberty, however, markedly increases their adipocyte content. A number of additional hormones promote secretory activity in the second half of pregnancy. Milk let-down as a result of contraction of mammary myoepithelial cells is elicited by oxytocin release from the posterior pituitary. Oxytocin can also elicit contractions of myometrial smooth muscle that are intense enough to bring about parturition.

Bibliography

General

Hafez ESE ed. Scanning Electron Microscopic Atlas of Mammalian Reproduction. New York, Springer-Verlag, 1975.

Johnson MH, Everitt BJ. Essential Reproduction, ed 4. Oxford, Blackwell Scientific Publications, 1995.

Ludwig H, Metzger H. The Human Female Reproductive Tract: A Scanning Electron Microscopic Atlas. New York, Springer-Verlag, 1976.

Norman RL, ed. Neuroendocrine Aspects of Reproduction. New York, Academic Press, 1983.

Van Blerkom J, Motta P. The Cellular Basis of Mammalian Reproduction. Baltimore, Urban & Schwarzenberg, 1979.

Ovaries, Follicular Maturation, Fertilization, and Gestation

Brodie AMH. Biosynthesis, metabolism, and secretion of ovarian steroid hormones. In: Serra GB ed. The Ovary. New York, Raven Press, 1983, p 3.

Centola GM. Structural changes: follicular development and hormonal requirements. In: Serra GB ed. The Ovary. New York, Raven Press, 1983, p 95.

Familiari G, Makabe S, Motta PM, eds. Ultrastructure of the Ovary. Boston, Kluwer Academic Publishers, 1991.

Kase NG. The microenvironment of the ovarian follicle. J Reprod Medicine 28:239, 1983.

Kemp BE, Niall HD. Relaxin. Vitam Horm 41:79, 1984.

Kotsuji F, Tominaga T. The role of granulosa and theca cell interactions in ovarian structure and function. Micros Res Tech 27:97, 1994.

Mathieu P, Rahier J, Thomas K. Localization of relaxin in human gestational corpus luteum. Cell Tissue Res 219:213, 1981.

Motta PM, Hafez ESE, eds. Biology of the Ovary. Boston, Martinus Nijhoff, 1980.

Newman-Hirshfield A. Development of follicles in the mammalian ovary. Int Rev Cytol 124:43, 1991.

Richards JS, Jahnsen T, Hedlin L, Lifka J et al. Ovarian follicular development: from physiology to molecular biology. Rec Prog Horm Res 43:231, 1987.

Schwabe C, Steinetz B, Weiss G et al. Relaxin. Recent Prog Horm Res 34:123, 1978.

Sidhu KS, Guraya SS. Current concepts in gamete receptors for fertilization in mammals. Int Rev Cytol 127:253, 1991.

Wassarman PM. Early events in mammalian fertilization. Annu Rev Cell Biol 3:109, 1987.

Weiss G. The physiology of human relaxin. Contrib Gynecol Obstet 18:130, 1991.

Placenta

Beaconsfield P, Birdwood G, Beaconsfield R. The placenta. Sci Am 243(2):94, 1980.

Boyd JD, Hamilton WJ. The Human Placenta. Cambridge, UK, W Heffer, 1970.

Kaufmann P, Sen DK, Schweikhart G. Classification of human placental villi: I. Histology. Cell Tissue Res 200:409, 1979.

Ogren L, Talamantes F. Prolactins of pregnancy and their cellular source. Int Rev Cytol 112:1, 1988.

Mammary Glands

Monaghan P, Perusinghe NP, Cowen P, Gusterson BA. Peripubertal human breast development. Anat Rec 226:501, 1990.

Pitelka DR, Hamamoto ST. Ultrastructure of the mammary secretory cell. In: Mepham TB, ed. Biochemistry of Lactation. New York, Elsevier Biomedical Press, 1983.

Vorherr H. The Breast: Morphology, Physiology, and Lactation. New York, Academic Press, 1974.

CHAPTER 18

Male Reproductive System

OBJECTIVES

With the information in this chapter, you should be able to do the following:

- Recognize spermatogonia, Sertoli cells, and interstitial cells in testis sections and state their main characteristics
- Specify the duration of spermatogenesis, list its main stages, and state two key differences between spermatogenesis and oogenesis
- List four major structural changes that characterize spermiogenesis
- Trace the route taken by spermatozoa from when they are produced to when they fertilize
- Discuss why cell junctions are needed between Sertoli cells
- List three features that the seminal vesicles and the prostate have in common

The principal functions of the male reproductive system are 1) to produce **spermatozoa** (male **germ cells**); 2) to produce **androgens** (male sex hormones, chiefly **testosterone**); and 3) to facilitate **fertilization** through the introduction of spermatozoa into the female genital tract (copulation). The paired **testes** (male gonads) produce the spermatozoa and androgens and several **accessory glands** deliver fluid constituents of semen. Long ducts store the spermatozoa and convey them to the penis, the organ of copulation (Fig. 18-1). The principal components of the male reproductive system are listed in Table 18-1.

Once the testes descend into the fetal scrotum they lie outside the abdominal cavity. This allows them to remain slightly below body temperature, a prerequisite for normal sperm counts. Spermatozoa are produced in the looped **seminiferous tubules** of the testes (Fig. 18-2). Between these tubules lie small groups of steroid-producing **interstitial (Leydig) cells**. In response to LH, interstitial cells produce **testosterone**, the androgen that promotes spermatozoon production (**spermatogenesis**), secretory activity in the androgen-responsive male accessory glands, and the acquisition of secondary male sexual characteristics. The seminiferous tubules in each testis are connected by a maze of anastomosing channels to the **ductuli efferentes** of the associated epididymis. These ductules lead to a long, convoluted **ductus epididymis**. The substantial duct emerging from the tail of the epididymis is the thick-walled **ductus (vas) deferens**. It ascends in the spermatic cord, passes along the inguinal canal, and enters the pelvis minor. It then passes posterior to the urinary bladder, where a tortuous

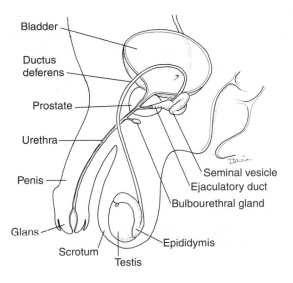

Figure 18-1
Principal parts of the male reproductive tract and
associated viscera.

TABLE 18-1

MALE REPRODUCTIVE SYSTEM

Main Components

Testes

Epididymides

Ducti deferentes

Penis (including urethra)

Accessory Glands

Seminal vesicles

Prostate

Bulbourethral glands

Urethral glands

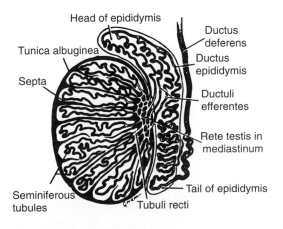

Figure 18-2
General organization of a testis and its associated
epididymis.

tubular gland termed a **seminal vesicle** opens into it. Leading from the junction between 1) the distal end of the ductus deferens and 2) the seminal vesicle that lies lateral to it is a common duct known as the **ejaculatory duct**. The ejaculatory ducts open into the **prostatic urethra**, which is the part of the urethra that traverses the prostate. The **prostate** is a substantial gland, medially situated, that consists of many compound glands. It surrounds the prostatic part of the urethra where this joins the neck of the bladder. Whereas the seminal vesicles provide a thick nutritive fluid, the prostate provides a thinner but more complex secretion. These two fluids substantially augment the volume of semen leaving by way of the urethra.

SPERMATOGENESIS

The term **spermatogenesis** broadly denotes the entire process leading to the production of spermatozoa. Two key differences exist between oogenesis and spermatogenesis (compare Tables 17-3 and 18-2). The first is a difference in timing, because primary oocytes, but not primary spermatocytes, form during prenatal life. Thus meiosis I starts before birth in females but not until after puberty in males. The second difference is that whereas meiosis I and meiosis II produce only one ovum in females, all four of the resulting progeny cells (spermatids) become spermatozoa in males.

Male **primordial germ cells** arise from the yolk sac endoderm, migrate to the developing testes, and become incorporated into the epithelial cords that will develop into seminiferous tubules. The primordial cells then differentiate into diploid **spermatogonia** that remain quiescent until late adolescence, when they proliferate by mitosis. By the onset of puberty, spermatogonia have begun to produce **primary spermatocytes**. Some spermatogonia, however, persist as **stem cells** capable of giving rise to further spermatogonia. Each new generation of primary spermatocytes enters the extended (but in this case, not protracted as dictyotene) prophase of meiosis I, and then goes on to complete the first maturation division. The haploid **secondary spermatocytes** thus produced promptly

TABLE 18-2

SPERMATOGENESIS STAGES

Primordial germ cells ($2n$)*
    Migrate from yolk sac to
    testes and differentiate
    into

Spermatogonia ($2n$)
    Proliferate by mitosis
    B type differentiates into

Primary spermatocytes ($2n$)
    Undergo 1st meiotic division
    (reduction division; 1st
    maturation division)

Secondary spermatocytes (n)
    Miss S phase and undergo
    2nd maturation division

Spermatids (n)
    Transform, without dividing,
    into

Spermatozoa (n)

* $2n$ denotes the diploid chromosome number; n denotes the haploid number.

undergo the second maturation division without first replicating their nuclear DNA, and their haploid progeny, known as **spermatids**, transform into **spermatozoa** without further division.

Additional details are given in the section describing the stages of spermatogenesis.

TESTES

Each testis is an ovoid, compact organ with a more or less crescent-shaped **epididymis** extending around its superior and posterolateral borders. Its outermost mesothelial covering represents the visceral layer of the **tunica vaginalis testis**, which is the membranous lining of a serous sac evaginated from the peritoneum. Beneath the mesothelial covering is a thick capsule of dense ordinary connective tissue that is known as the **tunica albuginea** because of its whitish appearance. From this capsule, fibrous septa extend inward and subdivide the interior of the testis into incomplete, roughly pyramidal lobules. The septa converge toward the midline of the posterior border of the testis, where they meet along a ridgelike thickening of the tunica albuginea called the **mediastinum testis**. Here, both ends of the component looped **seminiferous tubules** (up to four per lobule) open into a network of fine anastomosing channels called the **rete testis** (L. *rete*, net). This network leads into a number of **ductuli efferentes**.

Interstitial (Leydig) cells, present between seminiferous tubules, are active in secreting androgens in fetal life and then less active in childhood. The seminiferous tubules remain small, inactive, and without a lumen for the first decade of life. At puberty, which commonly occurs at about 14 years of age, rising luteinizing hormone (LH) levels elevate the testosterone level, and the action of testosterone together with follicle-stimulating hormone (FSH) promotes spermatogenesis. Scattered groups of interstitial cells become histologically recognizable and the seminiferous tubules acquire a lumen into which spermatozoa begin to be released.

Seminiferous Tubules

Sertoli cells, representing the **epithelial supporting cells** of seminiferous tubules, are derived from the epithelial sex cords of the developing gonads. They are tall simple columnar cells that span the entire epithelium from the surrounding basement membrane to the lumen (see Figs. 18-3 and 18-8). As well as harboring the proliferating and differentiating germ cell progenitors in peripheral pockets in their cytoplasm, Sertoli cells provide these cells with a special local environment, bring them

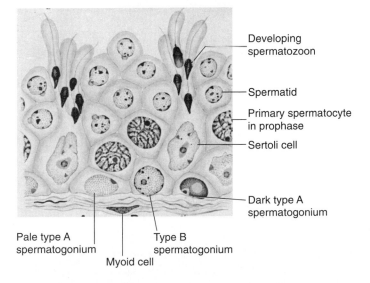

Developing spermatozoon

Spermatid

Primary spermatocyte in prophase

Sertoli cell

Dark type A spermatogonium

Pale type A spermatogonium

Type B spermatogonium

Myoid cell

Figure 18-3
Cellular composition of one of the cell associations found in the wall of a seminiferous tubule.

nutrients from nearby capillaries (since seminiferous epithelium, like any other epithelium, is avascular), and phagocytose excess spermatid cytoplasm not needed in forming spermatozoa. External to the basement membrane surrounding the tubules are collagen, elastin, and a few layers of flat **myoid cells** resembling smooth muscle cells yet squamous. Myoid cells are contractile and generate gentle peristaltic waves in these tubules.

A mixed population of differentiating spermatogenic cells (Plate 18-1) occupies the numerous interstices between Sertoli cells of the tubules (Fig. 18-3). Representing an intimate mixture of the following proliferative and nonproliferative stages of spermatogenesis, this diverse population progressively becomes displaced toward the lumen.

Spermatogonia

Although discrete patches of seminiferous epithelium contain distinctive combinations of spermatogenic cells, all regions of the seminiferous tubules have a basally situated population of **spermatogonia**. These large, rounded cells lie adjacent to the basement membrane of the tubule (see Fig. 18-3). They represent the diploid cells from which primary spermatocytes arise (see Table 18-2). Spermatogonia are a heterogeneous class of cells made up of pale type A, dark type A, and type B spermatogonia. The two subtypes of type A spermatogonia are distinguishable by the depth of staining of their respective nuclei. The nucleus in the dark type A cells has a darker appearance. Identifying the three types of spermatogonia, however, is not as important as understanding essential differences between them. The **pale type A spermatogonia**, relatively undifferentiated and with extensive mitotic potential, represent spermatogenic **stem cells** (see Chapter 2 under Cell Renewal). Some of their daughter cells remain undifferentiated as other pale type A spermatogonia. Such **self-renewal** (Table 18-3, [b]) counteracts depletion of the stem cell population. The other daughter cells, roughly equal in number, differentiate into progenitors known as **type B spermatogonia** (see Table 18-3, [c]) that on dividing produce primary spermatocytes. The **dark type A spermatogonia** are believed to represent quiescent or **reserve stem cells**. Unlike the pale type A spermatogonia (the **renewing stem cells**), they are held in reserve and go into cycle as renewing stem cells only if the latter become critically depleted (Table 18-3, [a]).

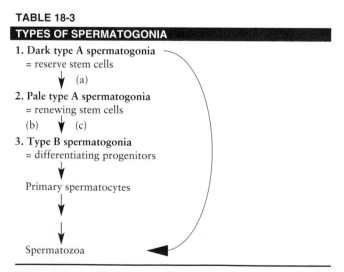

TABLE 18-3

TYPES OF SPERMATOGONIA

1. Dark type A spermatogonia
   = reserve stem cells

   ↓ (a)

2. Pale type A spermatogonia
   = renewing stem cells

   (b) ↓ (c)

3. Type B spermatogonia
   = differentiating progenitors

   ↓

   Primary spermatocytes

   ↓

   ↓

   Spermatozoa

Key: (a) emergency recruitment; (b) self-renewal; (c) differentiation.

Spermatocytes and Spermatids

The large dividing cells in the middle third or so of the walls of the seminiferous tubules are predominantly diploid **primary spermatocytes** at various stages of prophase I (see Fig. 18-3). The component stages of this prophase are listed in Table 17-2 and described under Oogenesis in Chapter 17. In males, however, diakinesis is not extended into a prolonged dictyotene as in oogenesis. Most of the smaller round cells on the luminal side of the tubular wall are haploid **spermatids**. Some spermatids have an elongated nucleus and are transforming into spermatozoa. The sequence of morphological changes that spermatids undergo when they transform into spermatozoa is termed **spermiogenesis**. The resulting **spermatozoa** are released into the lumen of the tubule. **Secondary spermatocytes**, the haploid, intermediate-sized parental cells of spermatids, are seldom seen because they do not persist for long. Without passing through an S phase they enter the second maturation division (see Table 18-2).

EM studies show that the clonal progeny of each spermatogonium remain interconnected by narrow **intercellular bridges**. Cytoplasmic continuity between differentiating spermatogenic cells probably explains why they develop in synchrony.

Cell Associations In Seminiferous Epithelium

Analysis of the detailed cellular composition of different patches of seminiferous epithelium shows that certain stages of spermatogenesis are consistently associated with certain other stages, constituting a particular **cell association**. Six different cell associations are recognized in human seminiferous epithelium. An example of such an association is shown in Figure 18-3. Each patch of seminiferous epithelium passes through all six consecutive associations in 16 days or so. This repeat period is therefore designated a **cycle** of the seminiferous epithelium. Every time a patch of this epithelium passes through approximately four cycles, a new crop of spermatozoa is finally produced, starting from pale type A spermatogonia. Spermatogenesis, like education, is an ongoing process, and for every "graduating class" of spermatozoa (graduating on a perpetual basis instead of once a year) a new generation of "freshmen" (pale type A spermatogonia) must be recruited for spermatogenesis to continue.

Radioautographic studies indicate that the duration of spermatogenesis, from stem cell to spermatozoon, is just over 2 months (64 $\pm$ 4 or 5 days). A widely accepted estimate of the total production time for mature human spermatozoa is 74 days.

Spermiogenesis

Without undergoing division, rounded spermatids transform into elongated spermatozoa. The organelles most involved are the spermatid's Golgi region, centrioles, nucleus, and mitochondria (Fig. 18-4A). First, a special membranous organelle known as the **acrosome vesicle** develops from the Golgi apparatus and adheres to one pole of the nucleus. A prominent rounded electron-dense granule known as the **acrosome** forms within the acrosome vesicle, which subsequently spreads around the anterior pole of the nucleus and becomes a flattened cup-shaped **head cap** (Fig. 18-4B). The acrosome contains hyaluronidase, lysosomal hydrolases, and a protease. These enzymes facilitate spermatozoal penetration of the corona radiata and zona pellucida at fertilization. Meanwhile, the paired centrioles have migrated to the caudal pole of the nucleus. Here, the axoneme of the **flagellum (tail)** develops in association with the more distal centriole, which later disappears. The nucleus elongates and flattens slightly when its chromatin continues to condense. Also, the head cap lengthens and proceeds to cover the anterior half of the nucleus (see Fig. 18-4C). The acrosomal contents become dispersed in the lumen of the head cap. Mitochondria associate with the proximal portion of the developing axoneme and then become arranged end to end in a tight helix as a collar-like

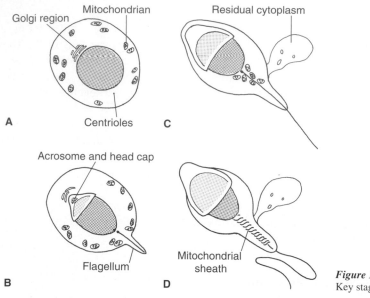

Figure 18-4
Key stages of spermiogenesis.

mitochondrial sheath that characterizes the **middle piece (midpiece)** of the spermatozoon (Fig. 18-4*D*). Residual cytoplasm (discarded between stages *D* and *E* in Fig. 18-4) is phagocytosed by the Sertoli cells.

Spermatozoa

Each spermatozoon consists of a head, midpiece (proximal portion of the flagellum), and tail (Figs. 18-5 and 18-6). The slightly flattened ellipsoidal head contains the nucleus, which is densely packed with condensed chromatin. Anteriorly, the nucleus is invested by the acrosomal head cap. The midpiece and the remainder of the tail constitute the flagellum. The midpiece incorporates the mitochondrial sheath and a small amount of cytoplasm. The remainder of the tail consists of a principal piece and an end piece. The arrangement of microtubules in the axoneme of the flagellum (nine peripheral doublets with a central pair of single microtubules) is similar to that found in cilia. Also, there is an outer ring of larger longitudinal **coarse fibers (outer dense fibers)**, the arrangement of which changes with the level along the tail. Proximally, there are nine interconnected coarse fibers. In the principal piece, two of these fibers are replaced by substantial **dorsal** and **ventral columns** that are interconnected by a series of circumferential **fibrous ribs**. The end piece is simpler, consisting of the flagellar axoneme and the surrounding region of cell membrane.

The mitochondrial sheath provides the ATP needed for flagellar motility. The fibrous sheath (coarse fibers and fibrous ribs) promotes propulsive lashing movements of the tail. Initially, however, such movements are feeble and ineffective, so spermatozoa are delivered passively to the epididymal ducts. While passing along these ducts, spermatozoa begin their maturation process, but capacitation, the final biochemical activation process leading to full attainment of fertilizing capacity, occurs only after they enter the female reproductive tract. A normal **sperm count** is at least 100 million spermatozoa per milliliter of semen, with an average ejaculate volume of 3 mL. The lower the sperm count, the smaller is the probability of successful fertilization, and men with sperm counts of below 20 million/mL are usually sterile. As many as 20% of the spermatozoa produced by fertile men may be morphologically imperfect without this affecting their fertility level. About 80% of the seminal volume represents combined fluid secretions from the seminal vesicles and prostate. Sper-

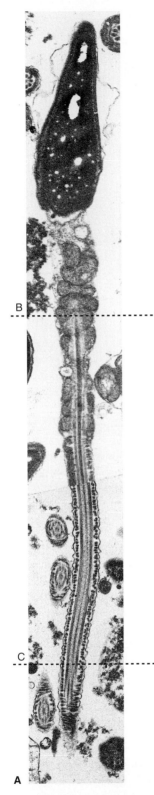

A

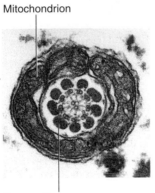

Mitochondrion

B

Coarse fibers
surrounding axoneme

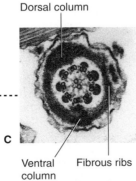

Dorsal column

C

Ventral   Fibrous ribs
column

Figure 18-5
Electron micrographs illustrating the fine structure
of a human spermatozoon. (*A*) Longitudinal
section. (*B*) Transverse section (at level B)
showing mitochondrial sheath of the middle piece.
(*C*) Transverse section (at level C) showing
fibrous sheath of the principal piece.

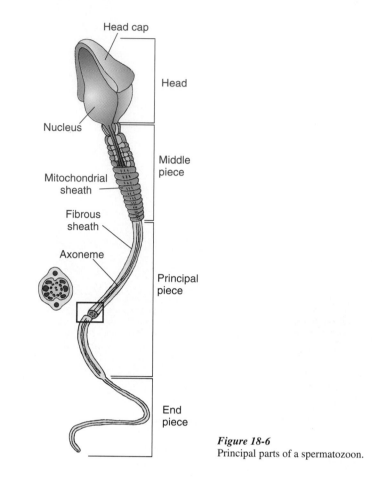

Figure 18-6
Principal parts of a spermatozoon.

matogenesis steadily declines with advancing age, but male reproductive capacity does not end suddenly in the same way as follicular maturation at menopause.

Interstitial (Leydig) Cells

Distributed as scattered islands in the stromal loose connective tissue between seminiferous tubules are the testosterone-secreting cells of the testis, hence the name **interstitial cells**. Lying in close association with blood capillaries or lymphatic capillaries, these steroid-producing cells are fairly large and have a more or less spherical nucleus (Plate 18-2). Their cytoplasm may appear pale because of its substantial content of cholesterol-containing lipid droplets. The first step in testosterone production from cholesterol (conversion to pregnenolone) is catalyzed by the mitochondrial cytochrome P450 enzyme, cholesterol desmolase. Subsequent steps are carried out in association with the sER, so this is extensive in interstitial cells (Fig. 18-7). Crystalloid inclusions of unknown significance also characterize the cytoplasm.

Hormonal Regulation of Testicular Function

Adequate plasma levels of both LH and FSH are necessary to maintain spermatogenesis. LH from anterior pituitary gonadotrophs stimulates the **interstitial cells** to secrete **testosterone**, a critical requirement for the early stages of spermatogenesis. The rising testosterone levels then suppress fur-

Lipochrome pigment

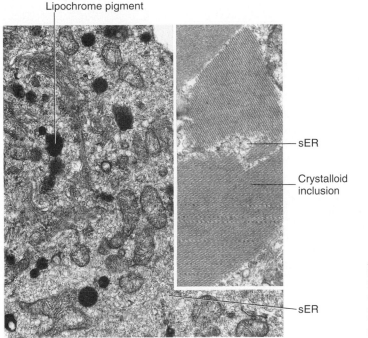

sER

Crystalloid
inclusion

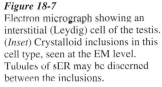

sER

Figure 18-7
Electron micrograph showing an
interstitial (Leydig) cell of the testis.
(*Inset*) Crystalloid inclusions in this
cell type, seen at the EM level.
Tubules of sER may be discerned
between the inclusions.

ther secretion of LH. FSH from the gonadotrophs stimulates the **Sertoli cells** to secrete an **andro-gen-binding protein** (ABP) into the luminal and lumen-associated compartment of the seminifer-ous tubules. By binding testosterone, this secreted binding protein maintains a sufficient local testos-terone concentration for spermatogenesis to proceed in the tubules. In the case of ABP, negative feedback is mediated by the polypeptide **inhibin**, which is also released by Sertoli cells in response to FSH. Rising inhibin levels suppress the further release of FSH. Final maturation stages of sper-matogenesis are particularly dependent on FSH.

Sertoli Cells

The simple columnar supporting epithelium of seminiferous tubules is made up of nonproliferating cells known as Sertoli cells. In LM sections, however, wide gaps seem to exist between these cells (see Fig. 18-3). The interposed gaps and highly irregular shapes of Sertoli cells result from the fact that successive generations of proliferating and differentiating male germ cell progenitors approach the tubular lumen by passing between the lateral borders of Sertoli cells. The spermatogenic cell population nestles in pockets in the peripheral cytoplasm of Sertoli cells (Fig. 18-8). Sertoli cells are characterized by a large, pale-staining nucleus that generally lies toward the base of the cell. Typi-cally elongated to ovoid, it may also be irregularly indented (see Fig. 18-3). Sertoli cells possess an elaborate Golgi complex, patches of rER, and an extensive sER. Lipid droplets and crystalloid in-clusions of unknown significance are also present in their cytoplasm.

Sertoli cells produce testicular fluid, a fluid secretion that enters the lumen of seminiferous tubules. In response to FSH, Sertoli cells also secrete ABP, the binding protein that effectively con-centrates testosterone in their immediate environment. Other functions generally ascribed to Sertoli cells are 1) nurture and nutritional support of their associated population of differentiating sper-matogenic cells, 2) translocation of these cells toward the lumen, 3) active delivery of newly-formed spermatozoa to the lumen (**spermiation**), and 4) phagocytic disposal of degenerating germ cells and surplus cytoplasm remaining from spermiogenesis.

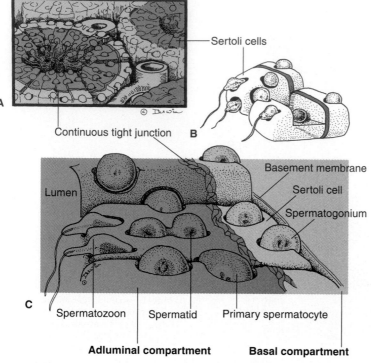

A

B

C

Sertoli cells

Continuous tight junction

Basement membrane

Sertoli cell

Spermatogonium

Lumen

Spermatozoon   Spermatid   Primary spermatocyte

Adluminal compartment   **Basal compartment**

Figure 18-8
Schematic diagram showing the structural arrangement by which Sertoli cells maintain the blood–testis permeability barrier. Interconnected by continuous tight junctions, Sertoli cells delimit two separate compartments containing different populations of spermatogenic cells. (*A*) Seminiferous tubules, showing the two separate compartments. (*B*) Sertoli cells (luminal view) showing the level where continuous tight junctions lie along their perimeters. (*C*) The two compartments, separated by tight junctions, with their contents.

Blood–Testis Barrier

A further characteristic of the Sertoli cells is that the basal regions of their lateral borders are interconnected by **continuous tight junctions** (see Fig. 18-8). These sealing junctions separate each seminiferous tubule into two distinct functional compartments. At the periphery of the tubule lies a **basal compartment** that extends inward to the level of the tight junctions. Then, extending inward from these junctions and including the lumen is an **adluminal compartment**. Most large molecules do not pass into the adluminal compartment from the basal compartment, and vice versa. In particular, potential access of large circulating molecules in the blood to the adluminal compartment is restricted. This permeability barrier is known as the blood–testis barrier.

Spermatogonia are basally situated in the epithelium, adjacent to its basement membrane (see Fig. 18-3). Hence, the mitotic proliferation of spermatogonia occurs in the basal compartment, comparable in interstitial composition to the intercellular environment in the rest of the body. By the time the differentiating progeny of spermatogonia begin prophase I, however, they have entered the adluminal compartment, occupying lateral pockets that lie nearer to the luminal border of Sertoli cells as depicted in Figure 18-8. Because of such progression, primary spermatocytes and all their progeny depend on nutrients reaching them indirectly from Sertoli cells. The seal effected by the zonular tight junctions of Sertoli cells enables these cells to provide a special microenvironment for spermatogenic differentiation. In particular, Sertoli cells play a key role in maintaining the necessary testosterone concentration in the adluminal compartment of seminiferous tubules through their secretion of ABP. When the successive generations of spermatocytes develop and pass into the adluminal compartment, new tight junctions form between the Sertoli cells at a level between the type A and the type B spermatogonia. Hence, progression of germ cell progenitors toward the lumen does not disturb functional compartmentalization of the tubule.

Confinement of the differentiating spermatogenic cells to their own special compartment has certain associated advantages. Because of genetic recombination in diplotene of prophase I, novel antigens may be expressed on the surface of these cells. In males, such antigens do not appear until puberty and as a consequence they have the potential to elicit a self-directed immune response (autoimmunity). Segregation of spermatogenic cells in the adluminal compartment restricts access of their "foreign" antigens to the immune system. Second, in the event that such an immune response does occur, passage of humoral antibodies into this compartment is restricted by the blood–testis barrier. The various ducts that lead from the testis, however, lack such a barrier, so protection is afforded only while the germ cells are forming.

The blood–testis barrier also helps to protect the differentiating spermatogenic cells from drugs, toxic chemicals, and mutagens (substances that cause mutations) that may enter the bloodstream. A third important feature of this arrangement is that it provides the specific environment for spermatogenesis by maintaining the appropriate hormonal and ionic requirements.

EFFERENT TESTICULAR DUCTS

The seminiferous tubules of each testis open by way of the **rete testis** into the 12 or so **ductuli efferentes** of the associated epididymis (see Fig. 18-2). Most of the epididymis consists of a long convoluted duct called the **ductus epididymis**, together with a thin fibrous external investment (corresponding to the tunica albuginea) with its covering visceral layer of tunica vaginalis testis. Each of the ductuli efferentes emerging from the upper pole of the testis is wound up into a small conical mass. The ductuli efferentes have a simple columnar epithelial lining made up of groups of tall ciliated cells alternating with groups of low absorptive cells that resorb some of the testicular fluid. Hence, ductuli efferentes may be recognized by their distinctive festooned (garland-like) appearance. External to the basement membrane of the epithelium lies a thin circular layer of smooth muscle.

Ductus Epididymis

Ciliary activity in the ductuli efferentes of each testis passively conveys spermatozoa to the **ductus epididymis**, a highly convoluted duct that together with its supporting connective tissue makes up the body and tail of the epididymis. The ductus epididymis and more distal male genital ducts lack motile cilia. Instead, the ductus epididymis has **stereocilia** (Gk. *stereos*, solid) each representing a group of immotile long microvilli. The ductus epididymis is lined by pseudostratified columnar epithelium with stereocilia (Fig. 18-9). The surrounding circular layer of smooth muscle increases in

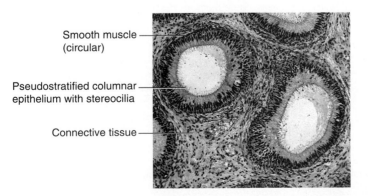

Smooth muscle (circular)

Pseudostratified columnar epithelium with stereocilia

Connective tissue

Figure 18-9
Ductus epididymis (epididymis, medium power).

thickness with distance along the duct. The ductus epididymis constitutes a **storage reservoir** for spermatozoa that begin their maturation and start acquiring fertilizing capacity while passing along this duct. It represents a major site of fluid resorption and has a partly secretory epithelium that produces the maturation-promoting factors necessary for spermatozoal maturation to commence.

Ducti Deferentes

Each **ductus deferens**, alternatively known as a **vas deferens**, is a substantial muscular-walled duct with three thick layers of smooth muscle in its wall and a relatively small lumen. The middle muscle layer is circular, whereas the others are longitudinal (Fig. 18-10). During emission, peristaltic contractions in these muscle layers transfer spermatozoa from the ductus epididymis to the urethra. The pseudostratified columnar epithelium of the ducti deferentes possesses stereocilia, except in the dilated distal portion of these ducts. The epithelium and the underlying fibroelastic lamina propria are corrugated with longitudinal folds. Within each spermatic cord, the ductus deferens is attached by its loose connective tissue adventitia to the accompanying arteries, pampaniform plexus of anastomosing veins, lymphatics, and nerves.

CLINICAL IMPLICATIONS

Vasectomy
Bilateral ligation of the ducti deferentes (vasa deferentia) has gained some acceptance as a relatively trouble-free means of birth control. This simple procedure, called vasectomy, prevents delivery of spermatozoa by way of the urethra. Instead, only the secretions of the accessory glands (seminal vesicles and prostate) are present in the ejaculate. Spermatogenesis nevertheless continues, producing spermatozoa that subsequently become resorbed without discomfort. In roughly 50% of the cases, however, fertility is not regained if circumstances change. In addition to the difficulty of restoring patency to the ligated ducts, autoimmunity may develop against postpubertally expressed novel spermatozoal antigens, and this may cause a permanent loss of fertility.

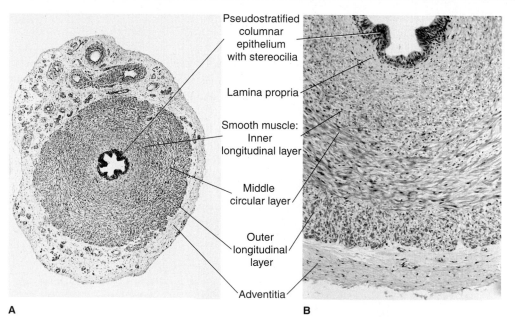

Pseudostratified columnar epithelium with stereocilia

Lamina propria

Smooth muscle:
Inner longitudinal layer

Middle circular layer

Outer longitudinal layer

Adventitia

A   **B**

Figure 18-10
Ductus deferens (vas deferens). (*A*) Very low power view. (*B*) Medium power view, showing the smooth muscle arrangement in the walls of this duct.

SEMINAL VESICLES

Each seminal vesicle is a tortuous, secretory tubular diverticulum bound by its adventitia into an elongated and compact vesicular mass. A section of a seminal vesicle accordingly shows many convolutions of the same tube, transected at various levels (Plate 18-3). This tube has substantial walls made of smooth muscle, with an inner circular muscle layer and an outer longitudinal layer. During emission, its smooth muscle contracts and adds stored vesicular secretion to the seminal fluid. The external adventitial coat of the vesicle is made of highly elastic loose connective tissue, which over the superior end of the vesicle is covered by peritoneum and constitutes a serosa. The glandular appearance of the vesicle is chiefly due to elaborate infolding of its secretory epithelium, which provides an extensive secretory surface and permits the vesicular lumen to distend when it fills with stored secretion. The lamina propria contains abundant elastin, and the epithelial lining, composed of tall columnar secretory cells, is partly pseudostratified and partly simple. Its copious secretion is viscid, slightly yellowish, and rich in nutrients. Secretory activity of the seminal vesicles requires adequate **testosterone** levels.

PROSTATE

The prostate is made up of many compound tubuloalveolar glands, arranged in three concentric regions around the **prostatic urethra** into which they open. Because the prostate surrounds the proximal portion of the urethra where this emerges from the bladder (see Fig. 18-1), prostatic enlargement has an occluding effect on the outlet of the bladder, a problem that is fairly common in men past middle age. If severe, benign obstruction may require partial prostatectomy to alleviate it.

The constituent glands of the prostate include small **mucosal glands** associated with the urethral mucosa, intermediate-sized **submucosal glands** lying peripheral to the mucosal glands, and large **main prostatic glands** situated toward the periphery of the gland (Fig. 18-11). The numerous mucosal glands are the ones that commonly overgrow, causing **benign prostatic hyperplasia** in older men. The subcapsular main prostatic glands have a higher probability of malignant change.

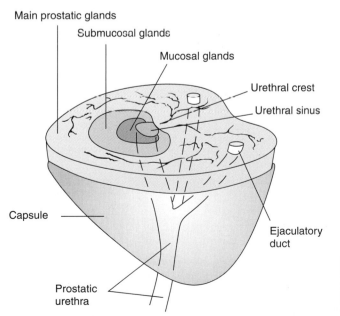

Figure 18-11
Schematic diagram of the inferior part of the prostate, showing the three groups of prostatic glands in relation to the prostatic urethra.

Each component gland of the prostate possesses a branched duct system and many irregularly shaped secretory units characterized by a tall columnar secretory epithelium that is highly folded (Plate 18-4). These folds allow the secretory units to distend when they fill up with stored secretion. The fibroclastic lamina propria is relatively vascular. Prostatic secretory epithelium is either pseudostratified or simple, depending on its level of secretory activity. Its thin, slightly acidic milky secretion contains several enzymes, notably acid phosphatase, and several other constituents. The stored secretion sometimes produces intraluminal calcified **concretions** in the prostatic secretory units, particularly in older men (see Plate 18-4*B*). The prostatic capsule and stroma lying between the secretory units consist of a distinctive mixture of dense fibroelastic connective tissue and smooth muscle, giving the prostate a firm consistency. The unique combination of this fibromuscular stroma, a markedly folded secretory epithelium, and concretions in secretory units (in cases where concretions have formed), is indicative of prostate sections. Forceful contractions of the smooth muscle component of the stroma and capsule express stored prostatic fluid from the gland during emission and this fluid, too, contributes to semen. Secretory activity of the prostate, in common with that of the seminal vesicles, requires adequate **testosterone** levels. If testosterone levels fall too low, the secretory tall columnar prostatic epithelium becomes nonsecretory and low cuboidal.

PENIS

The body of the penis contains erectile tissue arranged as three cylindrical **cavernous bodies (corpora)**, bound together and surrounded by elastic loose connective tissue with an outer covering of thin skin (Fig. 18-12). Paired **corpora cavernosa**, fused along their approximated medial borders, lie dorsal to a somewhat longer **corpus spongiosum** that surrounds the **urethra** and terminates as the **glans penis**. Penile skin moves freely over the underlying tissues and, unless trimmed by circumcision, extends over the glans as the **prepuce** (foreskin), a retractable protective fold of skin. Each cavernous body is encapsulated by a tough fibrous sheath called a **tunica albuginea** (see Fig. 18-12). The interior of each cavernous body consists of irregular vascular spaces, lined by endothelium, that are separated by intervening trabeculae (partitions) containing dense fibroelastic tissue

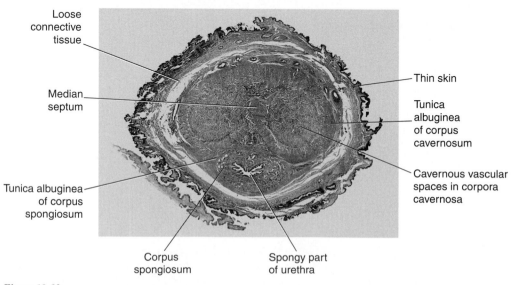

Figure 18-12
Body of penis (transverse section, very low power).

and smooth muscle. The penis, especially the glans penis, is abundantly supplied with various types of sensory receptors.

Before any response to sexual arousal, the penis remains flaccid because its cavernous bodies receive little blood. Erection is an involuntary response brought about by parasympathetic postganglionic efferent nerve impulses. It is a consequence of smooth muscle relaxation in the thick-walled distributing arteries supplying the cavernous vascular spaces. Parasympathetic impulses cause these arteries to dilate, allowing more blood to enter the spaces, and when each cavernous body distends it presses against the inextensible tunica albuginea that surrounds it. In the corpora cavernosa, such distention compresses the veins that drain blood from the vascular spaces, and resulting engorgement results in erection. The corpus spongiosum becomes less turgid because its tunica albuginea is more extensible, and this avoids undue compression of the penile urethra. After emission, which is a sympathetic efferent response, flaccidity returns when the arterial smooth muscle regains its former tonus.

MALE URETHRA

The male urethra has three parts. The **prostatic urethra** traversing the prostate is lined with a transitional epithelium that becomes pseudostratified or stratified columnar epithelium distally. The short **membranous urethra** traversing the urogenital diaphragm is also lined with stratified columnar epithelium. The **spongy part (penile urethra)**, the last and longest portion of the urethra, begins where the urethra enters the corpus spongiosum and extends as far as the external urethral orifice. Its epithelium is predominantly stratified columnar, but it becomes stratified squamous in the distal part of the navicular fossa, its terminal widening within the glans. Two **bulbourethral glands** opening into the proximal end of the penile urethra (see Fig. 18-1) are tubuloalveolar minor compound glands that produce a viscous lubricating secretion under conditions of sexual arousal. Minor mucus-secreting **urethral glands** are also closely associated with the distal part of the male urethra.

Summary

Spermatogenesis is summarized in Tables 18-2 and 18-3. For comparison with oogenesis, see Table 17-3.

Pocket-like surface invaginations in Sertoli cells (the supporting columnar cells of seminiferous tubules) contain proliferating and differentiating spermatogenic cells. Renewing spermatogenic stem cells (pale type A spermatogonia) lie within the basal compartment of the tubule, adjacent to its basement membrane. This compartment also contains dark type A spermatogonia (reserve stem cells) and type B spermatogonia (early differentiating progenitors). Spermatogonia are diploid cells with an extensive potential for mitosis. Primary spermatocytes, the diploid progeny of type B spermatogonia, enter an extended prophase I. Without passing into a prolonged (dictyotene) stage, they then undergo the meiotic reduction division, forming secondary spermatocytes. These haploid cells soon divide, forming spermatids. The clonal descendants of each spermatogonium, connected by intercellular bridges, divide and differentiate in synchrony. Successive generations of progenitors are produced on a continuous, overlapping basis, with about four waves of spermatogenesis proceeding concurrently at any given moment. Spermatozoa are generated from pale type A spermatogonia in approximately 2 months. Spermiogenesis involves development of the acrosomic system (acrosome and head cap) from the spermatid's Golgi region, along with flagellum formation, nuclear condensation and elongation, and mitochondrial rearrangement as a sheath. Head cap enzymes facilitate penetration of the oocyte coverings at fertilization. Most of the sperm tail has an outer fibrous sheath. Semen contains over 100 million spermatozoa per milliliter, together with fluids from the seminal vesicles and prostate. Capacitation of spermatozoa in the female reproductive tract is necessary for them to attain full fertilizing capacity.

Stromal interstitial cells secrete testosterone in response to LH. Testosterone promotes spermatogenesis and secretory activity of male accessory glands. FSH stimulates Sertoli cells to secrete ABP, the androgen-binding protein that maintains the requisite local testosterone concentration. In addition, Sertoli cells produce testicular fluid, and possess zonular tight junctions that seal off the adluminal compartment, with its distinctive internal composition, from the basal compartment. Sertoli cells also nurture germ cell progenitors nestling in their peripheral cytoplasm.

Spermatozoa pass by way of the rete testis and ciliated ductuli efferentes to the ductus epididymis, the pseudostratified columnar lining of which bears stereocilia and is both resorptive and secretory. Maturation of spermatozoa begins while they are stored in this duct. Leading from the ductus epididymis to the ejaculatory duct on each side is a ductus (vas) deferens characterized by thick muscular walls. Peristalsis in this duct propels spermatozoa into the urethra during emission. Its lining epithelium resembles that of the ductus epididymis. The tortuous, muscular-walled seminal vesicles, with tall columnar secretory epithelium (partly pseudostratified and partly simple), deliver their stored secretion by way of the ejaculatory ducts during emission. The prostate, made up of many compound glands, has an extensively folded tall columnar secretory epithelium, commonly with intraluminal concretions. During emission, its fibromuscular stroma and capsule contract, delivering stored prostatic fluid. The prostatic urethra is lined with transitional epithelium. Other parts of the male urethra are lined with stratified columnar epithelium.

Lying inferior to the dorsal paired corpora cavernosa of the penis is the medial corpus spongiosum traversed by the spongy part of the urethra. Under conditions of penile arterial dilatation, which is a parasympathetic response, more blood enters the vascular spaces of the corpora cavernosa. Resulting compression of the efferent veins restricts venous drainage from the corpora cavernosa and causes erection. Flaccidity is regained when sympathetic stimulation constricts the arteries.

Bibliography

General

Aumuller G, Seitz J. Protein secretion and secretory processes in male accessory sex glands. Int Rev Cytol 121:127, 1990.

Burger H, De Kretser, eds. The Testis, ed 2. New York, Academic Press, 1989.

Hamilton DW, Greep RO, eds. Handbook of Physiology, vol 5, sect 7. Male Reproductive System. Washington, DC, American Physiological Society, 1975.

Johnson MH, Everitt BJ. Essential Reproduction, ed 4. Oxford, Blackwell Scientific Publications, 1995.

Kerr JB. Ultrastructure of the seminiferous epithelium and intertubular tissue of the human testis. J Electron Microsc Tech 19:215, 1991.

Hafez ESE, Spring-Mills E, eds. Accessory Glands of the Male Reproductive Tract. Ann Arbor, MI, Ann Arbor Science, 1979.

Orgebin-Crist MC, Danzo BJ, eds. Cell biology of the testis and epididymis. Ann NY Acad Sci 513:1, 1987.

Riva A, Usai E, Cossu M, Scarpa R, Testa Riva F. The human bulbo-urethral glands: a transmission electron microscopy and scanning electron microscopy study. J Androl 9:133, 1988.

Russell LD, Ettlin RA, Sinha Hikim AP, Clegg ED. Histological and Histopathological Evaluation of the Testis. Clearwater, Fla., Cache River Press, 1990.

Trainer TD. Histology of the normal testis. Am J Surg Pathol 11:797, 1987.

Van Blerkom J, Motta P. The Cellular Basis of Mammalian Reproduction. Baltimore, Urban & Schwarzenberg, 1979.

Yeung CH, Cooper TG, Bergmann M, Schulze H. Organization of tubules in the human caput epididymides and the ultrastructure of their epithelia. Am J Anat 191:261, 1991.

Spermatogenesis, Spermatozoa, and Fertilization

Fawcett DW. The cell biology of gametogenesis in the male. Perspect Biol Med 2(Part 2):S56, 1979.

Fawcett DW, Bedford JM, eds. The Spermatozoon: Maturation, Motility and Surface Properties. Baltimore, Urban & Schwarzenberg, 1979.

Hafez ESE, Kanagawa H. Scanning electron microscopy of human, monkey, and rabbit spermatozoa. Fertil Steril 24:776, 1973.

Holstein AF, Roosen-Runge EC. Atlas of Human Spermatogenesis. Berlin, Grosse Verlag, 1981.

Matsumoto AM, Bremner WJ. Endocrine control of human spermatogenesis. J Steroid Biochem 33:789, 1989.

Sharpe RM. Follicle-stimulating hormone and spermatogenesis in the adult male. J Endocrinol 121:405, 1989.

Sidhu KS, Guraya SS. Cellular and molecular biology of capacitation and acrosome reaction in mammalian spermatozoa. Int Rev Cytol 118:231, 1989.

Sidhu KS, Guraya SS. Current concepts in gamete receptors for fertilization in mammals. Int Rev Cytol 127:253, 1991.

Tung K. Immunopathology and male infertility. Hosp Prac 23(6):191, 1988.

Wassarman PM. Early events in mammalian fertilization. Annu Rev Cell Biol 3:109, 1987.

Wassarman PM. Fertilization in mammals. Sci Am 259(6):78, 1988.

Interstitial (Leydig) Cells, Sertoli Cells, and Blood–Testis Barrier

Davidoff MS, Schulze W, Middendorff R, Holstein A-F. The Leydig cell of the human testis: a new member of the diffuse neuroendocrine system. Cell Tissue Res 271:429, 1993.

DeJong, FH. Inhibin. Physiol Rev 68:555, 1988.

Dorrington JH, Armstrong DT. Effects of FSH on gonadal functions. Recent Prog Horm Res 35:301, 1979.

Dufau ML. Endocrine regulation and communicating functions of the Leydig cell. Annu Rev Physiol 50:483, 1988.

Dym M, Cavicchia JC. Functional morphology of the testis. Biol Reprod 18:1, 1978.

Fritz IB. Sites of action of androgens and follicle stimulating hormone on cells of the seminiferous tubule. In: Litwack E ed. Biochemical Actions of Hormones, vol 5. New York, Academic Press, 1979, p 249.

Garde SV, Moodbidri SB, Phadke AM, Sheth AR. Localization of inhibin in human testes by immunoperoxidase technique. Anat Rec 222:357, 1988.

Gilula NB, Fawcett DW, Aoki A. Ultrastructural and experimental observations on the Sertoli cell junctions of the mammalian testis. Dev Biol 50:142, 1976.

Griswold MD. Protein secretions of Sertoli cells. Int Rev Cytol 110:133, 1988

Nagano T, Suzuki F. Cell junctions in the seminiferous tubule and the excurrent ducts of the testis. Int Rev Cytol 81:163, 1983.

Setchell BP. The functional significance of the blood–testis barrier. J Androl 1:3, 1980.

CHAPTER 19

Eye and Ear

OBJECTIVES

This final chapter should prepare you to do the following:

- Draw a simple diagram of an eye, showing its main features
- Describe photoreceptors and explain how their structure relates to function
- Name four types of retinal neurons that participate in collecting visual information
- Trace the path taken by sound waves when they enter the ear
- Explain what is meant by hair cells and state three of their functions
- Summarize the histological organization of the organ of Corti

EYE

The eyes are elaborate sensory organs necessary for the special sense of sight. By detecting intensities and wavelengths of light patterns entering them from the body's environment, the eyes enable the visual cortex to formulate an accurate impression of the surroundings, which under ordinary circumstances (adequate lighting and the use of both eyes) are perceived not only in color but also in three dimensions. For this purpose, the eyes have both an **image-forming mechanism** analogous to that of a camera and an **image-sensing mechanism** that employs two types of light-sensitive cells known as **photoreceptors**.

Each eye is situated in an orbit of the skull, with adipose and other tissues cushioning it from behind and the eyelids protecting it anteriorly. The surface of the eye is bathed by **tears** from the associated **lacrimal gland**. As shown in Figure 19-1, the eye is made up of an **anterior chamber**, a small **posterior chamber**, a **lens**, and a fairly large **vitreous chamber** occupied by a transparent gelatinous globular mass known as the **vitreous body**. Separating the anterior and posterior chambers is the **iris**, an adjustable circular diaphragm that regulates the size of the **pupil**. The wall of the eye is composed of three main coats. Outermost is an inelastic **fibrous coat** (Fig. 19-2A), which has a supporting function. The opaque white region of this coat is termed the **sclera** (Gk. *scleros*, hard), and its circular transparent window is known as the **cornea**. Internal to the fibrous coat lies a well-

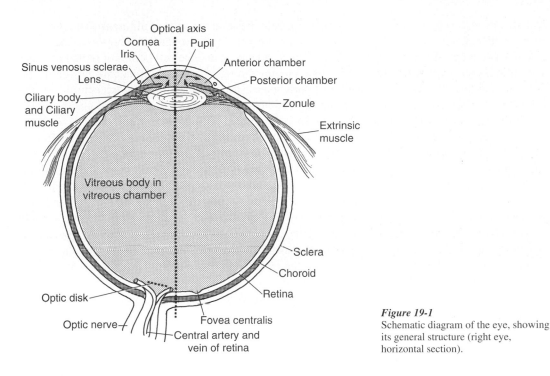

Figure 19-1
Schematic diagram of the eye, showing its general structure (right eye, horizontal section).

vascularized and heavily pigmented middle layer known as the **vascular coat** (see Fig. 19-2*B*). Anteriorly, the vascular coat is represented by 1) the **iris**, a pigmented area at the perimeter of the pupil that imparts particular eye colors according to the number and distribution of its melanin-containing cells, and 2) the **ciliary body**, an inwardly projecting, ring-shaped thickening of the vascular coat that lies at the corneoscleral junction and houses the **ciliary muscle**, the smooth muscle that focuses the lens. Posterior to the ciliary body, the vascular coat is represented by 3) the heavily melanized **choroid**, an intensely dark brown (almost black) yet richly vascularized nutritive layer that minimizes glare by absorbing scattered and reflected light. The innermost coat of the eye wall, termed the **retinal coat** (see Fig. 19-2*C*), is made up of an inner layer of **nervous tissue** (the **neural retina**)

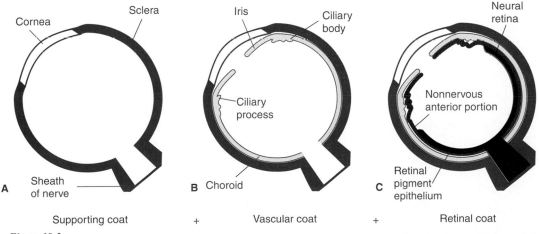

Figure 19-2
Three component coats of the wall of the eye.

bounded by an outer layer of simple cuboidal epithelium called the **retinal pigment epithelium** because of its melanin content. The **neural retina** represents the **light-sensitive** region of the eye. It contains two types of photoreceptors, termed **rods** and **cones**, and the cell bodies of retinal neurons. The **retinal pigment epithelium** absorbs light passing through the neural retina, thus preventing reflection back into the eye. Furthermore, it participates in upkeep of the photoreceptors and biochemical processing of their visual pigments. In addition, continuous tight junctions positioned between the cell perimeters in this epithelium constitute part of a **blood–retina barrier**.

Four components of the eye are transparent. One is the **cornea**, the clear window in the fibrous coat. Behind this lies a transparent watery medium called **aqueous humor**, formed by processes of the ciliary body. Aqueous humor provides nutrients for most of the avascular cornea and also for the third transparent eye component, the lens, which is similarly avascular. The fourth transparent component is the **vitreous body**, a highly hydrated gelatinous mass containing hyaluronic acid, dispersed type II collagen fibrils, and other proteins. The vitreous body is traversed from optic nerve to lens by a **hyaloid canal**, an indistinct channel that contains a vestige of the embryonic hyaloid artery. Besides transmitting light rays, this globular viscoelastic mass lies in contact with the inner aspect of the retina, gently holding it in place against the rest of the wall, and provides comparable support for the posterior border of the lens (see Fig. 19-1).

The following sections deal with the image-forming components of the eye and the image-sensing region, the retina.

Cornea

The cornea is the clear circular area that forms the anterior part of the supporting coat of the eye. It differs from the sclera in that it is both transparent and avascular. Also, its radius of curvature is slightly smaller (see Fig. 19-1). Its convex outer surface, the corneal—air interface, is the main site of refraction (light bending) that directs light rays on their convergent path toward the retina.

The anterior surface of the cornea is covered by a **stratified squamous nonkeratinizing epithelium** (Fig. 19-3) that contains pain receptors. Normally, this epithelium is kept moist by a film of tears without which the cornea tends to ulcerate. A basement membrane attaches the anterior epithelium to an acellular layer of stromal interstitial matrix termed **Bowman's membrane**. The bulk of the corneal stroma, the **substantia propria**, is made up of numerous flat interstitial layers containing type I collagen fibrils and proteoglycan, with fibrocytes sandwiched between them. The pos-

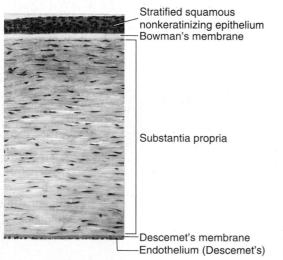

Stratified squamous
nonkeratinizing epithelium
Bowman's membrane

Substantia propria

Descemet's membrane
Endothelium (Descemet's)

Figure 19-3
Cornea, showing its histologic organization (*top*, anterior surface; *bottom*, posterior surface).

terior surface of the cornea is lined by a simple squamous epithelium and its associated thick basement membrane (**Descemet's endothelium** and **membrane**). By convention, the posterior epithelium is known as **corneal endothelium** even though it has nothing to do with the circulatory system. It appears to be responsible for transferring some of the water from the corneal stroma to the aqueous humor. Overhydration of the corneal stroma renders it cloudy.

CLINICAL IMPLICATIONS

Corneal Damage
Nutrients reach the cornea from the aqueous humor and scleral capillaries near the corneoscleral junction. Much of the oxygen, however, has to come directly from the air, and this has to be taken into account in the manufacture of soft plastic contact lenses of the permanent kind that may be worn for extended periods. Also, because the cornea is so exposed it is highly susceptible to abrasion or penetration by flying particles or projecting objects. The ensuing healing process may take several weeks to complete, and in severe cases it may lead to excessive scarring of the cornea and subsequent opacification requiring corneal transplantation to correct it.

Iris

Light passes to the interior of the eye through the pupil, the size of which is regulated involuntarily by the iris. By regulating the pupillary aperture through the **pupillary light reflex**, the iris optimizes the amount of light reaching the retina, compensating for a wide range of intensities. For this purpose, the iris is provided with a smooth muscle sphincter called the **constrictor pupillae** and an antagonistic **dilator pupillae** muscle composed of myoepithelial cells.

The concentration and distribution of melanin-containing cells in the loose connective tissue stroma of the iris determines eye color. Melanin that is limited to the two-layered cuboidal **pigmented epithelium** on the posterior surface of the iris can appear blue when seen through the stroma. The eyes appear brown if the melanin-containing cells are distributed throughout the stroma. The role of these light-absorbing cells is to block excess light, allowing only the right amount of it to enter by way of the pupil. Anteriorly, the iris is covered with a discontinuous layer of stromal cells. The constrictor pupillae is a circular compact band of smooth muscle that lies at the pupillary margin. The dilator pupillae is a less distinct single sheet of radially oriented myoepithelial cells that lies next to the posterior pigmented epithelium.

CLINICAL IMPLICATIONS

Reduced Drainage of Aqueous Humor in Glaucoma
Aqueous humor can flow around the pupillary margin of the iris through a valve-like arrangement where the anterior surface of the lens makes contact with the posterior border of the pupillary margin. When a pressure difference displaces the iris anteriorly, this one-way valve opens, admitting aqueous humor from the posterior chamber to the anterior chamber. The arrows in Figure 19-1 indicate the path taken by the aqueous humor. From the anterior chamber, aqueous humor drains by way of a circumferential venous canal called the **sinus venosus sclerae** (see Figs. 19-1 and 19-5), also known as the circular **Schlemm's canal**.

In a type of glaucoma known as **narrow-angle glaucoma**, the **angle of the anterior chamber (iridocorneal angle)** between the anterior border of the iris and the posterior border of the cornea is unusually acute. This angle is the site occupied by the sinus venosus sclerae (see Figs. 19-1 and 19-5). Drainage through the spaces leading to this venous canal may become restricted through narrowness of the angle, resulting in periods of elevated intraocular pressure. Because chronic elevation of intraocular pressure compromises retinal nourishment and is a cause of corneal opacification, it is recognized as a potentially avoidable factor predisposing to eyesight impairment.

Lens

The eye's biconvex lens, transparent and avascular like the cornea, is its image focusing component. To achieve this, the lens has to be highly elastic and its inherent tendency is to increase its own curvature (that is, to assume a more globular form). A unique capacity for changing shape enables the lens to bring into focus either the divergent rays from near objects or the more parallel rays from objects that are farther away. The lens consists entirely of modified epithelial cells that are arranged concentrically within an external **lens capsule** representing their substantial basement membrane (Fig. 19-4). Most of them are **lens fibers**, highly modified elongated cells that dispense with their nucleus and become transparent. Covering the anterior ends of the lens fibers, and merging with the smallest and most recently formed lens fibers at the **equator** (circumference) of the lens, is an anterior simple cuboidal epithelium. This additional layer of epithelial cells provides a circumferential **germinal zone** where new lens fibers may be added in adult life (see Fig. 19-4). Since the lens is totally epithelial, its nutrition depends on diffusion from both the aqueous humor bathing its anterior surface and the vitreous body behind it.

CLINICAL IMPLICATIONS

Accommodation
The equatorial region of the lens capsule is attached to the adjacent ciliary body by a circular suspensory ligament. This ligament, termed the **ciliary zonule** (see Fig. 19-1), is made up of bundles of fibrillin-containing fibrils having the same glycoprotein composition as the microfibrils present in elastic fibers. Elastin, however, is not present. When the eyes are in a rested, unstrained state, the inherent tendency for the lens to bulge because of its own elasticity is resisted by tension in the zonule. *Relaxation* of the **ciliary muscle**, a smooth muscle consisting of radial, meridional, and circular fibers that is situated within the ciliary body (Fig. 19-5), produces sufficient tension in the zonule to pull the lens into the more flattened configuration required for viewing distant objects. *Contraction* of the ciliary muscle pulls the ciliary body forward and toward the equator of the lens, easing the tension in the zonule and allowing the lens to assume its more convex shape. This mechanism, termed **accommodation**, brings near objects into focus. However, the capacity of the lens for regaining a more globular shape declines in middle age because of progressive *hardening* of the lens, which is why spectacles may then become necessary for reading small print.

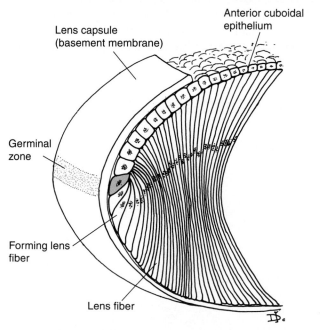

Figure 19-4
Lens, showing its histologic organization and circumferential germinal zone (horizontal section).

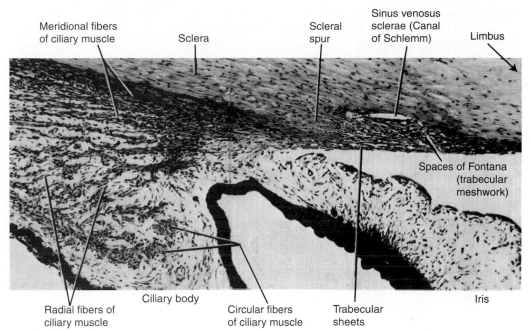

Figure 19-5
Structures present at the iridocorneal angle (angle of the anterior chamber). Aqueous humor drains into the sinus venosus sclerae (Schlemm's canal) from the anterior chamber, which lies to the right.

Retina

The image sensing region of the eye is known as the **neural retina**. This layer and its associated **retinal pigment epithelium** (the outer layer of the retinal coat) make up the retina. It should be understood that when applied to the retina, *inner* and *outer* still refer to the eye as a whole. Also, it should be realized that the light-sensitive portion of photoreceptors lies deep to (*external* to) other retinal neurons transparent enough for light to pass through them in reaching these receptors. The afferent nerve impulses relayed through the retina pass from its outermost to its innermost layer, that is, in the opposite direction to light (Fig. 19-6).

Representing the outermost layer of the retina is the **retinal pigment epithelium**. Then comes a layer containing the light-sensitive portion (**outer segment**) of the rods and cones (Figs. 19-6 and 19-7 and **Plate 19-1**). The inner part of this layer contains the **inner segment** of the photoreceptors.

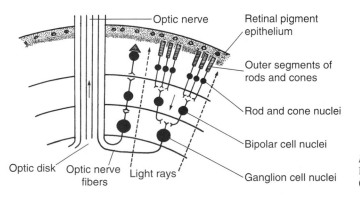

Figure 19-6
Basic organization of the retina (simplified).

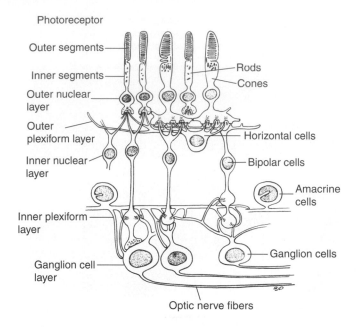

Photoreceptor

Outer segments

Inner segments

Outer nuclear layer

Outer plexiform layer

Inner nuclear layer

Inner plexiform layer

Ganglion cell layer

Rods

Cones

Horizontal cells

Bipolar cells

Amacrine cells

Ganglion cells

Optic nerve fibers

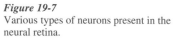

Figure 19-7
Various types of neurons present in the neural retina.

The next layer, called the **outer nuclear layer** (see Fig. 19-7 and Plate 19-1*A*), contains the rod and cone nuclei. In the next layer, the **outer plexiform layer**, the stubby axonic extensions of the photoreceptors synapse with the dendrites of a second order of neurons. The two types of neurons in the outer plexiform layer are 1) radial **bipolar cells** (see Figs. 19-6 and 19-7) that relay impulses to a third order of neurons called **ganglion cells** and 2) **horizontal cells** that interconnect the photoreceptors laterally. The **inner nuclear layer** that comes next (see Fig. 19-7 and Plate 19-1*A*) contains the nuclei of **bipolar cells** and horizontal **amacrine cells**. It also contains the nuclei of **Müller cells** (see Plate 19-1). These tall columnar radial supporting cells, the chief glial cells of the neural retina, span almost its full thickness. In the next layer, the **inner plexiform layer**, amacrine cells interconnect bipolar cells as well as ganglion cells. They also connect each bipolar cell with several ganglion cells. **Amacrine cells** (Gk. *a*, without; *makros*, long; *inos*, fiber) are unusual neurons because they seem to lack an axon. Their dendrites constitute the postsynaptic terminal of some synapses and the presynaptic terminal of others. Bipolar cells also synapse directly with ganglion cells in this layer. The next layer, termed the **ganglion cell layer** (see Fig. 19-7 and Plate 19-1*A*), contains the nuclei of ganglion cells (see Fig. 19-6). The innermost layer of the retina consists largely of the **optic nerve fibers** converging on the **optic disk**, the site of exit of the optic nerve (see Fig. 19-1). These unmyelinated nerve fibers traverse the sclera and acquire myelin sheaths in the optic nerve. The optic disk is penetrated by the central retinal artery and vein. Capillaries containing blood supplied by the central retinal artery provide nutrients and oxygen to the inner third of the neural retina. The outer third, which contains the all-important photoreceptors, depends on diffusion from the capillaries in the adjacent choroid (ie, the choriocapillaris) for its nourishment. The optic disk is devoid of photoreceptors and therefore represents a **blind spot**.

The retinal region with greatest visual acuity is the **fovea centralis** (L., central pit). The fovea lies close to the posterior pole of the eye, slightly lateral to the optical axis (see Fig. 19-1). The closely packed photoreceptors in this shallow retinal depression, free of covering blood vessels, are all cones responsive to color. The fovea centralis lies in the middle of a yellowish pigmented area termed the **macula lutea** (L., yellow spot).

Photoreceptors

Rods and cones are basically similar in design. Rods tend to be taller, however, and cones are slightly wider with a conical, instead of cylindrical, outer segment (see Fig. 19-7 and Plate 19-1). Also, whereas rods respond to low light intensities and produce visual images perceived in shades of gray, cones respond to higher light intensities, discern finer details, and, because they represent three populations each responsive to light over different wavelength ranges, produce visual images perceived in color.

Each photoreceptor is made up of an **outer segment** connected by a narrow stalk to an **inner segment**, a **nuclear region**, and a thick axonic extension terminating in a **synaptic body** (Fig. 19-8). The **outer segment** contains a stack of distinctive **membranous disks**, which are transverse flat saccules formed by infolding of the cell membrane. These disks are enclosed within a cylindrical extension of the cell membrane. The outer segment of the photoreceptor is considered a modified cilium because the narrow connecting stalk that joins it to the inner segment contains the nine peripheral doublet microtubules of a cilium, with a closely associated basal body. The companion centriole is present nearby. The **inner segment** contains abundant polysomes, some rER, a substantial Golgi region, and mitochondria. The club-shaped synaptic body (process) situated on the other side of the expanded nuclear region contains synaptic vesicles and mitochondria. It represents an expanded presynaptic terminal.

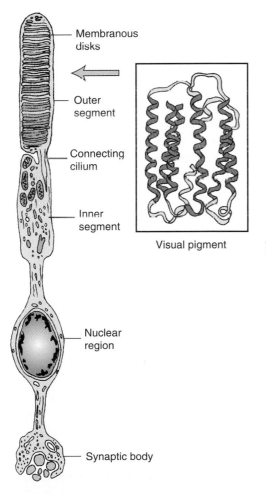

Visual pigment

Figure 19-8
Essential fine structure of a retinal rod.

Whereas rods have a cylindrical outer segment with membranous disks that are free-floating, cones have a conical outer segment and most (if not all) of their disks maintain continuity with the cell membrane.

Turnover Of Visual Pigments

Rhodopsin, a photosensitive visual pigment derived in part from vitamin A, is synthesized in the inner segment of rods. It becomes incorporated into their disk membrane at the stage when membranous disks invaginate at the base of the outer segment. Similar pigments (e.g., **iodopsin** in red-sensitive cones) are incorporated into the disk membrane of cones. Light absorption by these visual pigments leads to generation of receptor potentials, manifested as hyperpolarization of the cell membrane. Furthermore, the rod disks undergo steady turnover because a number of new disks forms each day. Disks produced at the bottom of the stack become progressively displaced by newer ones until they reach the tip of the outer segment, where they are shed as a disk stack remnant. The discarded part of the stack is then phagocytosed by the associated retinal pigment epithelium. In cones, comparable **disk shedding** occurs but membranous disk disposal is not compensated for by repetitive new disk formation as in rods. Instead, newly synthesized cone disk protein molecules are added at multiple sites to all the disks in the outer segment, not just those at the base. To some extent the resulting turnover of visual pigment compensates for lack of replacement of photoreceptors, which do not divide. Regeneration of new photoreceptors, other retinal neurons, and Müller glial cells nevertheless remains an exciting possibility, since the presence of adult mammalian retinal stem cells has recently been demonstrated in the pigmented ciliary margin overlying the ciliary muscle.

EAR

The ears house the unique sensory organs responsible for 1) the special sense of hearing and 2) producing the afferent nerve impulses involved in sustaining positional equilibrium (vestibular function). The body's discerning sense of balance is based primarily on detection of relative position and motion of the head. Both hearing and vestibular function involve similar receptor cells of the **inner ear**, the most protected part of the ear lying within the petrous (stone-like) portion of the temporal bone. The **middle ear** conducts sounds to the inner ear through three small bones (**ossicles**) arranged so that they transmit vibrations of the **tympanic membrane** (eardrum). Sound waves approach the tympanic membrane through the **external acoustic meatus** of the **external ear**. These main parts of the ear are illustrated in Figure 19-9.

The external ear is made up of three components. Its large **auricle** is supported by elastic cartilage with a minor amount of adipose tissue along its posteromedial border and inside its lobule. Leading from the auricle is the external acoustic meatus, a fairly short, air-filled canal lined by thin skin. The superficial (lateral) part of the external acoustic meatus is described as its cartilaginous portion because it is supported by elastic cartilage. This region is provided with hair follicles, large sebaceous glands, and modified sweat glands called **ceruminous glands** where ear wax is produced (L. *cera*, wax). The deeper (medial) part of the external acoustic meatus, termed its bony portion because it is enclosed by the tympanic region of the temporal bone (see Fig. 19-9), has fewer of these glands. Closing over the medial end of the external acoustic meatus is the third component of the external ear, the thin, fibrous **tympanic membrane** (eardrum) that vibrates when sound waves reach it (see Fig. 19-14*A*). The tympanic membrane is essentially a double layer of collagen fibers having a radial orientation in the superficial layer and a circular orientation in the deeper layer, with an external covering of extremely thin skin and an internal lining of simple, low cuboidal epithelium.

The **middle ear** consists primarily of 1) an air-filled **tympanic cavity**, lined by simple cuboidal epithelium, that extends posteriorly into the mastoid process of the temporal bone, and 2) a chain of three **auditory ossicles**, individually termed the **malleus, incus,** and **stapes**, traversing the cavity in a lateral to medial direction (see Fig. 19-9). The ossicles transmit vibrations of the tympanic membrane to the **fenestra vestibuli** or **oval window**, a tiny oval aperture in the medial wall of the tym-

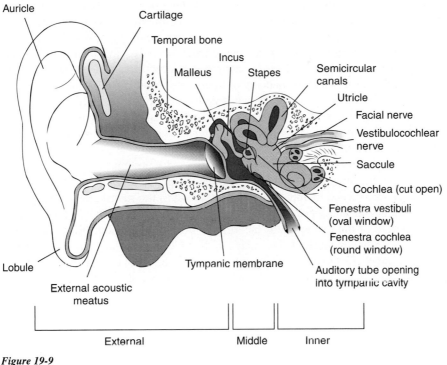

Figure 19-9
Principal parts of the ear.

panic cavity (seen in surface view in Fig. 19-10). The fenestra vestibuli is closed over by the base of the **stapes**, the circumference of which is attached to the perimeter of its associated oval window by a ring-shaped **anular ligament**. By transmitting vibrations to such a small area, the auditory ossicles amplify the effect of pressure variations impinging on the tympanic membrane. In the lower part of the medial wall of the tympanic cavity lies a small round aperture called the **fenestra cochleae** or **round window** (Figs. 19-9 and 19-10). This second aperture is closed over by an epithelially covered, fibrous **secondary tympanic membrane**, a flexible diaphragm that dissipates the sound waves after they have stimulated the sensory receptors in the inner ear (see Fig. 19-13A). Interconnecting the tym-

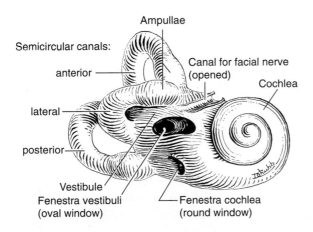

Figure 19-10
Bony labyrinth of the inner ear (right ear, lateral view).

panic cavity with the nasopharynx is the **auditory** (eustachian) **tube** (see Fig. 19-9), the role of which is equalization of the air pressure on both sides of the tympanic membrane. Leading from the bony canal representing the tympanic end of the auditory tube is a wider medial section with walls supported by cartilage. This more flexible region can be opened temporarily by yawning or swallowing.

The **inner ear** contains 1) the organ of hearing, housed in a structure called the **cochlea**, and 2) the organ of vestibular function, which is made up of three **semicircular ducts**, the **utricle**, and the **saccule** (see Fig. 19-9). These vestibular components lie within the petrous portion of the temporal bone, where they constitute a system of interconnected bony channels and cavities known as the otic **bony labyrinth**. The four bony channels are the **anterior, lateral,** and **posterior semicircular canals** and the **cochlear canal** (see Fig. 19-10). The substantial bony cavity, or **vestibule**, with which they individually communicate contains two interconnected membranous sacs, the **utricle** and **saccule**. These sacs and the three semicircular ducts lying within the semicircular canals represent the vestibular portion of a closed membranous system known as the **membranous labyrinth**. The **cochlear duct** represents the auditory portion of this labyrinth. The space between the walls of the bony labyrinth and those of the membranous labyrinth is filled with **perilymph**, a fluid fairly similar in composition to cerebrospinal fluid. The lumen of the membranous labyrinth is filled with **endolymph**, a different fluid characterized by its having a relatively high potassium and low sodium content. All the sensory receptors of the inner ear lie within this endolymph-filled lumen.

Cochlea

The cochlea is situated in the spiral bony **cochlear canal**, the base of which opens into the vestibule (see Fig. 19-10). The name cochlea is derived from its distinctive shell-like appearance (L. *cochlea*, snail shell). Its central bony axis, the **modiolus**, houses the **cochlear** (spiral) **ganglion** and the **cochlear nerve**. Much as the thread winds around a tapered screw, a spiral bony shelf termed the **osseous spiral lamina** (Fig. 19-11) winds around the modiolus. This spiral rigid shelf supports the stationary parts of the organ of Corti. The **cochlear duct**, which is the spiral, endolymph-containing part of the membranous labyrinth extending along the cochlear canal, looks triangular in transverse section because its roof and floor converge toward its axial (inner) border. Attached to its higher circumferential (outer) border is the **spiral ligament**, a spiral thickening of the periosteum lining the cochlear canal. Extending outward from the osseous spiral lamina to the spiral ligament is the **basilar membrane**, the fibrous partition-like floor of the cochlear duct (see Figs. 19-11 and 19-12). The basilar membrane supports the spiral organ of Corti on its upper surface and has a layer of simple columnar epithelium on its undersurface. The thin roof of the cochlear duct, the **vestibular (Reissner's) membrane**, is even thinner because it consists of only two layers of apposed simple squamous epithelium with their associated basement membranes. Above and below, between the cochlear duct and the bony walls of the cochlear canal, lie substantial perilymph-containing chambers, the top one known as the **scala vestibuli** and the bottom one, the **scala tympani**. Hence, an alternative name for the cochlear duct situated in between them is the **scala media**. The three parallel contiguous spiral compartments, with their interposed membranous partitions, extend the full length of the modiolus. At the apex of the modiolus, the scala vestibuli communicates with the scala tympani through a tiny opening called the **heliocotrema**. The functional significance of the three parallel fluid-containing compartments in the cochlea is discussed in the next section.

Organ of Corti: Role in Hearing

The detailed organization of the organ of Corti, structurally adapted for detecting a broad band of frequencies, is shown in Figure 19-12. This organ consists primarily of sensory receptors called **hair cells** and their supporting columnar epithelial cells. The epithelial supporting cells along the

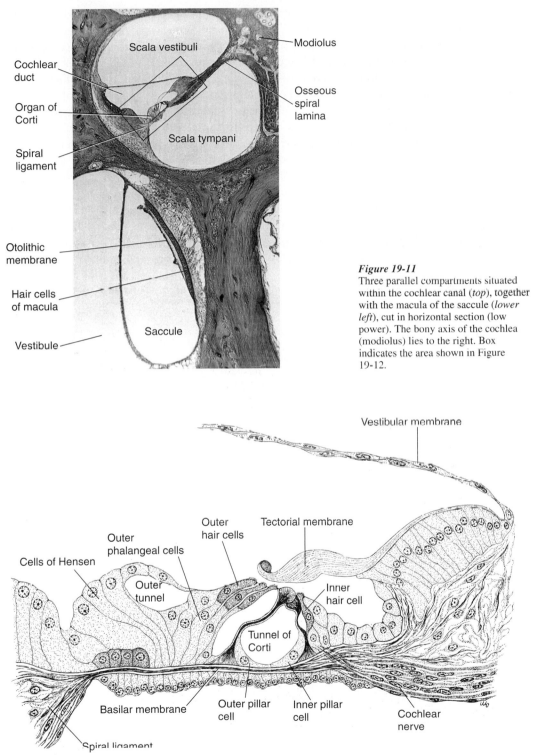

Figure 19-11
Three parallel compartments situated within the cochlear canal (*top*), together with the macula of the saccule (*lower left*), cut in horizontal section (low power). The bony axis of the cochlea (modiolus) lies to the right. Box indicates the area shown in Figure 19-12.

Figure 19-12
Histologic organization of the organ of Corti (guinea pig cochlea). The spiral ligament is on the left and the modiolus is on the right, as in Figure 19-11.

circumferential (outer) edge of the osseous spiral lamina produce a resilient cuticular sheet known as the **tectorial membrane** (L. *tectum*, roof). This membrane forms a roof over the hair cells. Because the tectorial membrane is keratin-like, it is highly susceptible to fixation artifact, hence its shape and relation to underlying hair cells are usually distorted in sections. Other supporting cells known as **phalangeal** and **pillar cells** are reinforced with microtubule bundles, providing support and rigidity to the free surface of the hair cells (see Figs. 19-12 and 19-13). Cylindrical and flask-shaped hair cells are arranged as inner and outer groups. Whereas the inner hair cells form a single row, the outer hair cells constitute three rows, with an extra row or two toward the heliocotrema. Synapsing with the base of each hair cell, which is accommodated within a recess in a phalangeal cell, are afferent and efferent nerve endings. On the free surface of each hair cell, and strongly reinforced by a dense terminal web, is a W-shaped row of tall, specialized straight microvilli called **stereocilia**. Positioned in the notch of the W is a vestigial cilium that is represented solely by its basal body. This notch faces outward, toward the spiral ligament. The stereocilia on the outer hair cells are arranged in several rows of graded height. The tips of the stereocilia in the outermost, tallest row are embedded in the tectorial membrane. Each stereocilium is narrower at its base than at its tip and contains an axial bundle of crosslinked microfilaments extending down to the dense terminal web.

Whereas perilymph and endolymph act as incompressible fluids, the vestibular and basilar membranes are flexible and slack. The vibrations transmitted to the oval window by the base of the stapes enter the scala vestibuli as pressure waves in the perilymph. They pass through the floor of this chamber (i.e., traverse the vestibular membrane), enter the endolymph of the cochlear duct (the scala media), and then become transmitted through the basilar membrane to the perilymph in the scala tympani. After this, they dissipate through the round window (Fig. 19-14A). The effect of the pressure waves passing across the scala media on their way from the scala vestibuli to the scala tympani is to make the basilar membrane oscillate. Different regions of this membrane are designed to oscillate at different resonant frequencies, with resulting frequency discrimination along the length of the organ of Corti. Displacement of the basilar membrane is detected by the shearing stresses that it creates between 1) the tectorial membrane and its affixed tips of hair cell stereocilia and 2) the remainder of the hair cell, which is rigidly supported by the strongly reinforced phalangeal and pillar cells of the organ of Corti (see Figs. 19-13 and 19-14B). Resulting displacement of the stereocilia causes hair cells to depolarize, contributing to the complex pattern of afferent impulses reaching the auditory cortex by way of the vestibulocochlear nerve.

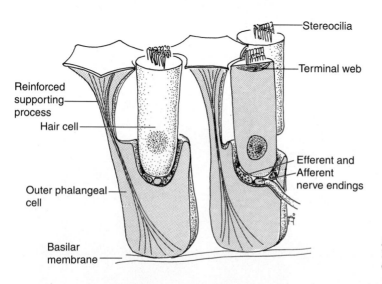

Figure 19-13
Hair cells and phalangeal cells in the organ of Corti.

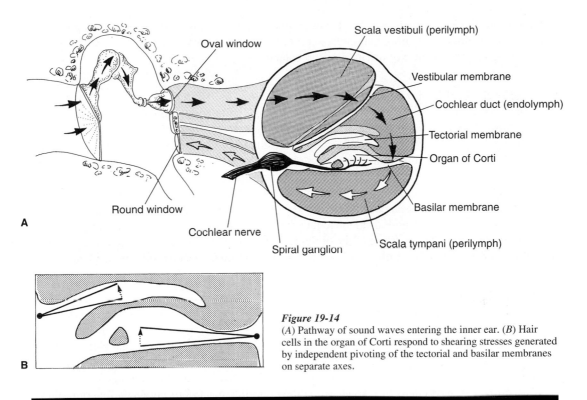

Figure 19-14
(*A*) Pathway of sound waves entering the inner ear. (*B*) Hair cells in the organ of Corti respond to shearing stresses generated by independent pivoting of the tectorial and basilar membranes on separate axes.

CLINICAL IMPLICATIONS

Hearing Losses
Age-related permanent hearing loss is attributed to a combination of 1) depletion of responding cochlear hair cells and 2) neuronal degeneration, with resulting transmission impairment in the auditory pathways. Persistent exposure to unnecessarily loud noise levels and, in some cases, the administration of certain antibiotics, can also be injurious to cochlear hair cells. Potentially reversible episodes of deafness often reflect a temporary hindrance to the conduction of sound waves (e.g., dampened oscillation of wax-encrusted eardrums; substantial occlusion of a narrow external acoustic meatus by accumulated ear wax). Fibrosis of the eardrums following an infection and damage to auditory ossicles may lead to a more extended hearing loss. Temporary hearing losses that are associated with variations in altitude (e.g., during air travel) often reflect delayed equalization of the air pressures on the two sides of the eardrum. Such equalization is brought about independently in each ear by way of the auditory tube connecting the tympanic cavity with the nasopharynx (see Fig. 19-9). If partial collapse or occlusion of the flexible region of the auditory tube impedes air movement, oscillations of the eardrum are subject to dampening as a result of any existing pressure difference.

Vestibular Labyrinth

The **vestibular portion** of the membranous labyrinth in the inner ear consists of the utricle, three semicircular ducts, and the saccule. Both ends of each **semicircular duct** open into the **utricle**, a membranous sac filled with endolymph. Each semicircular duct lies in a different plane, and it incorporates an expanded region known as its **ampulla** near one end (see Fig. 19-10). Another membranous sac called the **saccule** is filled with endolymph that is in free communication with that filling the utricle, semicircular ducts, and cochlear duct. The saccule, utricle, and semicircular ducts are suspended within the bony labyrinth by strands of loose connective tissue. Their thin connective tissue walls are lined with simple squamous epithelium. The sensory regions of the utricle and saccule are known as **maculae**, whereas those of the semicircular ducts are termed **ampullary cristae**

(cristae ampullaris) because they lie in the ampullae. In both cases, the receptive regions are patches of epithelium containing hair cells, and the vestibular impulses that the hair cells generate contribute to an overall sense of orientation and balance.

Maculae In the Utricle and Saccule

Maculae are spotlike areas (L. *macula*, spot) in which the lining epithelium consists of stereocilia-bearing hair cells with columnar supporting cells. These sensory areas of the epithelial lining are covered over by an extracellular layer of glycoprotein studded with calcium carbonate crystals (Fig. 19-15A). Termed **otoliths (otoconia)**, these crystals are relatively heavy. The layer of gelatinous material in which they are embedded is known as the **otolithic membrane** (see Figs. 19-11 and 19-15A). The utricle is characterized by a patch of sensory epithelium that lies almost in a horizontal plane, whereas the saccule has a patch that is almost vertical. Depending on the position of the head, the heavy otoliths of one or both of the maculae may apply shearing stresses to the hair cell stereocilia embedded in the undersurface of the otolithic membrane (see Fig. 19-15B). Because of the inertia of the substantial otoliths, macular hair cells also detect linear acceleration or deceleration.

Ampullary Cristae

The membranous wall of the ampulla of each semicircular duct projects inward as a transverse ridge or crest called a **crista** (L., crest). The ampullary crista has a connective tissue core and an epithelial covering made of hair cells and columnar supporting cells (Fig. 19-16A). The hair cell stereocilia of the ampullary crista are embedded in a thick flap-like mass of extracellular glycoprotein called a **cupula** (L., cup). This flap projects into the ampullary lumen and acts like a swing-door (see Fig. 19-16B). Highly susceptible to shrinkage artifact, the flap-like gelatinous cupula is free of otoliths. Because it hinges freely on the crista, the cupula readily becomes deflected when the endolymph moves. Rotational acceleration or deceleration involving the head is detected in any given plane by the crista of the corresponding semicircular duct. This is because the endolymph content of the duct tends to remain stationary as a result of inertia, resulting in deflection of the cupula.

Ampullary cristae and the utricular and saccular maculae are all characterized by hair cells of two slightly different kinds. Also, unlike the hair cells in the organ of Corti, these hair cells have a single cilium known as a **kinocilium** that lacks independent motility. It lies to one side of a conical bundle of stereocilia of graded height that are tallest next to the kinocilium. Deflection of the kinocilium—stereocilia complex toward the kinocilium triggers depolarization of the hair cell and increases the number of vestibular impulses generated.

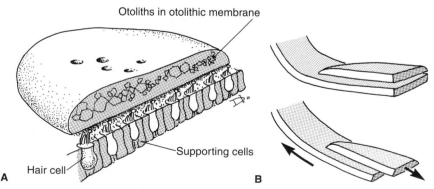

Otoliths in otolithic membrane

Supporting cells

A   Hair cell   B

Figure 19-15
(*A*) General structure of the utricular and saccular maculae. (*B*) Macular hair cells respond to movement of otolithic membranes.

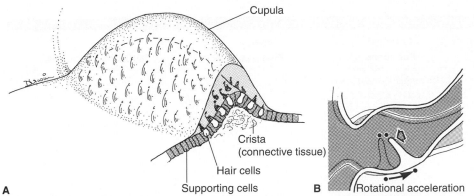

Figure 19-16
(A) General structure of the ampullary crista in a semicircular duct. (B) Ampullary hair cells respond to deflection of the cupula.

Summary

Essential features of the eye and ear, respectively, are summarized in Tables 19-1 and 19-2.

TABLE 19-1

CHIEF FEATURES OF PRINCIPAL PARTS OF THE EYE

Part	Principal Functions	General Features	Distinctive Features
Cornea	Main site of light refraction	Part of the fibrous coat; posterior border lies next to aqueous humor	Transparent; avascular; substantia propria with stratified squamous epithelium anteriorly and endothelium posteriorly
Iris	Regulates pupillary aperture, blocking excess light	Part of the vascular coat; aqueous humor passes anteriorly around pupillary margin	Pigmented; vascular loose connective tissue; constrictor pupillae muscle at pupillary margin, dilator pupillae posteriorly; pigmented epithelium on posterior surface
Lens	Focuses image on retina	Epithelial origin; nourished by diffusion from aqueous humor and vitreous body; attached by zonule to ciliary body	Transparent; avascular; elastic; made of lens fibers with simple cuboidal epithelium anteriorly; enclosed by lens capsule (basement membrane)
Retina	Detects all parts of image focused by lens	Constitutes retinal coat; inner neural retina + outer retinal pigment epithelium (RPE)	RPE (phagocytic, lightproof); photoreceptive rods (night vision) and cones (color vision); neurons (bipolar, ganglion, horizontal, and amacrine); Müller cells; optic nerve fibers; fovea with cones only

TABLE 19-2

CHIEF FEATURES OF PARTS OF THE EAR

Part	Principal Functions	General Features	Distinctive Features
External ear	Conducts sound waves toward tympanic membrane	Air-filled, opens onto body surface	Auricle with elastic cartilage; cartilaginous and bony portions of external acoustic meatus with ceruminous glands; fibrous tympanic membrane with external thin skin and internal simple low cuboidal epithelium
Middle ear	Transmits tympanic membrane vibration to inner ear through ossicles	Air-filled, communicates with nasopharynx through auditory tube	Tympanic cavity with simple cuboidal epithelial lining; malleus, incus, and stapes; base of stapes transmits vibration to fenestra vestibuli (oval window); sound waves dissipate through fenestra cochleae (round window)
Inner ear	Hearing	Bony labyrinth containing perilymph lies external to membranous labyrinth containing endolymph; organ of Corti lies in cochlear duct	In spiral cochlear canal lies endolymph-containing cochlear duct (scala media), with perilymph-containing scala vestibuli above and scala tympani below; vestibular membrane (= roof of cochlear duct) has a double layer of simple squamous epithelium; basilar membrane (= floor of cochlear duct) is the fibrous partition under the organ of Corti; hair cells, supported by phalangeal and pillar cells, have sterocilia embedded in the tectorial membrane; hair cells detect local resonant oscillation of the basilar membrane
	Vestibular function (balance and orientation)	Maculae in endolymph-containing utricle and saccule; cristae in ampullae of endolymph-containing semicircular ducts	Utricle, semicircular ducts, and saccule have connective tissue walls and a simple squamous epithelial lining; maculae have hair cells with an otolithic membrane; hair cells respond to gravity and detect linear acceleration; cristae have hair cells and a cupula; hair cells of cristae detect rotational acceleration and have a kinocilium as well as stereocilia

Bibliography

Eye: General

Augusteyn RC, Rogers KM. The Eye, vol 1. Montreal, Eden Press, 1979.

Hogan M, Alvarado J, Weddell J. Histology of the Human Eye. Philadelphia, WB Saunders, 1971.

Jakobiec FA, ed. Ocular Anatomy, Embryology, and Teratology. Hagerstown, MD, Harper & Row, 1982.

Kessel RG, Kardon RH. Nervous tissue—eye and ear. In: Tissues and Organs: A Text-Atlas of Scanning Electron Microscopy. San Francisco, WH Freeman, 1979.

Lens and Vitreous Body

Bloemendal H, ed. Molecular and Cellular Biology of the Eye Lens. New York, John Wiley & Sons, 1981.

Swann DA. Chemistry and biology of the vitreous body. Int Rev Exp Pathol 22:2, 1980.

Retinal Photoreceptors, Stem Cells, and Other Components

Besharse JC. The daily light-dark cycle and rhythmic metabolism in the photoreceptor-pigment epithelial complex. Prog Retinal Res 1:81, 1982.

Bok D. Retinal photoreceptor—pigment epithelium interactions. Invest Ophthalmol Vis Sci 26:1659, 1985.

Borwein B. The retinal receptor: a description. In: Enoch JM, Tobey FL, eds. Springer Series in Optical Sciences, vol 23. Vertebrate Photoreceptor Optics. Berlin, Springer-Verlag, 1981, p 11.

Borwein B. Scanning electron microscopy of monkey foveal photoreceptors. Anat Rec 205:363, 1983.

Cunha-Vaz JG, ed. The Blood—Retinal Barriers. New York, Plenum, 1980.

Daw NW, Jensen RJ, Brunken WJ. Rod pathways in mammalian retinae. Trends Neurosci 13:110, 1990.

Hollenberg MJ, Lea PJ. High resolution scanning electron microscopy of the retinal pigment epithelium and Bruch's layer. Invest Ophthalmol Vis Sci 29:1380, 1988.

Masland RH. The functional architecture of the retina. Sci Am 255(6):102, 1986.

Tropepe V, Coles BLK, Chiasson BJ, et al. Retinal stem cells in the adult mammalian eye. Science 287(5460):2032, 2000.

Young RW. Visual cells and the concept of renewal. Invest Ophthalmol 15:700, 1976.

Zinn KM, Marmor MF, eds. The Retinal Pigment Epithelium. Cambridge, MA, Harvard University Press, 1979.

Ear: General

Friedmann I, Ballantyne J, eds. Ultrastructural Atlas of the Inner Ear. London, Butterworths, 1984.

Kessel RG, Kardon RH. Nervous tissue—eye and ear. In: Tissues and Organs: A Text Atlas of Scanning Electron Microscopy. San Francisco, WH Freeman, 1979.

Organ of Corti and Vestibular Receptors

Ashmore JF. The electrophysiology of hair cells. Annu Rev Physiol 53:465, 1991.

Corwin JT, Warchol ME. Auditory hair cells: structure, function, development, and regeneration. Annu Rev Neurosci 14:301, 1991.

Holley MC, Ashmore JF. A cytoskeletal spring in cochlear outer hair cells. Nature 335:635, 1988.

Hudspeth AJ. The hair cells of the inner ear. Sci Am 248(1):54, 1983.

Kimura RS. The ultrastructure of the organ of Corti. Int Rev Cytol 42:173, 1975.

Lawrence M, Burgio PA. The attachment of the tectorial membrane revealed by scanning electron microscope. Ann Otol Rhinol Laryngol 89:325, 1980.

Lim DJ. Functional structure of the organ of Corti: A review. Hear Res 22:117, 1986.

Lindenman HH. Anatomy of the otolith organs. Adv Otorhinolaryngol 20:405, 1973.

Parker DE. The vestibular apparatus. Sci Am 243(5):118, 1980.

Roberts WM, Howard J, Hudspeth AJ. Hair Cells: transduction, tuning, and transmission in the inner ear. Ann Rev Cell Biol 4:63, 1988.

Soudijn ER. Scanning electron microscopy of the organ of Corti. Ann Otol Rhinol Laryngol 86(Suppl):16, 1976.

Index

Page numbers in bold face indicate major discussions; t following a page number indicates a table. Plate numbers refer to color plates.